Psychiatric Nursing Skills

A patient-centred approach
Second edition

Graham Dexter

Formerly Principal Lecturer at the University of Teesside, UK
Freelance Lecturer and Trainer

and

Michael Wash

Consultant to the Health Service and Private Sector on
Quality Management and Strategic Team Building

CHAPMAN & HALL

London · Glasgow · Weinheim · New York · Tokyo · Melbourne · Madras

Published by Chapman & Hall, 2–6 Boundary Row, London SE1 8HN, UK

Chapman & Hall, 2–6 Boundary Row, London SE1 8HN, UK

Blackie Academic & Professional, Wester Cleddens Road, Bishopbriggs, Glasgow G64 2NZ, UK

Chapman & Hall GmbH, Pappelallee 3, 69469 Weinheim, Germany

Chapman & Hall USA, One Penn Plaza, 41st Floor, New York NY 10119, USA

Chapman & Hall Japan, ITP-Japan, Kyowa Building, 3F, 2-2-1 Hirakawacho, Chiyoda-ku, Tokyo 102, Japan

Chapman & Hall Australia, Thomas Nelson Australia, 102 Dodds Street, South Melbourne, Victoria 3205, Australia

Chapman & Hall India, R. Seshadri, 32 Second Main Road, CIT East, Madras 600 035, India

Distributed in the USA and Canada by Singular Publishing Group Inc., 4284 41st Street, San Diego, California 92105

First edition 1986

Reprinted 1987 , 1990, 1991

Second edition 1995

© 1986, 1995 Graham Dexter and Michael Wash

Typeset in Times 10½/12 pt by Saxon Graphics Ltd, Derby

Printed in Great Britain at the Alden Press, Oxford

ISBN 0 412 553201   1 56593 098 3 (USA)

A catalogue record for this book is available from the British Library

Library of Congress Catalog Card Number: 94-68797

Printed on permanent acid-free text paper, manufactured in accordance with ANSI/NISO Z39.48-1992 and ANSI/NISO Z39.48-1984 (Permanence of Paper).

N464
1769
IRF W (Dex)

Psychiatric Nursing Skills

Contents

Preface

In this book we have attempted to identify skills which are needed by the psychiatric nurse, and in doing so to identify a body of knowledge unique to the professional psychiatric nurse. The book has been written to demonstrate the basis of a skills approach for both the experienced and the inexperienced nurse to build upon, for we believe that psychiatric nurses, due to both their training and their particular mixture of interests, are well equipped to be in the forefront of psychiatry as a developing art and science. We hope that this book in some small way helps this development.

Some of the more recent advances in psychiatric nursing have been reinforced by the publication of a training syllabus for mental nurses (English and Welsh National Boards, 1982). This document highlights the need for a change from a medical model to a social model and from a task-oriented learning experience to a skills approach. We have attempted to reflect this change in emphasis by including such aspects as personal development and self-awareness, human sexuality, the nursing process and counselling skills.

As it is our earnest wish for this book to be widely read, we have tried to make it simple in text and illustrative in case material and dialogue. The case histories we have cited are an amalgam of various experiences and people we have met and are in no way a true reflection of any particular individual; they are constructed to illustrate and facilitate understanding of the concepts involved in the care of particular individuals and any similarity to anyone is purely coincidental.

It is our intention to stimulate interest and pride in the psychiatric nursing profession, knowing that its unique body of knowledge is embodied in the skilled application of an eclectic armoury, i.e. counselling, behavioural and applied psychological techniques.

Finally, we sincerely hope this book reaches not only psychiatric nurses, but all other people interest in helping those in need.

Acknowledgements

We would like to thank all our students, for they have taught us much of what we know and present as ours in this volume. As Mike and I are no longer full-time mental health nurse teachers, (Mike Wash is currently a very successful management consultant, and Graham Dexter teaches nurses only as a part of a wide range of freelance work), we are pleased to thank all those splendid friends, colleagues, ex-students and general supporters who have made this edition possible. A very special thanks to Janice Russell, who is the one person I can definitely say made this edition happen. Particular gratitude is owed to those contributors who have edited, reviewed, rewritten and generally added their expertise, specifically: Andy Betts (Chapter 24); Eddie Byrnes (Quality management); Barry Ford (Chapters 10 and 12); Vivien Markham (Chapter 18); Janice Russell (Chapters 20, 21 and 23, and work on Chapters 1, 3 and 4); Rod Walsh (Chapters 16 and 17); Pete Turner (Chapter 3); and Terry Wilson (Chapters 5, 6, 7, 8 and 9). Thank you all most sincerely.

Graham Dexter

Introduction

Whether you are seriously interested in mental health nursing or are simply a browser who has selected this volume at random, we hope the contents will be of interest to you and you will continue to read. For this very reason, we have tried to keep a wide range of contents, from light and stimulating to sobering and thought-provoking. We think it appropriate at this point to share with you our views, orientations and attitudes towards mental health nursing, and finally to reveal the map which may help you negotiate this book.

The old days of the psychiatric hospitals which were rigid institutions with high walls and predetermined routines are all but gone. To replace them we have 'community care' which, although superb in principle, is already frayed at the edges: the idea has not quite taken reality by storm. Mental health nurses find themselves fighting for resources and not always receiving the support they deserve. Patients, now referred to as clients, find themselves in a community not always as welcoming as the politicians would have us believe, and for this very reason in need of support and skilled help from the caring professions. We do not mourn the psychiatric hospital, but perhaps we can remember some of the good things it offered: the sanctuary, the peace and the spirit of nurturing which in its best forms it offered to everyone non-judgementally. Let us hope that with 'community care' the baby has not been thrown out with the bathwater.

The mental health nurse's task was traditionally a custodial role, to ensure that the public was protected and isolated from psychiatric patients and, equally, that psychiatric patients were protected from themselves. It was the early to mid 1970s before all the high-walled courtyards were removed, and along with these some concrete attitudes of the staff also fell. Now, in the middle of the 1990s, we seem to have a harder edge to caring, a competitive commercial aspect that the nurse must face. The first cohorts of Project 2000 nurses will soon begin to take up senior posts, and hopefully they will have been prepared to compete for resources with the new managers, articulate their caring views more effectively and argue their clients' position as good advocates should. This second edition has tried to move with the current trends: it is for this reason that the new chapters on research, supervision, sexual abuse and quality management have been included. Hopefully, both new and old readers will find the volume some use, either as refreshment or as new insights. This is the sole reason for a second edition. We have tried to leave the best of the old and incorporate the new; we think we have succeeded, but you the reader will be the best judge.

The new era for mental health nursing should therefore encompass the knowledge which has been built upon by decades of professionals in mental health, and embrace the new optimism of helping patients become more independent and self-directed.

The mental health nurse of the future must have the skills of interpersonal relationship formation in much the same way a counsellor has, but – much more – she must have a knowledge of the abnormal mind and be able to adapt her interactions to ensure a skilled approach. Together with this ability she must have at her fingertips an armoury of strategies and techniques from which she can choose which, when directed appropriately, will 'help' the client in every sense of the word. The ability to do this requires sound judgement based on an awareness of needs which, when fulfilled, will enable patients to function as independently as possible. This task is much more difficult for today's mental health nurses, for it is no longer simply enough to protect, care for and entertain the patient. The modern nurse has to learn to judge when it is appropriate to withdraw, and help the patient by not helping and forging new independence.

Although the authors' main orientation has been within traditional mental hospitals, much has been added to this new edition to encompass the different demands of community care. Throughout the book, the reader may notice that we have not differentiated between serious mental health problems and the less debilitating problems of living. It is true that some authors and clinicians would have classified the chapters in a much more traditional style. However, our intention is to present our material in an uncomplicated way, based on clients being individuals with various problems. It is our hope that by presenting client issues as separate chapters, readers may be able to amalgamate the single symptom and behaviour pattern in any combination to form their own picture of the clients being nursed. We hope that the result of this system will be that nurses come to appreciate that each client is an individual.

A significant percentage of the book consists of what can only be described as counselling skills, modified and applied to mental health problems and issues: mental health nurses should not, however, try to be full-time counsellors or believe that they are counsellors, for much the same reason as they are not doctors, psychologists, occupational therapists or behaviour therapists. The good mental health nurse is partly an amalgam of all these professionals, without such an intensity of specialism but having a broad knowledge base of significant insight. This should not be interpreted as 'Jack of all trades and master of none', for she is a practitioner in her own right. She is the professional implementor, the functioning component pulling together all these theoretical approaches to plan and return appropriate care for her client.

To help the reader, the book is set out in three parts as follows: Part I sets out what we believe to be 'core skills and strategies', the essence of skills that are imperative to the sound practice of mental health nursing. Chapter 1 focuses upon the mental health nurse as a person, her interactive skills of approach, awareness and development. Chapter 2 describes a complete model of counselling, beginning with an orientation of qualities (which we believe apply to mental health nurses as perfectly as they do to counsellors) and details basic and advanced skills of counselling, from non-verbal communication to challenging skills and problem-solving strategies. Chapter 3 attempts to explain behavioural theory as described by Pavlov and Skinner in a simple and understandable way, using examples and analogies. We hope this approach will potentiate its helpfulness for individuals who may have found other texts more complex and difficult to work through. The chapter ends with a discussion of some therapies associated with behavioural theory currently used in mental health practice. Chapter 4 demonstrates our high regard for and the importance of supervision, and gives a simple model to enable practitioners to supervise and be supervised systematically and effectively. This is an absolute must for the modern mental health professional.

Part II deals with the practical application of the core skills to particular client behaviours and situations. Case illustrations, theoretical concepts and implications for the nurse are included to enable the reader to visualize a complete picture of the patient, and examples of dialogue are offered to illustrate appropriate skilled responses. The reader is invited to read Part II in any order, as each chapter is self-contained.

Much of Part II is compiled from our experience with patients throughout our clinical experience, and is consequently composed simply of our views and ideas. This new edition has also benefited from a second generation of skilled practitioners. We are proud to acknowledge that some of the nurses we trained ten years ago have participated in revitalizing and renewing these sections. Aspects of community care have been inserted or amalgamated into these chapters to give them a flavour of the real world in the 1990s.

As many of the chapters in Part II are the subject of entire books by other authors, it is apparent that our discussion of them may at times be cursory in comparison. Readers who wish to know more are referred to the Further Reading sections.

Part III seeks to add a further dimension to mental health nursing by extending skills and knowledge in other specialized areas. The chapter on sexuality has been extensively rewritten by Janice Russell, and now includes a section on HIV and AIDS. Janice also contributes chapters on research and working with the sexually abused; these excellent contributions enhance the book and maintain the reader-friendly style which we tried to make the hallmark of the first edition.

Andy Betts, a friend and colleague, adds a chapter on Groups. This subject had been intended for inclusion in the first edition, but was not written in time for publication. We are indebted to Andy for bringing his expertise to bear on this subject essential for modern mental health nurses.

The other three chapters within Part III, 'Community skills', 'Creative skills' and 'Management principles and skills', are intended to offer some brief insights into complex areas. The idea of including these areas is to stimulate interest and further reading; they are not an exhaustive in-depth study, but simply an appetizer to areas of complex study. The final section on quality management, including the appendix, is largely the work of Eddie Byrnes, who helps us bring the flavour of modern management to this essential skill for contemporary nurses.

Graham Dexter

Core Skills and Strategies

Personal skills | 1

Mental health nursing is the practice of caring for people who have mental illness, potentiating their independence and restoring their dignity. In order to fulfil this arduous occupation, the mental health nurse must possess a sound knowledge base and the requisite skills of good nursing practice. The ideal nurse must be able to look after the physical needs of the client, understand the social and psychological function of the individual, both normal and abnormal, and have the necessary ability to direct her skills appropriately.

QUALITIES AND ATTITUDES FOR THE MENTAL HEALTH NURSE

The ability to adapt

The mental health nurse needs to be adaptable to a variety of different settings and cultures. Working within the residential setting, for example, may demand different attitudes and roles from those needed when working in the community, as in the former setting the nurse may have an authority or a supervisory role that she does not have in the community. This may be different again, and perhaps exaggerated, when the nurse is working in a forensic setting, where clients have also been convicted of criminal behaviour.

The mental health nurse will also need to cope with a variety of social and cultural settings. Social settings involve the class and the status of individuals; you may feel differently working with, for example, an architect, than with a canteen worker. You may feel more or less intimidated or comfortable, and may bring various different assumptions to bear on the working relationship.

Similarly, the mental health nurse may work in a diverse range of cultural settings. Significant features here are race, ethnicity and gender. All of these categories have a 'dominant' group, so that mental health norms, for example, have been traditionally fixed by western, white, male theorists and practitioners. Some research goes so far as to suggest that these limited norms themselves contribute to the production and diagnosis of mental illness. Littlewood and Lipsedge (1982) argued that alienation through racism stimulates high stress levels, which in turn contribute to mental illness. Broverman, Broverman and Clarkson (1970) showed that clinical practitioners conceptualized a mental health norm which correlated with how they saw a healthy male, while being different from how they expected females to act. Mental health nurses need to be sensitive to such issues, so that their attitudes and values do not further alienate their clients.

Moreover, they may need to be familiar with the issues that arise in cross-cultural mental health nursing, such as religious or cultural practices and norms, so that they may respect such practices. They may need to be aware of the dilemmas which exist between immigrant parents and British-born children, and sensitive to differences of language and non-verbal communication. The nurse may need to be aware of what dress norms are acceptable to different cultures, such as whether it is seen as insulting to wear a hat, or to reveal the shoulders. The subject is too lengthy to go into in detail here, but suffice it to say that the mental health nurse needs to be adaptable to a range of settings.

Individualism (self as a therapeutic tool)

One of the prime qualities in a mental health nurse is individualism, i.e. those qualities that make a person unique. Bearing this in mind, we will endeavour to describe what we think are desirable qualities and attitudes for this rather demanding profession.

Someone once said to one of us, 'You must be mad working in that loony bin!' The reply at the time was, 'I sometimes wonder myself.' We still wonder today: not that we might be mad, but are we fulfilling a personal need by working in this type of place? Could it be a basic need to help others? One could look further and deeper to explore various theories that may explain this situation, but we feel that it suffices to say that yes, in some people there does tend to be a desire, drive or motivation to help others.

Ideally this is not to satisfy a personal need, as mental health nursing involves the giving of yourself in order to muster the resources available, thereby being free of selfish motives which may be distracting within the helping process. In saying this, we recognize that helping is rarely completely altruistic and that some reward may be gained from a better understanding of others, which may generate personal insight and understanding. It is often helpful for the mental health nurse to recognize her own issues and concerns. The point is that the helping process must focus on the needs of the client.

Many people wish to help others but do not have the 'personal equipment', such as adequate intelligence, an appetite for reading in order to gather more ideas and having respect for the ideas of others, but also having a sense of reality. The nurse must be a practical person, a person who uses knowledge and skills in a practical way for the benefit of others. She must be a good learner, have an open mind and be willing to listen to anything that may help another to live more effectively. She should be sensible and socially intelligent. The mental health nurse should feel comfortable with her own emotions and also the emotions of others in any given situation. A good mental health nurse views helping as hard work and a heavy responsibility, which may involve entering and influencing the life of another. She should be a good listener, both physically and psychologically, i.e. know what her own body is saying non-verbally as well as verbally, and she should also be sensitive to the client's non-verbal communication. She must work hard to understand her client, to be able to see the world through the client's eyes without emotional entanglement, thus being able to stand back to help in an objective way.

A mental health nurse is not afraid of giving something of herself, disclosing experiences and feelings if this will enhance the client's self-understanding. She is not afraid to challenge clients, albeit with care and respect; equally, she is not afraid to challenge herself. Having helped the client to identify his problems, the nurse is then prepared to offer support and guidance to move the client forward in finding solutions. In doing so she will use any resource that will add to or enhance the effectiveness of the helping process. She will use and master the necessary skills, making them work for her rather than being limited by them. The ideal mental health nurse will be living effectively, and by doing so demonstrating this process to the client. No-one is free from problems, but the major difference between the non-effective person and the person who is living effectively is that the latter is able to utilize self-resource in order to solve or cope with problems, whereas the former finds this extremely difficult.

Core values and attitudes

We have suggested that the mental health nurse needs to be respectful of a diversity of cultures, and integrated and skilled enough to offer something of herself within the helping process while retaining an objective stance. These aspects of the job come together when she is able to accept an individual without judgement, respecting that person's right to be himself. She genuinely cares, is non-defensive and at all times honest with herself, which enables her to help the client explore feelings, experiences and behaviour in order to identify problems and ways of achieving solutions to them.

In order to do this, the nurse needs to be able to offer value-free listening; that is, listening without judging. This may be challenging when the nurse does not agree with the values of the client. The nurse may be politically anti-marriage for example, yet be able to respect the importance of marriage for her client. Even if accepting marriage, she may find the concept of an arranged marriage rather alarming, whereas this may be desirable for the client. It is important that she can listen to the client without distortion and without interfering with his right to self-determination. One exception to this is when the client's judgement is mentally impaired, when the nurse must make a carefully considered clinical judgement of her own. Another exception is where the client is a danger to others, as with violence or abuse, particularly where this involves minors and there are statutory and moral regulations to be met.

Many of the skills, attitudes and qualities described above are the ideal, but they are also realistic in that they can be achieved given the appropriate 'foundation' and training. Once the initial development commences, then the personal growth will continue with skill acquisition and experience.

There are some experiences that even the most skilful person will find disturbing and/or difficult, and the mental health nurse will experience situations that require much thought. Certain issues revolving around personal ethics will be explored and, hopefully, any conflicts resolved during training. These issues may centre on topics such as death and dying, the quality of life, the rights of an individual and certain treatments. By being open-minded and willing to learn, the nurse is able to balance realistic attitudes with personal acceptance. Other situations include those for which the nurse is unprepared, e.g. a sudden death, a personal attack or the sudden realization of a sense of hopelessness. These and others will require not only personal strength at the time, but also an inner strength to recover afterwards.

Mental health nursing is a demanding profession: it is both mentally and physically tiring; it requires strength and dedication. If these are given, the sense of satisfaction in not only being able to do the job but also to be seen to be doing it is immense. The rewards are not always obvious and they are often intermingled with frustration and resentment. Gratitude is sometimes shown in a peculiar fashion, if at all, and often personal satisfaction is experienced only when some subtle response or improvement is shown by the client. For example:

> Concern had been expressed about Mr Jones. Although he had readily agreed to join in the group, for the past three weeks he had not participated at all. Mr Jones was 83. He had been in the unit for six months and had a history of progressive confusion. Over the past month he had become less aware of his surroundings, incontinent and non-communicative. The group consisted of fellow clients, all of whom were elderly and experiencing various degrees of confusion. The therapy consisted of reminiscing about the old days, as the memory for past events was often relatively intact, and stories, pictures or music enabled the clients to embark upon a reasonably orientated discussion. However, Mr Jones would not talk and rarely moved. The therapist was considering leaving Mr Jones out of future groups as she thought he had deteriorated beyond help. At the final group meeting, one of the nursing staff interrupted the session and placed an object on the table in the middle of the group. There was silence, and expressions of surprise, as Mr Jones stared at the object, moved towards it and picked it up. A tentative smile appeared on his face and an overall expression that seemed to be saying, 'Yes, I'm still here, and this I know is part of me.' The object was an old miner's lamp. Mr Jones had been a miner all his working life.

This moment of reality experienced by Mr Jones convinced the therapist that he was not a hopeless case and resulted in tremendous satisfaction for the nurse in her attempt to reach a part of Mr Jones that had not been lost.

Instantaneous peaks of satisfaction such as the one just described are rare. It is said that 'patience is a virtue'; if one relies on waiting for success, as indicated by improvements in a client's lifestyle, then patience is a virtue the mental health nurse must have. It can be said that for the majority of long-stay clients, permanent changes in behaviour are minimal and gradual over the years. Clients often experience setbacks and relapses when for the nurse it must seem like an endless and hopeless struggle to guide the client towards a better quality of life. Equally, the nurse may see a client readmitted to the acute ward after yet another suicide attempt, or in the community apparently making no progress despite lengthy intervention programmes.

We can see clients we have nursed, helped to dress, shave, bathe and escorted back and forth from the Occupational Therapy Unit living today without that degree of help, surviving with a certain amount of independence, enabling them to be considered for holidays, outings and, for the future, part-supervised accommodation. We also, from time to time, see the client who no longer needs to make suicide attempts but has found some insight or safer strategy, and those who respond positively to community nursing and counselling. Whether such changes have been due to a combination of persistent rehabilitation programmes, counselling interventions, reduction in the intensity of the illness or more effective medication, the role of the nurse–client relationship in this progression from dependence to relative freedom cannot be ignored. It is the observation and awareness of this progression to a better quality of life that results in another aspect of personal satisfaction.

To generalize as to where personal satisfaction is experienced is somewhat trivializing the uniqueness of the individual mentioned earlier. Everyone's experience is different; consequently, the moments of satisfaction will vary, depending upon the individual nurse and not necessarily upon the experience.

Finally, the mental health nurse must be someone special, someone who can attempt to satisfy the needs of others by selflessly utilizing her personality in order to give some meaning to their life. This is done mainly by:

- Listening with understanding;
- Responding with care and respect;
- Supporting with trust and confidence;
- Reassuring with explanation and honesty;
- Physically nursing the helpless with compassion;
- Skilfully carrying out procedures;
- Working within personal and ethical boundaries;
- Overcoming the distaste that would be experienced by most, by concentrating on the feelings of the person, and not on the nurse's personal experience.

The skills required of a mental health nurse are indeed varied and many, and in order to be proficient in them the nurse must be a specialist, a specialist in people.

SELF-AWARENESS

Complete the following sentences:

I see myself as ...

My friends see me as ...

My family see me as ...

What I like about myself is ...

What I dislike about myself is ...

One thing other people like about me is ...

One thing other people dislike about me is ...

One aspect within me I would like to change is ...

The aspects about me that other people would like to change are..

The sentences you have just completed may reflect your present level of self-awareness. By this we mean acknowledgement of your own feelings and behaviours and accepting and understanding, or attempting to understand, their presence. The amount of self-awareness may reflect the congruity between how you see yourself and how others see you. The following is a verbal account from a first-year nurse, describing how she thinks her first ward experience has been:

> I've really enjoyed this allocation; it took me a while to get into it, but after a few weeks it seemed all my worries were unfounded. I enjoy talking to the clients and I think they enjoy talking to me, even though there have been a couple of dodgy moments, but that's to be expected on this ward. The staff have been really good: the charge nurse I find really thorough, I respect him a lot, and I think he likes me for that. Yes, I've enjoyed this allocation, I think I've done quite well.

On the nurse's ward report were the following comments by the charge nurse:

> After a very slow start, Nurse Davis seemed to jump from one extreme to another, i.e. treading carefully at first followed by overconfidence and taking the job less than seriously. Her eagerness to relate to certain clients was not welcomed, and even after several guidance sessions she persisted in her over-zealous manner, which resulted in several dramatic episodes which required considerable intervention by the qualified staff. She certainly has a lot to learn.

From these two accounts there appears to be a considerable difference in opinion in the evaluation of this nurse's experience. The question of which of the two is most accurate is irrelevant; the main principle is that the nurse's account of herself is incongruent with how others see her. The nurse implies in her account that she took everything in her stride, coped well and was liked by the staff. The charge nurse's account implies that she did not take the job seriously and was a hindrance at times.

If the report comes as a shock to Nurse Davis, it is likely that she was not aware of how her behaviour was perceived by others. However, if the report does not surprise her she may be quite self-aware and her 'incomplete' sentences in this case might read something like:

'I see myself as a keen, conscientious and respectful learner.'

'Others see me as over-eager, sometimes flippant and a bit of a crawler.'

Therefore, it is not necessary to see yourself as others see you, but to be aware of both perceptions. However, if the perceptions are different then you need to ask why. What are the reasons for this discrepancy? If you are conscious of this behaviour and its effect on others, can something be done about it? It is not that easy: you can be aware at the level of knowing how your behaviour affects others, but the reasons behind that behaviour require a deeper understanding. How you acquire this deeper understanding stems initially from having 'role awareness'. Being aware of how you act in the different roles of life and how your behaviour affects others is as far as many people are prepared to look. It takes a certain amount of courage to look at yourself in an honest and purposeful way, for it may result in your finding something that the 'self' does not like.

This is in fact usual, but finding something is one thing, whereas admitting and accepting it is another. People will often make excuses for, or deny, negative behaviour they find within themselves, for example:

'One thing I dislike about myself is that I'm not always honest.'

Excuse: 'There are sometimes occasions when honesty is not the best policy.'

Denial: 'No, this can't be true, I must be honest at all times in this sort of job.'

Mental health nurses need to go beyond this superficial role awareness in order to become effective helpers. Within society there exist stereotypes of mental disorders, such as the alcoholic vagrant, the drug abuser, the sex offender and many more that people generally find difficult to understand, and consequently wish to leave to people specifically trained to deal with them. As an alternative to condemning such individuals, the mental health nurse must know her own feelings towards them if she intends to help them. If she is negative in any way, then it will hinder her effectiveness as a helper, mainly because personal emotions will prevent her listening objectively and make it difficult to achieve any form of understanding. Negative feelings towards types of behaviour, race or religion are usually based on prejudice. Self-awareness involves not only awareness of how others see you, but also awareness of your own attitudes and values in respect of other people.

Give your personal rating of the following statements, from 0 = 'Don't agree' to 4 = 'Agree strongly' and add up your scores for each individual statement:

1. Gay men should not be allowed to teach in primary schools.
                    0   1   2   3   4

2. The Irish tend to be of less than average intelligence.
                    0   1   2   3   4

3. Women tend to be poorer drivers than men.
                    0   1   2   3   4

4. Jews tend to be miserly with their money.
                    0   1   2   3   4

5. Black people tend to be better dancers and sports people.
                    0   1   2   3   4

These particular statements relate to prejudices common in our society today. If you rated the statements honestly and your score is above 0, then you have some element of prejudice within yourself which may compromise the care that you give. For example, if you scored at all on statement 1, then you are probably assuming something about homosexual behaviour, whereas we cannot assume that a particular form of sexual expression will be detrimental. Even knowing this, people with this prejudice will still find it difficult not to rate the statement. This is primarily because knowledge is only one of three components that make up an attitude.

This does not mean that if you are prejudiced it is impossible to be a mental health nurse. The significant factor is that you must be aware of your prejudices in order to understand your feelings towards particular people. Once this awareness is established and the feelings are accepted, then you can work towards being less prejudiced, especially in situations where the effectiveness of the helping relationship may be affected.

Once you begin to understand your own attitudes and values, you can then begin to realize how important they are to you and how difficult they are to change. This will help you to accept other people's attitudes and values, which are as important to them as yours are to you. The acceptance of an individual within a therapeutic relationship is essential in order to listen objectively with accurate understanding.

Self-honesty is also a facet of awareness. It enables you to look purposefully at self-behaviour and the reasons behind it. Once the contract to be honest with yourself has been made, then the discoveries can be enlightening. By self-honesty, we mean the admission and acceptance of your own behaviour of feelings, however positive or negative they may be, thus avoiding the use of excuses, rationalizations or denials, e.g. 'The thing I like about myself is the way I readily accept any particular individual.' 'The thing I dislike about myself is my inconsistency in being me, i.e. variations in my mood and outlook.' By being honest and avoiding superficiality, the rest of the incomplete sentences, once filled, become very personal and meaningful statements about yourself.

How often do people look inwards? Is it necessary to do so in order to live effectively? Can being too self-aware actually inhibit you? We believe that the right to enter into the world of another must be earned by looking into your own world first.

The incomplete sentences at the beginning of this section gave you an opportunity to look at yourself. It may be appropriate now, after dwelling on the subject, to look at them again. Once you have made the necessary changes, if any, it may be useful to complete the following sentences, which should guide you further as to what we mean by self-awareness.

The things in my life that are going right are ...

The things in my life that are going wrong are ...

The occasion when I am most likely to blame other things or people for my behaviour or circumstances is ...

The situations when I tend to lose control are ...

My main 'strengths' are ...

My main 'weaknesses' are ...

The reasons I am uncomfortable in certain situations are ...

The reasons why I decided to commence nurse training are ...

I believe that I look ...

How I appear to other people is ...

Self-awareness is not acquired instantaneously, but develops gradually over a period of months or years. It may be argued that achieving total self-awareness may result in 'stripping' a person of all defences. Everyone requires personal defences to protect themselves from conflicts and anxiety. These defences give us time to adjust to certain ways of thinking, feeling or behaviour. We are not proposing that such defences be dropped, but that you should be aware of how behaviour and feelings are affected in any interaction. Some defences may be helpful: they can enable the nurse to feel secure in therapeutic situations, giving an air of confidence which is conveyed to the client, allowing him to feel able to relax and relate. The nurse who has been honest with herself, and who has experienced self-searching with courage and purposefulness, can feel secure in the fact that she has indeed earned the right to propose herself as a helper. In order to be effective and help the client to develop, she may have to enter his world and return unscathed.

Self esteem

Much of the above refers to the requirement of the mental health nurse to esteem others, offering them acceptance and respect. It is equally important that the nurse hold herself in esteem. Look at the following statements and rank them according to whether you mostly agree or mostly disagree:

My opinion is as important as that of my elders.

I am confident enough to express my opinion in most situations.

I am attractive and likeable.

I am competent in my job.

I am fairly intelligent.

It is important to make myself a priority at times.

I can say no to requests for favours when I'm busy.

I take care of my body.

If you mostly agree with these, then you are likely to have a reasonable level of self-esteem, seeing yourself as worthwhile and valuable, whereas if you found yourself disagreeing then you may be experiencing a low self-esteem. Most people fluctuate in their levels of self-esteem at different times, although they will be generally on one side of the line or the other.

When an individual regularly or continually holds themselves in low esteem, then they are more likely to suffer stress and, at the extreme end of the scale, burnout. This can happen when the need to be helping others at the expense of oneself becomes paramount, or when the nurse takes no real care of herself when off duty. It is important, then, to recognize that you are a worthwhile human being who also needs to be looked after by yourself and others. Ways of looking after yourself may range from spending two hours a week in the steam bath or treating yourself to a relaxing meal, to asking others for help when you need it. With the stress of training, nursing others and sometimes playing hard, it is not surprising that some mental health nurses find that the whole process takes its toll and that their self-esteem can become low.

For some student nurses, training may be the first time that they have left home, whereas for others it may require a juggling of responsibilities at home. Adult learning is sometimes demanding of or threatening to relationships and partnerships. In other words, mental health nursing training can represent a period of transition and it is possible for this to threaten one's self-esteem, particularly if you have been encouraged through early influences, at home or at school, to see yourself in a poor light. At such time, help from a personal tutor or counsellor can be extremely valuable.

Handling feelings

The demands on the mental health nurse are many, and in the process of nursing she is likely to experience a whole gamut of emotions. These may occur in several different ways.

Identification

On occasion, the material the client is using or the circumstances they describe may remind the nurse of her own experience. For example, the nurse who is in the middle of separating from a partner might identify with a client in a similar position. It is important here not to contaminate the listening by assuming that you know what it is like for the client, or by trying to 'make it better', as you might like to do for yourself.

Care and concern

The caring individual is likely on occasion to feel sadness or helplessness for the plight of the client. While such feelings are not particularly useful, they are nevertheless a human response to suffering and should not be ignored in the nurse's self-care.

Interpersonal issues

In every nurse–client relationship there will be some interpersonal element. For the most part this will be at a comparatively low level, given that the nurse demonstrates some level of care for the client. Sometimes, however, the nurse may feel much stronger emotions, such as extreme attraction, of a platonic or a sexual nature, or extreme revulsion or fear. In the last instance it is important that there is a bottom line of safety, so that if a nurse is afraid of her client it would clearly be undesirable for her to make home visits, for example. In less dramatic scenarios, however, it is important that the nurse is able to acknowledge her feelings, with support, and to find a way to work through them so that her client receives the best-quality care.

Where the nurse is subject to harassment or violence, again she needs space and support to vent her feelings and to discover ways of continuing her work with confidence. One nurse who was forcibly struck and marked by a client, said: 'I felt doubly betrayed. He's a difficult lad, and I was the only one left who offered him positive regard. I doubt myself now and whether I should have invested so much. I was also disappointed in how my colleagues handled it, and felt unsupported. I don't know if I can work back in the unit.'

This nurse had complex emotions of fear, disappointment, irritation, self-doubt and confusion, for which she needed support, as well as validation of her courage and sensitivity in the work she had done. This is an extreme situation, but similar emotions might be felt in other situations where a nurse has invested a sense of self and optimism in working hard with her client. There is also a sense of involvement which can occur when a nurse particularly likes a client, and this can lead to strong emotion when there is change of any kind.

Intrapersonal issues

Occasionally, the nurse may be confronted by issues that stimulate emotions in her which are to do with her self. For example, a nurse who has been bereaved at some time in the past may feel emotions which are tied up with her own experience. This may be at a conscious or an unconscious level, and is different from identification in that the situation does not have to be the same, but rather triggers an old scenario for the nurse. She may not identify directly with the client.

Looking after yourself

Just as it is important to take care of yourself in terms of self-esteem and value, so it is important to find means of ensuring support in debriefing emotions and gaining insights which will be useful to practice. We see peer debriefing as an important part of mental health nursing: an opportunity to offload events and feelings before going home. We also see supervision as an important part of the job. Supervision allows for reflection on practice, including taking space for the kind of emotional issues illustrated above (see Chapter 4). Although supervision is not yet recognized as an automatic part of psychiatric nursing, some authorities have accepted it as an effective strategy towards better practice and staff support and development.

It is also important to find ways of relaxing and getting away from the pressures of the job. Learning to balance the demands of work and home is important. Many mental health workers give their all to the job, only to feel depleted when they get home. This can be seen as an early warning sign that the emotional toll is too wearing.

Each individual will find their own ways to look after themselves and seek support. The important thing is to recognize that to give selflessly does not mean to be totally selfless. If you do not look after yourself, not only will your quality of life diminish, but you will no longer be an effective mental health nurse.

SUMMARY

We have tried to introduce many complex issues involved in human relationships. The ability to interact appropriately is mainly dependent upon your understanding of the person-to-person situation. This includes being sensitive to the client's needs, showing interest and motivation to understand, and being aware of your own internal 'messages' during any given situation: anxiety, anger, embarrassment and confusion are just some of the feelings you may experience during your interactions with clients. Being aware of these and acknowledging them is the first step towards understanding yourself and thus reducing the likelihood of your feelings compromising the care you give to the client.

Finally, we recognize that we have described what may be to some the ideal requirements for the mental health nurse. It is not necessarily the achievement of these ideals that is the measure of success, but the willingness, motivation and efforts made in striving towards them.

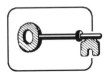

KEY CONCEPTS

1. Interaction skills involve the exchange of behaviours within any given situation. It is essential that the nurse uses these skills appropriately, as many clients are either incapable, insensitive or oversensitive in their use and interpretation.
2. They involve:
   - Being sensitive to the reaction;
   - Being aware of her own non-verbal communication and sensitive to the client's non-verbal communication;
   - Reacting appropriately to the client's feelings.
3. Within the behaviours that make up interaction skills are the personal qualities and attitudes to be an effective helper.
4. A mental health nurse is someone who can attempt to satisfy the needs of others by selflessly utilizing her personality to give some meaning to the client's life. This is done mainly by listening with understanding, responding with care and respect, supporting with trust and confidence and reassuring with explanation and honesty. She is also someone who can physically nurse the helpless with compassion and skill, and carry out procedures that are essential to maintain or improve the client's quality of life.
5. To be able to demonstrate these attributes, self-understanding is necessary, i.e. the nurse must know and accept her own feelings and behaviours, and understand or attempt to understand their presence.
6. For the mental health nurse to help the individuals that society rejects, she must know her own feelings towards them so that personal emotions do not prevent accurate and objective listening, thereby making it difficult to achieve any form of empathy.
7. She needs to be aware of her own prejudices, in order to understand her feelings towards particular people.
8. Before entering into the world of another, the right to do so must be earned by looking into her own world first.
9. The skills of the mental health nurse are acquired alongside the development of personal growth, i.e. self-awareness and the use of the essential qualities become an integral part of her own personality.
10. The mental health nurse needs to be aware of her own self-esteem needs and how to prevent 'burnout'. She needs to be able to value and care for herself.
11. This includes handling feelings that occur throughout your personal and professional life.

FURTHER READING

Argyle, M. and Trower, P. (1979) *Person to Person: Ways of Communicating, A Life Cycle Book*, London, Harper and Row.

Burnard, P. (1984) Developing self-awareness. *Nursing Mirror*, 158.

2 | Counselling skills

INTRODUCTION

Nurses are not counsellors, despite the view of some notable celebrities in nursing, who assert: 'We are all counsellors. Anyone who works in one of the health professions and comes into contact with people who are distressed in any way, whether psychologically, spiritually or practically, offers counselling help' (Burnard, 1989, p.1). We would have to disagree. In fact, nurses of all descriptions seem to do badly in the evaluation of counselling skills (see Connor, 1986). Some research (e.g. Hardin and Halasis, 1983) suggests that in empathy scales mental health nurses appear to rate very poorly. This remark is not aimed at attacking or demoralizing the reader, but is perhaps a challenge for the interested and determined nurse to break this unfortunate mould. It is not surprising that nurses are poor at counselling, for despite its introduction as a core element in the 1982 syllabus it has not found the support in training that it deserves. Very few nurse tutors are trained and supported in teaching counselling effectively, and there is some resistance to 'buying in' the necessary expertise due to budgetary constraints.

Counselling is a term that is currently used in all sorts of situations and circumstances. In some ways this is pleasing, for it shows that there is more interest in and recognition of a subject that until quite recently was almost entirely confined to the USA. Unfortunately its wider use in current expression has produced a negative side; the term is used in contexts quite outside its original meaning and, alarmingly, it is frequently linked with disciplinary action.

It is very important, in our opinion, to have a clear idea of what is meant by counselling, and how the skills associated with its practice can help all mental health professionals, if employed intelligently. The definition of 'counsellor' and 'counselling', as laid out quite simply by the British Association for Counselling, best suits our purpose. The Association defines it thus:

> The overall aim of counselling is to provide an opportunity for the client to work towards living in a more satisfying and resourceful way. The term 'counselling' inclues work with individuals, pairs or groups of people often, but not always, referred to as clients. The objectives of particular counselling relationships will vary according to the client's needs. Counselling may be concerned with developmental issues, addressing and resolving specific problems, making decisions, coping with crisis, developing personal insight and knowledge, working

through feelings of inner conflict or improving relationships with others. The counsellor's role is to facilitate the client's values, personal resources and capacity for self-determination. (BAC, 1990, p.2).

The purpose of this chapter is to inform the committed, interested or simply curious, about counselling and its appropriateness in nursing. Our objective is to help the reader to discover a skilled approach to fulfil the definition, and additionally to identify specific areas of interest to mental health workers, especially the mental health nurse, and assist her clinical practice.

In addition to the British Association for Counselling's definition, we want to add that certain qualities, and at least basic skills, should be possessed by an individual before she considers herself a 'counsellor' or purports to be practising 'counselling'.

To have an honest intention to help, a desire to promote growth within the client and a reluctance to offer advice or judgement are in our opinion precursors to effective counselling. Even these alone are insufficient. An understanding and a proficient ability to perform the skills of listening, paraphrasing, reflecting, questioning, clarifying, summarizing and challenging are essential. These skills cannot be acquired by simply reading, but are gained by practice. Practising the skills after studying the text requires courage, not just in the personal risk involved, nor in commitment to a role, but also the courage required to ask for guidance, to accept constructive criticism, to be sufficiently self-aware to observe yourself and admit your mistakes. The individual who seeks skill acquisition needs to be aware enough when dealing with a client to see the dangerous areas and pitfalls, and avoid harming him. In order to do this you need to be resourceful enough to change direction when feeling out of your depth, and confident enough as an individual to share with the client your feelings, misgivings and uncertainties.

In short, it is our view that you must earn the right to counsel others by acquiring the skills, owning the qualities and understanding yourself. We are aware that this is no mean feat. One of the most important facets of good 'counselling' is good 'supervision'. It is the opinion of both BAC and ourselves that counsellors should not practise without contracting supervision. To go even further, we would add that mental health nurses, in either residential or community settings, should not practise without regular supervision (see Chapter 4).

Carl Rogers, who is considered by many to be the father of counselling, coined the term 'client-centred therapy'. We shall now consider some of the concepts that Rogers and other leading authorities suggest are important in the field of counselling based on client-centred therapy.

CLIENT-CENTRED

This is the linchpin of many counselling models, at least in the initial stages. The idea is based upon the belief that the client is the important person in the relationship, and that he has the resources and the ability to help himself if given the opportunity. The counsellor facilitates the client's seeing himself more clearly, and does not advise, suggest, persuade or in any way interfere

the client's view of himself. Initially, to operate in this manner may mean
~~~eviously trained health workers have to shed their preconceived ideas
~~~emselves and their clients, i.e. relationships based on the idea that 'I
~~~pert, you are the client – you tell me what is wrong and I will tell you

~~~nt-centred therapy suggests that the client will, given the correct climate,
~~~iagnose, prescribe and treat himself. It is therefore implicit in the client-
centred approach to have a trust in human beings, that all people have inner
resources, and above all are motivated to improve.

UNCONDITIONAL POSITIVE REGARD/NON-JUDGEMENTAL APPROACH

The expression of 'unconditional positive regard' is a fundamental principle of
counselling without which it is difficult to imagine how a therapeutic relationship can be maintained. Although the term sounds difficult, the idea is really
quite simple. Rogers explains that, before a client can really understand
himself clearly, he must be able to accept himself. One way of assisting this
process is for the counsellor to show that she accepts him unconditionally. It
has been our experience that all effective and therapeutic mental health nurses
have this quality to some degree. To have faith, trust and respect for another
human being, despite his behaviour, is probably one of the most difficult things
a nurse can be asked to do. She has lived to the age of 18 years at least, during
which time she has been bombarded with values and judgements, all playing
their part in shaping her personality and character. Parents, friends, the law,
society, teachers and colleagues have continually influenced her to believe
certain things, to act in certain ways and to think in an 'acceptable' way. Now,
in this specific therapeutic relationship, she is asked to accept an individual
without any kind of judgement, without criticism and without reservation.
Additionally, she is being asked not just to accept but to respect her client,
without necessarily knowing what his previous behaviour has been, or who he
is, because he is another human being.

To be effective the counsellor has to dispense with her own values, beliefs,
prejudices and stereotypes. She must positively – i.e. in a 'friendly' manner –
accept and try to understand the other person's values, ideals and beliefs, even
if these are totally opposed to her own and are prejudiced, stereotyped and
uncaring.

The advantage this has in the relationship is tremendous, for the client is
confronted with another person who does not reject, ridicule or argue with him.
He feels that the counsellor is interested, not, as so many people are, in herself,
but in him.

She is genuinely interested, wants to really know him and how he thinks and
feels, and still does not judge him. The realization of this fact engenders in the
client the feeling that if someone else is interested, thinks he is worth something, and cares, then perhaps he too should take some time to look at himself
more closely.

The practical application of this is, of course, extremely difficult for the inexperienced, and it is our experience that it is sometimes only after a series of successful counselling sessions that the counsellor's fundamental beliefs are changed. Ask yourself these questions and answer them honestly:

1. Do you believe that most human beings are capable of helping themselves if facilitated by skilled counsellors?
2. Could you counsel a person convicted of rape, child murder or some other crime that you find heinous, trying to put his past out of your mind and accepting him with a positive attitude, respecting his values and not judging him for his behaviour?
3. Do you have enough trust in yourself and your client to be open and honest, and not feel exposed to exploitation by the client?

We would guess your response to at least one of these will be negative, and indeed some of you may have answered 'No' to them all. Indeed, neither of the authors could have honestly answered 'Yes' to them all a few years ago. Moreover, it is not expected that to be an effective counsellor you have to answer 'Yes' to all of them unequivocally in every circumstance and at all periods of your life. It would be foolish, for example, to take on a client who had murdered a child if your own child had just been murdered, just as it may not always be the best practice to take on a bereavement client shortly after a personal bereavement. Despite this, we can assure you that our unanimous answer to the questions now would be 'Yes'. It is only with the acquisition of counselling skills, practice in counselling situations and observation of results in effective interactions that our faith in the process has gradually increased to a certain, unshakeable belief.

When you can look back at the three questions and answer them all in the affirmative, we are sure you will be capable of entering into a helping relationship with your client and expressing unconditional positive regard.

Before we leave this area, it is perhaps sensible to state that some workers and therapists recognize a danger in this concept. To accept without question any goals, behaviours or attitudes in a client may be positively colluding with immoral, antisocial or evil intent. We do not believe this was Rogers' original suggestion, and would clarify that it is possible to accept a person unconditionally without necessarily condoning or agreeing with his or her behaviour. In certain situations it may be necessary for the therapist to refer to someone else if there is potential for postive regard to be lost.

Understandably, some workers will only offer positive regard 'conditionally'. If a client insists that what they want is to change for the 'worse' in what is reasonably evaluated, e.g. 'I want to become a 'better' murderer, rapist or exploiter of others', this may clash so radically with the counsellor's personal values that they will not continue with the helping relationship. We have no argument with this position. In such situations, our expressed view to the client might well be: 'Although I can accept you unconditionally as a human being, and offer you warmth and understanding simply on those terms, your behaviour is totally unaceptable! Until your stated aims (of endangering or exploiting others) change, your attitudes, values and behaviour clash so much with my own that I cannot continue to offer help'.

[handwritten margin notes:] criticism of Rogers idea of UPR + way of getting round it

what to do if you can only offer conditionally

EMPATHY, WARMTH AND GENUINENESS

Another concept accepted almost universally by counsellors is that of the 'core conditions'. Carkhuff and Truax (1979) identify these as empathy, warmth and genuineness. Here we will try to explore briefly what is meant by these terms.

Empathy

Most authorities on counselling agree that this is perhaps the most important quality the counsellor must own. It refers to the ability to understand the client, not superficially but in an accurate and meaningful way. It must be carefully distinguished from sympathy, and is probably the concept most misunderstood by the inexperienced person interested in counselling. Egan (1994) helps to clarify the idea of empathy by suggesting that it is not an all-or-nothing quality, and that it can be achieved on different levels. He suggests two: 'accurate empathy' and 'advanced empathy'.

Accurate empathy

The first is some kind of verbal or non-verbal indication that the helper is right. That is, the client nods or gives some other non- verbal cue, or uses some assenting word or phrase (such as 'that's right' or 'exactly')....The second and more substantive way in which clients acknowledge accuracy of the helper's response is by moving forward in the helping process; for instance, by clarifying the problem situation more fully (p.115).

To do this the helper must respond to the client in a way that shows she has listened to and understands how the client feels: she must see the client's world from the client's frame of reference; she must communicate her understanding.

Advanced empathy

...as skilled helpers listen intently to clients, they often enough see clearly what clients only half see and hint at (p.180).

Here, then, the counsellor is no longer merely responding to the client, but is demanding that the client take a deeper look at himself. Egan argues that a counsellor using advanced accurate empathy can use genuineness, respect, understanding and rapport as a power base, where the power is used to influence the client to see his problems from a more objective frame of reference.

Empathy is built up by using skills rather than a quality that a person either has or has not developed. We have noticed, however, that some nurses tend to be extremely quick in establishing advanced empathy, while others need far more time. The time factor is not particularly important, whereas accuracy is absolutely vital: nurses should not be too eager to compliment themselves on their speedy attainment of empathy. On many occasions we have observed nurses responding to a client's remarks and receiving swift results by saying something quite profound and very accurate. The client has an overwhelming feeling of relief that at last someone understands, and a great advance in the relationship occurs. Although this is wonderful and no doubt very helpful, all may not be well. For instance, this reaction might have been achieved by a wild and lucky guess, not by accurate observation, skilful listening and thoughtful consideration. It might have been disastrous if the nurse had guessed wrongly. Our advice in this area is to take the slow accurate route, and not to go for wild stabs in the dark which may have poor overall results.

Probably the most frequent problem in establishing accurate empathy occurs when the counsellor is unable to enter the client's world and understand it from the client's perspective. This difficulty exists because commonly the nurse becomes overwhelmed by her own feelings of sorrow, or perhaps fear, and contaminates or confuses her understanding of the client's world with her own thoughts and emotions.

Sundeen (1976) takes a more systematized view of empathy as a four–stage process. Here empathy is broken down into identification, incorporation, reverberation and detachment. The general idea (simplified) is that the empathic counsellor is able to lose consciousness of self (identification) and become engrossed in the client (incorporation). A process of mental interaction between the feelings of the client and the counsellor then follows (reverberation). Finally, the counsellor returns to her own reality (detachment), combining all this and previously gained information into an objective knowledge about the client.

It is perhaps important at this point to clarify a general misunderstanding or confusion about empathy. To do this it is important to say what empathy is not. Empathy is not listening to the client and imagining what it would be like to be them, or how you would feel in a similar situation, and it is certainly not trying to be them. These approaches are all likely to miss the point and result in a sympathetic response, i.e. sharing your vision and potential feelings. Empathy is the objective acknowledgement of the client's feelings, situations and experiences from their position.

The final word goes to Rogers (1967). He describes achieving empathy as 'sensing the feelings and personal meanings which the client is experiencing in each moment, when he can perceive these from 'inside', as they seem to the client, and when he can successfully communicate something of that understanding to his client.'

Genuineness

This quality is based on the individual's ability to be himself: he does not have to play a role; he can 'afford' to be transparent; he can own his feelings and express them honestly.

An individual throughout his life may play many roles in different situations and circumstances – father, teacher, friend, husband. As a counsellor he has to be himself, putting away all the prejudices and stereotypes that make him an individual, because he needs to be aware that they are just that. Having a sincere belief in human beings and their potential for 'growth' and improvement, he will not have to pretend. He will concentrate all his energies on understanding the client fully and accurately, in the knowledge that he will be challenged about himself. He can honestly share what is appropriate, because he understands himself fully. On the occasions when he becomes unhappy with the client he will say so, and it will probably help him to understand the client better in the long term. However, when the counsellor shares his feelings with the client on these occasions, it will be done skilfully to enable further insight for the client.

For example, Robert, an imaginary client, goes round and round in circles, evading the real issue of his problem. At some point, in order to prevent the counsellor feeling his time is being wasted, and to move the client forward, the counsellor may say something along these lines: 'Robert, I'm not sure we're really getting anywhere – it seems to me that whenever you reach the point of understanding what the problem might be, you steer away from it. Apart from this being rather irritating, I'm not sure we will accomplish much if we carry on like this!'

Although this may temporarily inhibit the client, it shows that the counsellor is real – a person too – that he is not prepared simply to go along with everything and anything. In a way, we feel it would devalue the relationship if the counsellor did not occasionally disclose his own feelings. It may be helpful to create a feeling of mutuality between client and counsellor, i.e. they both have a shared purpose, they are going somewhere together, they are sharing an experience, an adventure. Genuineness is important. We are sure that not only will it help the client, it will also help the counsellor. Without it we would both have experienced impossible situations when dealing with clients.

To summarize, genuineness means being 'yourself', not being like anybody else or trying to live up to or become another sort of person. It involves you as a person being that person in every situation. 'You' as a nurse should be no different from 'you' as a brother, sister or friend. That is to say, fundamentally you do not change your values or attitudes towards people just because of another role. You take on different responsibilities and you may be expected to behave in certain ways to suit that role, but within that role it is still you. This involves a certain amount of self-awareness, awareness of your own feelings, not presenting a facade. It requires honesty and courage to allow yourself to be seen as a real and authentic person. To hide behind a uniform and to misuse a position of status in order to avoid explanations and difficult situations can be an easy option for people who have not looked at themselves with any degree of honesty. To have any genuineness, you need to know yourself.

Warmth

Warmth is a quality that hardly needs explaining, especially to anyone interested enough in people to read this text. Warmth is so closely connected to the principles of unconditional positive regard that if you have accepted the concept you already have warmth.

One necessary highlight in this area that perhaps deserves attention is ensuring that your natural warmth is conveyed to your client. While earnestly and actively listening to your client, try not to become so tense and anxious about listening that the human expressions of warmth, such as smiling, gesturing and posture, are lost in the intensity of the moment. Clients need to have your warmth transmitted to them, to encourage them to continue. A smile costs nothing and is seldom misinterpreted, but can mean everything to the client.

'Warmth' is an appealing term associated with attraction, comfort and safety. To possess it is to be able to demonstrate the acceptance of others as individuals. This acceptance involves adopting non-judgemental attitudes, respecting the feelings and behaviours presented by the client non-defensively, and being open and having a respect for the individual, thereby communicating an approachable manner. To emphasize this concept, contrast these qualities with the components of a 'cold' person, i.e. one who is rigid in stance and attitude, stern and upright, unsmiling and glaring. From this description, it can be seen that non-verbal communication plays a major part in conveying these qualities. Possession alone is insufficient, and demonstrating warmth and genuineness is essential to form the basis of a therapeutic relationship.

It is worth adding that the therapeutic warmth addressed to an individual is of a 'non-possessive' type. The warmth for your client should not encompass the additional component that one might expect from a personal relationship with a friend or lover. The client must not be smothered in the kind of warmth often connected with the possessive pronoun 'my', as this position of ownership is often invested with directiveness; it often makes for a claustrophobic component, and consequently leads to a diminished self-determination.

VALUES

One area we cannot over-stress is the uniqueness of the individual and how important it is to maintain that uniqueness. The client will hold many experiences, people, possessions, beliefs and attitudes as valuable – these are his. Do not try to steal them from him.

A most fundamental and yet frequently met problem in the inexperienced counsellor is the tendency to reinforce or criticize the individual client's values. The counsellor's values in this context are unimportant, and should not interfere with or contaminate the client's values. If, for instance, a client is pregnant and has decided to seek an abortion, it may suggest to the counsellor that the client places a low value on life. This is presumptive and may be completely wrong. However, even if it is so, it should not influence the counsellor's interactions. It would be fundamentally wrong to condemn the client for her values, and no attempt should be made to bring them into line with your own. As in any situation, the counsellor would perhaps want to stay in this particular area of the client's values and try to form some accurate understanding in order that both the client and the counsellor understand the true situation, and if the counsellor is successful in this, logical decisions could be made from the client's point of view.

CONFIDENTIALITY

Finally, a very important aspect of counselling is confidentiality. Nurses and health professionals are constantly being reminded of the need to respect confidences, but the implications of this for the counsellor are more difficult. If the counsellor is working independently in a private consultation, confidentiality poses little problem, although total confidentiality may still lead to problems for any counsellor. It is necessary to know your own personal boundaries and to make these clear to your client. In our practice the boundaries of confidentiality are still limited by the disclaimer that disclosures indicating that clients are intending to exploit or endanger others may breach the confidential boundaries. Although you may wish to reassure your client that no action would be taken in any regard without opportunities for discussion, and at the very least for the client to be informed, there may be some circumstances when regard for others has to be your concern as well. For instance, one of us, early on in his counselling practice, was told by his client that his problem was one of a sexual nature. It emerged that the client was sexually abusing his young daughter. Had this situation arisen in a contract of complete confidentiality, the counsellor would have found himself very limited in terms of acting according to his own professional and personal values. Indeed, it is hard to conceive of situations in practice where total confidentiality is realistic, if for no other reason than the need of the counsellor for supervision and the consequent sharing of case material with at least one other person. Although anonymity can often be maintained, it is still important that the client knows that they will be discussed with someone else.

In most health organizations it is extremely rare for one person to have sole responsibility for care, and to some degree a transfer of information is expected and necessary for the rest of the team to function efficiently. This has caused many problems in nurse counselling, for an implicit trust and a feeling of being able to disclose information of a sensitive nature without fear of the counsellor breaking the confidence are essential for a successful outcome. The counsellor does not have to decide simply whether to break confidence to people outside the normal caring professionals, but also how much to disclose to colleagues. Although this is a very sensitive area, and one in which people hold strong views, it is our hope that common sense and professional attitudes will prevail. After much discussion and debate, we consider that the following suggestions may be helpful:

1. Begin any formal session with a statement of exactly what confidentiality means, so that both parties clearly understand its personal implications, e.g.:

   - 'I cannot guarantee completely that what you say to me will be in confidence, but what I disclose to the other members of the team will be only in your interests.'
   - 'There are certain areas we may discuss that I will feel bound to convey to my colleagues so that they can offer you help as well.'
   - 'If I feel during our talks that other staff need to be given some of the information you disclose, I hope you will understand.'
   - 'There may be certain facts that I would have to share with other staff: for instance, if you told me you were contemplating suicide.'

These areas should be clearly identified and, if possible, definite policies about such areas discussed and agreed by the team before counselling is undertaken.

2. In case of difficulties in these areas, be prepared with alternative courses of action, e.g.:

   • Stop the conversation until the client understands the implications of what he is saying.
   • Be honest: say you are sorry, but you will have to disclose that.
   • Seek permission to disclose, even if this requires active persuasion.
   • Be genuine and say how you are feeling.

To conclude this short introduction to counselling, we would like to emphasize that the model we are recommending in this chapter is a developmental style, i.e. its basis and essence are a client-centred approach, developing in the later stages towards strategies for helping the client set and achieve goals (see Figure 2.1). The emphasis is on helping the client help himself. The following analogy may clarify this statement.

explains the differences between CCA + helping + achieve goals!

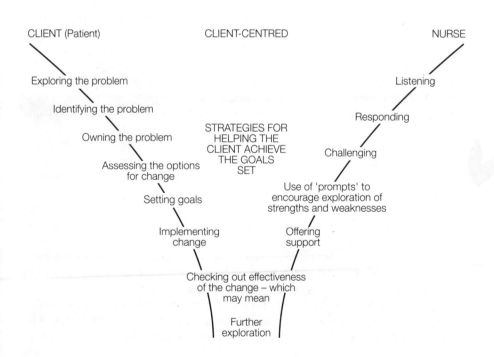

CLIENT (Patient)   CLIENT-CENTRED   NURSE

Exploring the problem   Listening

Identifying the problem   Responding

Owning the problem   STRATEGIES FOR HELPING THE CLIENT ACHIEVE THE GOALS SET   Challenging

Assessing the options for change

Setting goals   Use of 'prompts' to encourage exploration of strengths and weaknesses

Implementing change   Offering support

Checking out effectiveness of the change – which may mean

Further exploration

Figure 2.1   Illustrating the developmental style of this counselling model

Life itself may be considered a journey, and from time to time the participant may well hesitate, rest a while and wonder which direction to take. This must be his choice and his alone, but if someone offers him some spectacles to help him see more clearly, so much the better. Having explored his options, seen much more clearly, and having finally decided to continue in a particular direction, if he should be offered speedier transport and accepts the lift, the journey may be made more easy. In a true client-centred approach the counsellor should seek only to be the spectacles. When the model takes on a behavioural approach, the counsellor should offer the speedy method after the goals have been decided by the client, who needs help in reaching them.

It should be noted that counselling cannot be a compulsory therapy. By its very nature, compulsion would prevent an open and honest interchange. It should not, therefore, be considered the answer or the suitable approach to any client's problems. Perhaps some people do not have any definite goals to be driven towards, but are simply here to enjoy the scenery. If this is true, and it is what they hold valuable, who are we to direct them?

NON-VERBAL COMMUNICATION

Non-verbal communication is communication other than the spoken word. It is not necessary to verbalize words in order to communicate: thoughts and feelings can be effectively transmitted by the slightest gesture or other movement of the body. Such gestures and movements often accompany the spoken word, adding to or even changing the literal meaning of what is said, or they may occur in isolation. The human being is such a complex set of moving signals that it is extremely difficult to be anywhere without 'saying' something.

The impossibility of not communicating is explored in great detail in a paper by Watzlawick, Beavin and Jackson (1968). It is suggested that communication is constant and continual and that non-communication is impossible. However, what is important to the counsellor is that the communication is congruent, i.e. that the message sent is the message received, with little room for error or misinterpretation.

In reality, even the intention of saying nothing is still communicating something to those who choose to judge people on appearance alone. Walking, talking and gesticulating are all signals given within an environment comprised of people who are complex 'senders' and 'receivers'. It is the degree of complexity in this environment that determines whether or not the message sent will be the message received, or how many distortions will occur.

In order to be an effective counsellor, the nurse requires a depth of understanding that goes beyond superficial requests and information exchange. This understanding is partially gained by the nurse being sensitive to the client's non-verbal as well as verbal messages. The complexity of the individual and the environment in which we live gives rise to the possibility of misinterpreting or ignoring the non-verbal message. Within any human interaction there is potential for the expression of thoughts and feelings to be dramatically misinterpreted. This is particularly so within the caring relationship between the mental health nurse and her client, due mainly to the existence of extremes experienced by the client in psychological and physical states. The nurse who wishes to understand her clients needs to be sensitive to the meaning of their communication and must use her own non-verbal signals appropriately.

NON-VERBAL SENSITIVITY

Sensitivity to non-verbal communication requires an appreciation of the various components that create the wealth of signals we continually convey to each other throughout our lives. These components are the face, posture and body space, gestures, touch and tone of voice.

The face

The human face has a great potential for expression, and each part of the face can be observed as a potential communicator. It is extremely difficult to speak without changing facial expression. Some messages are conveyed by nodding, shaking, frowning, or simply by using eye contact, mouth and eyebrow movements. The most powerful of these signals involves the eyes. They have been called the 'windows of the soul' and can convey quite clearly the powerful emotions of aggression, fear, concern and love. Observing the state of clients' eyes alone can be very informative. Some examples include:

forms of non verbal on face

	Possible emotion
Redness/tearfulness	Sadness
Dull, lack of movement	Depression
Lack of eye contact	Insecurity/unsure/uncomfortable/ depression
Eye contact/staring/fixed	Accusing
Staring with movement	Excitement

If the nurse relied upon single observations it is possible that the interpretation would be wrong, as few non-verbal signals occur in isolation. It is the additional signals that can build up the obvious picture, for example, red and tearful eyes can be symptomatic of happiness but the accompanying behaviours confirm the picture of sadness: lack of body movement, head stooped, drooping mouth and speaking in monosyllables with a dull tone.

Posture and body space

Posture alone can convey certain emotions and attitudes. Try matching the following stick diagrams to the list of terms given:

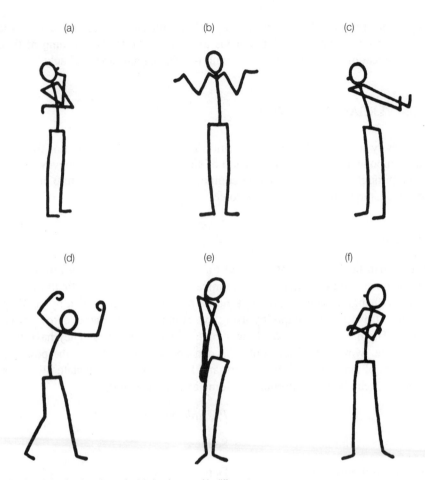

(a)   (b)   (c)

(d)   (e)   (f)

rejecting / dominating / puzzled / shy / angry / indifferent

(From Argyle, 1975).

posture expresses certain emotions + attitudes.

The distinct positioning of the body, arms and legs seems to be universal for expressing certain emotions and attitudes. Observing the posture of clients could indicate expressions of mood, e.g.:

leaning forward head bowed legs and arms closed inwards	could be indicating depression
tense, rocking and generally rigid	anxiety
bizarre, agitated movements	possible reaction to delusions or hallucinations.

Posture alone does not allow an accurate perception of the client's feelings. Confirmation of the meaning of any communication from the client arises out of taking note of all non-verbal signals. Probably the most significant aspect of observing a client's posture is related to postural change during an interaction. These changes are frequently quite subtle and often involve the client either moving towards the nurse or turning away. Moving towards the nurse could indicate that the client accepts the nurse and is ready to disclose, especially if this approach is made in a relaxed manner. However, if the client turns or leans away, it could indicate that he is not prepared for the interaction or that he feels uncomfortable talking about the topic in question. If the nurse is sensitive to this, she can act appropriately. However, if she is not aware of what the client is communicating, she may inadvertently persist in pursuing an interaction that is one-sided and subsequently spoil her chances of the relationship developing in a therapeutic manner.

It is important to be sensitive not only to how the body is positioned, but also to where it is positioned, especially in relation to others. Like many animals, people have a desire for a personal territory or personal space. The behaviour of people on a crowded beach illustrates this, where they mark out 'their' space with towels, deckchairs and windbreaks, positioning them in a situation mutually acceptable to all concerned considering the space available. Invasion of this space causes anxiety and discomfort. The same principles apply in a crowded ward, but this time the client has his locker and a few personal effects instead of beach equipment. A major difference between these two situations is that the client in the ward experiences many infringements of his space, either by another client or by a nurse who is insensitive to his need. The nurse may sit close to the client on his bed, or 'barge' into the bathroom, or lean forward with enthusiasm during an interaction. If these situations occur without mutual respect for each other's personal space, withdrawal, defensiveness and resentment could be the client's response. It is therefore necessary to avoid taking the nurse–client relationship for granted and to approach the client with respect and sensitivity.

Gestures

Observation and subsequent sensitivity to hand, head and body movements can be useful aids to assessing the client's emotional state. A clear example of this is the ceaseless hand-wringing or fidgeting observed in anxiety, or the clenched fist seen in anger and tension. Many of the conventional gestures are used in everyday life by all, for example:

head nod/shake	agree/not agree
shaking fist	anger
rubbing palms	anticipation
beckon	come
extended hand	invitation
shrugging shoulders	do not know/uninterested.

Some long-term clients, due to the course of their illness, will use gestures rather than words. The pointing finger, the banging of furniture, the broken cup, the persistent pacing up and down or the tightly folded arms can all be observed as gestures. It is sensitivity to these within the context of knowing the client that creates the possibility of the nurse approaching the situation appropriately and consequently increasing the likelihood of understanding the gesture and the reasons for it.

Touch

This is probably one of the most primitive and powerful forms of communication. The amount of touch between individuals varies with culture and the type of relationship. Touch is often used in extreme emotional states such as love, anger or distress. On the one hand it can be soothing and reassuring, but on the other hand it can be threatening. It is probably more appropriate to talk about sensitivity to the non-use of touch, as people in our society are generally quite inhibited about touching each other. This facet of our culture seems to be accentuated among mental health clients, making it essential for the nurse to respect and appreciate the client's readiness to accept, or not accept, various forms of touch. This applies particularly when attempting to communicate with clients who may be suspicious or paranoid, for they tend on occasions to misinterpret physical contact and may perceive what was intended to be a reassuring touch as a threat, thereby putting the success of the relationship at risk.

Nurses are expected to touch any part of the client's body, if necessary, and the nurse should therefore appreciate that some people react to touch with anxiety, discomfort and defensiveness, because it becomes an intrusion upon something very private. This appreciation can be attained by examining your own feelings about being touched, which will depend upon how and where you are touched and in what circumstances. Generally, the closer the relationship the more bodily contact there is. So how much bodily contact is acceptable to clients? Obviously, during physical care the amount of contact given is directly concerned with the procedure. However, during counselling the general principle is to use that which comes spontaneously and naturally, e.g. the reassuring hand on or round the shoulder and the holding of hands are frequently used for a variety of reasons, and are very effective if performed in a genuine way.

Tone of voice

This is included in a section on non-verbal communication because how something is said is as important as its literal meaning. In order to receive the spoken word accurately, the nurse must listen to the way it is said; it is possible to perceive how someone is feeling by the way they speak: the tone, speed, pitch and intensity of the voice are all factors that influence the spoken word. While listening to the client, it is important to be sensitive to his tone of voice in order to detect true and often hidden feelings, thus confirming or even contradicting the verbal communication. Some mental health problems include symptoms of thought disorder which cause clients difficulties in verbal communication. In these situations, listening to the tone and theme rather than the actual content is probably of more value in determining what the client is trying to say; subtle changes in tone can often give the nurse an additional clue to how the client is feeling. If these observations are linked to other aspects of non-verbal communication, as well as listening to the words, there is a likelihood of the nurse achieving empathy.

It is important that the nurse focuses upon the whole picture rather than the spoken word alone. One major reason for this is that non-verbal communication can contradict the verbal message; an example is the client who responds to the question 'How are you today?' with: 'OK, not bad!' while at the same time shaking his head, shrugging his shoulders and lifting his hand. A possible interpretation of this could be:

shaking head: 'I'm not all right.'

shrugging shoulders: 'I'm not sure.'

lifting hand: 'Can you help?'

The detailed analysis of this reply is not important. What is important is the nurse's sensitivity to the client's reply, 'not bad'. Many clients use very little non-verbal expression, particularly the depressed and long-term dependent clients, and when they do the changes in expression are subtle; mental health nurses need to be aware of this.

> These expressions last about one fifth second and can be seen on slow motion film and by mental nurses but may be missed by many others. (Argyle, 1975)

Individuals do not consciously control every body movement. Many of the gestures that are made are subconscious reactions to thoughts and feelings.

NON-VERBAL ATTENDING

Not only is it essential to be sensitive to the client's non-verbal communication, but sensitivity to and awareness of your own body signals is also vital. One major reason for this is that certain mental health problems are manifested in such a way that the client may be oversensitive to, or misinterpret, any non-verbal communication. An example of this can be seen in the person experiencing persecutory ideas who, seeing two nurses talking and gesticulating to each other in the corner, interprets it as referring to him, and rushes up to them shouting abuse and threats. A general awareness of the fact that you are continuously emitting signals and that they may be interpreted from different perspectives may help when nursing this type of client. However, general awareness is not enough, and nurses must be able to use non-verbal communication effectively within the helping relationship. This is what we mean by non-verbal attending. Using your body language appropriately in a helping relationship will facilitate the client's trust and confidence in you. The use of tone of voice, eye contact, touch, facial expression and posture can convey to the client the qualities of genuineness and warmth.

Attending to the client in a physical way is saying, 'I'm interested, and listening', thus forming the basis of a relationship whereby the client can perceive the nurse as someone who will accept what he has to say, in a non-judgemental manner. Physical attending is orientating yourself towards the client. Egan (1982) summarizes this by using the acronym SOLER:

S   -   facing the client 'squarely' as opposed to turning away is usually considered to be a posture of involvement.

O   -   adopting an 'open' posture as opposed to a closed one. Crossed arms and legs can be a sign of defensiveness and unwillingness to give or receive.

L   -   'leaning' towards the client usually conveys interest and willingness to be involved. Contrast this with leaning back; here the posture could be interpreted as boredom, or, at its extreme, 'sleep'.

E   -   maintain appropriate 'eye contact'. It can be seen when observing people in intense conversation that eye contact is established most of the time. Avoidance of eye contact could signify insecurity, defensiveness and lack of confidence, all of which are non-productive for the nurse as a counsellor. The nurse should be aware that constant unwavering eye contact, i.e. staring, can be interpreted by the client as threatening. Looking away occasionally is natural and quite acceptable, but if you catch yourself looking away frequently, this may have something to do with your feelings rather than the client's.

R   -   'relax' within any given therapeutic relationship and many of the behaviours described will come naturally. It also diminishes the likelihood of your fidgeting, which can be distracting for the client, and often your nervousness will reflect on to the client, which is hardly conducive to relaxed and thoughtful communication.

This description of appropriate non-verbal behaviour is only a guideline, and should not be viewed as a rigid formula for non-verbal attending. However, it would be unfortunate if the nurse's internal state of warmth and genuineness was contradicted by the her non-verbal communication, causing difficulties in the relationship. So it may be useful for the nurse to look at herself and her approach and ask herself whether, when listening to the client, she is non-verbally communicating: 'I'm interested' and 'I'm with you'.

The importance of non-verbal attending can be appreciated when you consider that it conveys not only that you are interested and are listening effectively, but also the qualities of warmth and genuineness. Smiling and nodding appropriately, moving in a relaxed and natural way and using touch naturally and spontaneously are all extremely effective and often enable the client to relax and feel secure, thus increasing the likelihood of him exploring his problems effectively within a relationship based on trust and confidence.

Non-verbal responding

Using non-verbal communication can be as effective as a verbal reply if used appropriately. Thus the non-verbal response not only shows the client that the nurse is listening, but also that she is responding, e.g.

Non-verbal response	Possible verbal equivalent
Head nod	'Go on, I understand.'
Smile appropriately	'You're safe, I accept what you are saying.'
Raised eyebrow	'That's particularly interesting.'
Frown	'I'm not sure what you're saying.'
Touch	'Reassure, console, accept.'

You can tell from the tone of voice alone whether a person is 'warm' and accepting, or 'cold' and judgemental. A calm, non-threatening, clear tone of voice will usually have a positive effect on the relationship, as opposed to a harsh, abrupt, loud response.

One non-verbal response that can be considered in this context is silence. This can be very positive if the timing and length are judged appropriately and if it is client-centred rather than nurse-centred. By this we mean that the silences should be natural ones based on the client's thought processes, giving him time to think, as opposed to being based on the nurse's need for time to think of something to say or her anxiety to say something. The nurse should never feel threatened by a silence. She should be sensitive to the feelings of the client during silences, judging whether it would be advantageous or not to the client for her to break the silence and continue the verbal exchange.

It is not uncommon for learners, having studied non-verbal communication, to feel awkward and self-conscious during the initial stages of learning these skills. The question often arises: 'How can I be genuine when I am purpose-fully engineering my body signals to a position I would not normally adopt'? The answer is simply that genuineness is an attitude, which is held firmly and not contradicted by the effective use of non-verbal communication. The awkwardness and self-consciousness are natural responses experienced by anyone who sets out to master new skills. Eventually, once your awareness of your own non-verbal communication is achieved, it will be possible to correct any negative use. Progress is made from there to using appropriate non-verbal communication naturally, spontaneously and effectively. By studying non-verbal communication you can increase your self-awareness in order to be sensitive to your own and your client's 'messages' and their subsequent exchange. It is then more likely that the client will be given every opportunity to express himself, and the nurse will have every likelihood of hearing what has been said, accurately.

EXPLORATORY RESPONDING

Throughout the counselling process it is imperative that the nurse 'listens'. This means not only passively sitting and responding with appropriate non-verbal communication, but also actively listening, i.e. showing the client, by your verbal as well as your non-verbal responses, that you understand. These responses are extremely important, particularly in the initial stages of a rela-tionship, for it is the nurse's ability to empathize with the client that facilitates the building of trust and confidence, establishing a sound foundation for counselling. The importance of these 'initial responding skills' becomes clear when you consider that this is a very early stage in the helping relationship: the problem or problems have yet to be identified. It is through your use of these skills that the client can 'explore' his feelings, behaviour and circumstances and come to see his problems clearly. It is therefore vital that the exploratory responding stage is totally client-centred. The skills required at this stage are:

- Paraphrasing
- Reflecting
- Clarifying
- Summarizing.

Paraphrasing

This involves listening to what the client says and putting the essential meaning into other words, which are then repeated back to the client without adding or subtracting anything. In essence, what this is actually doing is acting as a 'sounding board'. By paraphrasing, the nurse shows the client that she is listening accurately and helps the client hear what he has just said, thus allowing for further thought on the subject if necessary. Repeating the essential meaning back to the client in a 'tentative' way allows an element of inaccuracy to be acceptable, and permits the client to correct the nurse's paraphrased response:

Client: 'I find it difficult to concentrate, I'm not sure whether it is the ward, clients or just the way I'm feeling.'

Nurse: 'So your concentration difficulties could be due to several factors or just the way you're feeling at the moment.'

This single paraphrase is virtually word for word what the client said. This is acceptable, especially early on in the relationship. It is important to earn the client's trust and confidence by showing him that you are listening accurately. However, there are different ways of paraphrasing which are more or less appropriate, depending upon the nurse's understanding of the client's position. In the above exchange it could be that the nurse detects from the client's emphasis and non-verbal communication that his feelings are of equal or greater importance than his stated 'difficulty in concentration'. The repeating or 'parroting' of a word or phrase allows the client to expand upon it, as appropriate. The nurse could reply in a tentative, questioning way: 'Just the way you're feeling?', which would allow the client to think about the way he feels in order to explore this area if it is important to him at the time. Paraphrasing can be useful in allowing the client to explore his own feelings, encouraging him to talk freely and expand upon what is important to him.

Client. 'I can't stand the way my wife continually harasses me, it makes me so angry.'

Nurse: 'Angry?

Here the nurse repeats just one single word on the basis that she feels this is the area that is probably important to the client. As it is repeated in a tentative way, it is a 'safe' paraphrase. On the other hand, the nurse may paraphrase thus:

Nurse: 'Harasses you'?

This would probably allow the counselling to take the direction of exploring the wife's behaviour, which is only acceptable if it is important to the client to do so. It is the client's choice to pursue this theme or not. However, it is important to bear in mind that throughout the counselling process it is the 'here and now' and its effect on the client that is the crucial issue.

Client: 'The burden...I can't cope with it, it seems endless, how is it going to end, what is going to become of me, is there any hope?'

Nurse: 'You think you can't cope with this never-ending burden and you're questioning the outcome of it all.'

Here the paraphrase involves repeating back to the client the essence of what he has just said. This is particularly useful in cases where a client's thoughts are somewhat clouded or confused by extremes of emotion, such as anxiety or depression.

Paraphrasing is the first stage of actively showing that you understand what the client has said. This understanding has so far focused upon paraphrasing experiences, behaviours and insights, derived from what the client has stated. However, within any circumstances or behaviour there exist feelings which may not be overtly stated. Detection and communication of clients' implicit and explicit emotions is called 'reflecting'.

Reflecting

In order for you to understand the thoughts, attitudes and behaviour of a client, you must also understand how he feels. Because of the very personal nature of feelings, reflecting is essential in order to achieve mutual understanding of the expressed feeling. What you mean by sad, happy or fearful may be completely different from what another person means. This partly depends upon the context in which such feelings are experienced, and how they are expressed at the time. Reflecting allows the nurse and the client to choose a mutually acceptable 'feeling term' that best conveys the emotion felt at the time (see Table 2.1), e.g.:

Nurse: 'It sounds as though you might feel a bit resentful, then, towards your wife'?

Client: 'Not exactly, it's more that I am disappointed with her.'

Here the nurse has detected a feeling of resentment, and reflected this in a tentative way. This allowed the client to focus upon his feelings, helping him look at the situation more clearly and helping the nurse to understand further how he feels. Another example is:

Client: 'The trouble with me is that every time something goes wrong, I have to resort to the bottle. It just seems that I can't see any alternative. I wonder if it is just me or the situation I find myself in.'

We suggest that you try to explain the feelings this client is expressing. From the written word only, it is difficult and rather presumptuous to do so because

Table 2.1   Feeling vocabulary

Positive Feelings

Mild	Moderate	Strong
relaxed	content	at peace
at ease	carefree	serene
comfortable	secure	fulfilled
untroubled	safe	
patient	independent	determined
smart	intelligent	strong
	capable	sure
	worthy	brilliant
regarded	appealing	affirmed
encouraged	popular	loved
	attractive	adored
	wanted	worshipped
	approved	idolized
sensitive	concerned	pity
sympathetic	protective	
	tender	
regard	trust	admiration
	appreciation	worship
	respect	adoration
	gratefulness	awe
freindly	affectionate	loving
benevolent	caring	in love
warm	like	infatuation
interested	turned on	enchantment
tempted	desirous	ardour
alert	excited	amazed
wide awake	keen	vibrant
aroused	eager	alive
	brave	daring
optimistic	anticipating	zealous
hopeful	enthusiastic	inspired
		intoxicated
good	great	fantastic
amused	jolly	stupendous
pleased	glad	delighted
	happy	elated

Negative Feelings

Mild	Moderate	Strong
indifferent	listless	sick
resigned	bored	hopeless
lethargic	apathetic	futile
tired	weak	impotent
fatigued	worn out	exhausted

Mild	Moderate	Strong
timid	inhibited	paralysed
shy	inadequate	useless
bashful	ineffectual	helpless
self-conscious	stuck	trapped
disturbed	troubled	threatened
puzzled	baffled	shocked
perplexed	confused	bewildered
	mixed up	horrified
nervous	edgy	in dread
unsure	tense	terrified
apprehensive	worried	petrified
	afraid	frantic
suspicious	jealous	contemptuous
wary	envious	disdainful
cynical	bitter	scornful
sullen	spiteful	disgusted
	resentful	hatred
	vengeful	
moody	upset	crushed
unhappy	depressed	destroyed
disappointed	gloomy	miserable
discontented	dismal	awful
dissatisfied	dejected	disconsolate
unpopular	unloved	ashamed
regretful	alienated	worthless
embarrassed	hurt	hated
dependent	rejected	humiliated
impatient	indignant	outraged
irritated	angry	furious
annoyed	vexed	infuriated

Source: Egan, G., *Training the Skilled Helper* (Brooks/Cole, Monterey, California, 1982).

there are no accompanying non-verbal clues. However, the feelings we think that this client may be expressing are related to frustration and confusion. He seems frustrated because of his losing battle against alcohol and he is confused about the cause of his problem. Whether we are right or wrong does not matter; what is important is to reflect back these observations to the client so that he can think about what he has said, focus upon his feelings and confirm or deny the accuracy of the reflection, e.g.:

Nurse (reflects): 'So you feel frustrated because of your inability to cope with crises without having to resort to drink.'

    or

'It seems that you're in a dilemma and maybe feel confused because you're not sure what the reasons are for your drink problem.'

[handwritten margin note: eg of what I could have done.]

[handwritten margin note: If the client mentions 2 feelings - then reflect both + allow them to choose]

In both these replies the nurse reflects back circumstances that the client has already stated, and the feelings that he appears to be expressing. Both may be effective in allowing the client to explore further the area that is particularly important to him. Where the feelings of confusion are more important than the feelings of frustration, the first response may delay the counselling process, as the client may spend time talking about something that is not the crucial issue; the second response would be a more accurate reflection. The safest reply in this situation, where several feelings have been expressed in one phrase, is to reflect those feelings back to the client and allow him to choose which to elaborate or comment upon, e.g.:

Nurse: 'So you're feeling frustrated because you are unable to cope with crises without drink and confused because you're not sure what the reasons are for your drink problems.'

This allows the client to choose in which direction the counselling should go. One possible direction this may take is:

Client: 'That's right. Maybe my frustrations will be reduced if I could understand how I find myself in these situations in the first place'.

Nurse: 'Situations?'

Client: 'Yes: the situation of stress, the marriage, the job, the kids, it all adds up and drinking my problem away seems to have caused another problem.'

Nurse: 'So your drinking problem seems to be just one on top of many others.'

From this short dialogue it can be seen how the simple paraphrase and the reflecting back of feelings allow the client to explore his own world in order to achieve and communicate insight into his own problems. It enables the nurse to understand accurately not only the client's situation but also how he feels about it. This accurate understanding is part of what we mean by empathy. An empathic response combines the skills of paraphrasing and reflecting, as seen in the italicized response of the nurse to the client with a drink problem. It involves the element of feelings and the possible reasons for those feelings.

[handwritten margin note: PARAPHRASING + REFLECTION MUST BE DONE WITH UNCONDITIONAL POSITIVE REGARD! TO PROMOTE EMPATHY]

For the skills of paraphrasing and reflecting to be effective, thereby achieving empathy, they need to be closely related to the quality of 'unconditional positive regard' (see p. 18). If this is not present within the nurse, her listening will be inaccurate because her own feelings and attitudes are serious 'barriers'.

Clarifying

There are times when listening to what a client is saying is difficult because of all the detailed complications of feelings and circumstances conveyed, often in one uninterrupted sentence. In this situation, and in any other circumstances where confusion may occur, the nurse must convey her genuineness, be honest, and admit that she is confused.

[handwritten margin note: IF YOU DON'T UNDERSTAND, BE GENUINE + SAY SO]

Client: 'We used to understand each other, have a respect for each other, now we don't seem to talk to each other. It doesn't seem fair that she should punish me like this.'

Nurse: 'I'm not quite sure what you're saying. You seem to be saying there's no communication between you and also that she is punishing you.'

This admission by the nurse allows the client to focus back on what he has said in order to communicate more accurately, thus helping not only the nurse's understanding but the client's as well. The example given was a specific request to clarify something that was ambiguous. Often a client will say several things in an attempt to explain the situation, and in doing so will convey quite conflicting experiences.

Client: 'I can't understand it, what happened just amazes me, it was fantastic yet it's so soul destroying that the stimulation and satisfaction I achieved at the time barely seem worth it now'.

Nurse: 'Am I right in saying that the experience was a positive one at the time, but now you're wondering whether it was worth it?'

It can be seen from the last two examples that clarifying can be just an extension of paraphrasing and reflecting. The main difference is that the nurse picks out the part that is confusing and asks directly whether her understanding is correct. This portrayal of honesty and subsequent genuineness will often be reciprocated by the client. If the nurse happens to say anything that he finds confusing, because she has previously admitted difficulties in initially understanding, the client will also find it easier to admit confusion.

Another use of clarification occurs when a client states several factors that at the time seem equally important to him.

Client: 'It's not just the financial aspects that are involved, I mean, I can't ignore the marriage, the kids, and my involvement with this other man, they are all part of it, not to mention me being here.'

Nurse: 'You have mentioned many factors that are affecting you at this present time. I'm wondering which one of these is the one that you may wish to talk about further.'

Allowing the client to choose increases the likelihood that the counselling will progress to a crucial area affecting him in the 'here and now'. On the other hand, he could choose an area that he feels safe in and is able to talk about. In this situation further skills are required, such as challenging (see p. 41). Note that the nurse is not asking the client which of the factors is most important to him. This would involve much more exploration before he could decide, as it requires him to disclose his value orientation. Thus it can be seen that the skill of clarifying gives an opportunity to correct any inaccurate understanding on the part of either the client or the nurse.

Summarizing

This involves bringing together the main issues and feelings that the client has conveyed to the nurse so far. It is a skill that involves very accurate listening and empathy, for it could have a negative effect on the counselling process if, in her summary, the nurse were to leave out what the client thought was a major issue. If the summary is accurate, it conveys to the client that the nurse

WHEN TO SUMMARIZE

understands. Summarizing to convey understanding is an extremely useful skill to use at the beginning and end of any counselling session. It helps form a basis on which to proceed, it checks progress and avoids the temptation to go round in circles. At the end of any session it acts as a stopping point, but one that can be picked up next time. In doing this it often acts as a form of reassurance to the client that the nurse understands, that progress has been made and that it will be picked up again later. It is also useful during a session, especially when there is a temptation to 'backtrack' or dwell on certain issues that have already been covered. Summarizing during counselling often helps to focus upon scattered thoughts and feelings. It is often useful here to ask the client whether he is able to say 'where we have got so far'. This involves the client checking back on his thoughts, feelings and behaviours and communicating the crucial facts to the nurse, which can be very useful in a situation where the nurse suspects that the client is having difficulty in bringing together his feelings and circumstances and may too readily accept the nurse's summary. Asking the client to summarize too often, however, may reduce the nurse's credibility to demonstrate the skill in question.

'Let me see if I've got this right so far' summarizing can be a useful skill at the beginning, during and after a counselling session. It involves bringing together ideas and feelings in order to focus upon scattered issues or to check progress so far. In doing this it checks understanding and often acts as a form of reassurance: 'Would you say that sums it up?' or 'Have I left anything out?'

ASKING AT END OF SUMMARY "IS THAT RIGHT?" KEEPS IT CLIENT CENTRED.

Notice again the tentative statement: 'Have I got this right?' 'Is there anything else?' This is very important in order for the counselling at this stage to remain 'client-centred', i.e. the counselling does not follow the direction of the nurse's ideas but purely the client's perspective. It says to the client also that 'I am trying to listen and I accept that it is possible for me to leave something out or get something wrong.'

After a summary, especially during or at the beginning of a counselling session, a reminder of the helping contract established can be very useful. This is often stated in terms of:

Nurse: 'Where do you see us progressing from here?'

Reader: 'Well, it may be useful for me to look at some of the 'key concepts' involved with this chapter so far.'

PROGRESSIVE RESPONDING

The preliminary skills previously described, and the development of the necessary qualities discussed in the introduction, combine to ensure that the nurse is able to create a closeness, a rapport, an empathic relationship. When this is achieved, the nurse may be able to help the client to find solutions to his problems.

Progressive responding is the final stage of our counselling model. The previous skill of exploratory responding should have helped the client begin to understand what problems he may have and generally to see himself much more clearly. Now it is necessary for the nurse to help change occur. It is essential to understand that these skills should not be used until an empathic relationship has been developed, or the nurse may be in grave danger of advising, directing or prescribing for the client from her own perspectives.

The imaginative reader may have already discovered the limitations of the skills so far. They are, of course, extremely potent for engendering self-awareness, and this in itself may be all that is necessary to stimulate change. Some clients may become aware of themselves and decide that they want to change, but are unable to find effective methods of doing so. Some clients may have developed such sophisticated defences that, although they see problems in their situation, they are unable to connect them with themselves and continue to disown responsibility for them. In this type of situation, the nurse who is able to use only preliminary skills may begin to feel frustrated as the relationship of trust and self-awareness becomes deeper and greater, but without seeming to resolve any of the difficulties.

It is our belief that in order to move forward from this situation, to facilitate change in clients that seem entrenched in their helplessness, and in order to help effectively, more advanced skills may be needed. These are the skills of problem solving from a client-centred approach. It is our contention that this is chiefly facilitated by the use of skilled and effective challenging.

Challenging

What is challenging? Connor, Dexter and Wash (1984) had this to say about it:

> In order to identify problems, the nurse may need to helpfully challenge the client. Challenging is one of the most important skills used when responding, and particularly at this stage of problem identification.

> Sometimes the nurse will notice that there are certain discrepancies in what the client is saying. These need to be challenged. The client may seem to be evading the problem, perhaps by blaming other people for his predicament. If this is reflected back to the client in a positive way it will help him to challenge himself about the way he is responding to his own situation.

> Challenging is a very powerful way of helping people, but because of its power it can be either helpful or harmful. Attempts at trying to shock clients into changing their attitudes may have the negative result of anger and resentment.

> Good challenging helps the client to think carefully and positively and it often helps the client to see exactly where he wants to make changes in his life.

> Sometimes, very sensitive areas of thoughts, feeling or behaviour require great courage from the client. In such situations, the client sometimes finds it easier to escape from reality. It is the responsibility

of the nurse to be sensitive to this and to encourage the client to face his problems rather than turn away from them. Challenging can remotivate the client, persuade him not to give up, and help him find what strengths he needs in order to face a problem.

The skill of challenging is the skill of giving honest feedback to a client in a sensitive way, with the intention of introducing new ideas or new ways of looking at a situation. An effective nurse tries to enable the client to begin to challenge himself in a way that encourages positive and realistic goals to be set before trying to change specific behaviour.

The authors go on to suggest that challenges can be graded from very good to bad and negative, with consequent feelings engendered:

Type of challenge	*Effect on client*
1. Very good challenge	Client feels enlightened
2. Good challenge	Thought-provoking
3. Average challenge	Confused
4. Negative challenge	Resentful
5. Bad negative challenge	Very resentful.

CASE ILLUSTRATION

Maggie is talking to a nurse about her problems related to alcohol. The dialogue here may help you to see how challenging may help the client fulfil the prerequisites of problem solving (the initial steps).

Maggie: 'There doesn't seem much point staying sober around here, nobody listens to me until I'm drunk – then at least I get an injection to help me calm down.'

Nurse (challenges discrepancy and the genuineness of the remark): 'You say staying sober is pointless as no one listens to you unless you're drunk [paraphrase] and yet you also seem to be saying that when you're drunk you become excited and you need calming down with an injection [reflection and paraphrase]. I'm a bit confused about this: are you saying the drink makes you excited and you want to be calm, or am I right in suspecting what you really mean is you think no one listens to you?' [clarification].

This example illustrates that the skilled nurse may be able to use various skills as a response, all showing empathy but each one having a different depth, and subsequently the client's reaction may differ accordingly. It seeks to challenge the client to look more closely at what she means.

The next example illustrates the nurse attempting to enable Maggie to identify the real or main problem by challenging. Note the contrasting styles of challenging and decide which one is the most helpful.

Maggie: 'My husband is having an affair, I know he is, he's a rat, no wonder I drink such a lot.'

Nurse: 'It's nothing to do with your husband; so maybe he is being unfaithful, perhaps he's fed up with living with a drunk. If you stopped drinking maybe he'd be more faithful.'

or (carefully, tentatively and with genuine puzzlement)

'You appear to be very angry with your husband, but I'm wondering exactly how much you can blame him for what's happening to you?'

We hope it can be seen in the second example that the nurse allows the client to challenge herself about the real problem. The first nurse can only be presumptive, she cannot know which event came first, neither should she assume that the drinking is the main problem. The second nurse allows a more open-ended challenge, which may result in the client not only looking closely at which of her own statements contains the major problems, but also which is her fault or problem, which can then be owned and dealt with effectively.

Staying for a while with Maggie's problem, it may be helpful to see that once the problem is identified and owned it can be expressed more clearly and the next step attempted, i.e.:

Maggie: 'I see what you mean, my problem is that I deal with my feelings about my husband by drinking, but what can I do to stop him behaving like he does?'

Nurse: 'I think you are now saying it's your feelings that are the main problem, but I still sense you are planning on trying to change your husband. I wonder if that's very realistic; for instance, if your husband heard you say that what would he say?'

Maggie: 'Well, he'd probably say it's my life and I'm going to enjoy it; if that makes you unhappy I'm sorry, but I have to be me.'

Nurse: 'I'm wondering if 'stopping him behaving like he does' is very realistic, then?'

Maggie: But what else can I do?'

Nurse: 'Perhaps you could try to imagine how you would like to see yourself in three months' time as realistically as possible, and work towards that in small steps.'

Although this appears to be directive, in fact the nurse is suggesting a structure, almost like offering a journey rather than prescribing a desti-nation. From this position the nurse can help structure the journey but should not push in any particular direction. For instance, the nurse may challenge the client when his goals are vague and unspecific, i.e. 'I want to be better'. The nurse is correct to challenge also when the client is being unrealistic, or when the methods chosen are ineffective or inappropriate. Care should be taken not to direct but to challenge in a way that allows time for the client to reflect carefully. These follow-ing examples of challenges, we believe, emphasize this point.

Client not owning problem and being vague

Client: 'Life has really kicked me around.'

Nurse (challenge): 'You seem to be saying you have no control over life. Perhaps we ought to talk specifically about what it is in life that kicks you around.'

Client has unrealistic goals

Maggie: I'm going to discharge myself today, go out and get myself a job.'

Nurse: 'It's great to see you so energetic, Maggie. Have you any specific ideas about this job?'

Client may have chosen ineffective or inappropriate methods to reach her goal

Maggie: 'I'm sick of feeling so frustrated and angry with him, I'm just going to slap him in the face when he visits tonight.'

Nurse: 'You feel very angry because you believe him to be the root of your frustration. Are you saying hitting him will help you reach your goals?'

Maggie: 'I'll just kill myself.'

Nurse: 'Killing yourself may be a solution to this particular frustration, but how is that going to help you reach the goal we discussed earlier?'

PRINCIPAL SKILLS OF CHALLENGING

Summarizing

This skill centres around the counsellor's ability to pick out common themes and recurring issues and feed them back in an accurate, non-judgemental way. Elucidating feelings associated with each idea without adding or subtracting material may enable the client to see contradictory ideas and emotions and challenge himself to sort these out.

Confrontation

This is an invitation to the client to confront himself with discrepancies he holds within himself. For example, he says he wants to give up drinking but he hides alcohol in his locker, or states, 'I get bad chest infections but I continue to smoke'. The nurse here simply feeds back this information in one sentence, when previously it was separated by other material. It is, however, much better if strengths rather than weaknesses are challenged, e.g. 'You have told me how difficult life is for you – you are unemployed, your wife has left you, you are in financial difficulties – and yet you are still able to smile about it. I think you have many untapped resources if only you could reach them.'

Games and smokescreens may need to be confronted, as these are often used by clients to keep the roundabout turning and prevent the nurse helping. When the climate of the relationship is secure, this confrontation is easy, e.g. 'I'm really trying to understand how you are feeling, but it seems to me that every time you talk to me about your mother you become uncomfortable and change the subject.' 'You seem to feel tired or bored with these sessions whenever I sense we're really starting to get somewhere.' 'I hear you saying something you feel very uncomfortable with, but at that point you make a joke and laugh; I'm not really sure I understand you.'

Immediacy

This skill is to do with having an appreciation of what is happening between nurse and client at times throughout interactions, and is characterized by nurse statements such as 'I sense you are feeling disappointed with me.' 'I seem to have upset you when I said that.' 'You're annoyed because I got that wrong', and by clients' statements such as 'I don't think I really meant that. I think I said it because I thought you'd like it.' 'I'm having problems concentrating because I want to tell you how much I appreciate you trying to help me.'

These potentially highly emotional interactions need to be explored before the business of counselling can continue. They require to be confronted by both parties so that purposeful client-centred therapy can continue.

Data-based hunches

These are made from a position of deep understanding of the client and, as suggested, are based on data. They begin with an empathic response such as 'You seem to be feeling puzzled about that' and continue with the hunch 'and I sense that you may be feeling angry over the way you've been treated'. This has to be data-based because not only may it be insulting to be considered so transparent, but without data you may be a long way from the truth. Consider this client response to this last statement:

Client: 'Why do you say angry?'

Nurse: 'Well, because when I see that puzzled look appear I also notice you clench your fists and your lips tighten.'

as opposed to:

Nurse: 'Oh, just a lucky guess, I suppose.'

or, more mystical:

Nurse: 'I just feel these things.'

The response should also be tentative, as there is probably no greater sin in counselling than telling someone what they are feeling, except perhaps not allowing them to feel at all. For example:

Client: 'I just can't cope, I feel terrible.'

Nurse: 'Oh, I'm sure you can, it's not that bad.'

Self-disclosure

This is useful to show the client that you too are a real person with feelings and experiences. It encourages disclosure from the client, and may as a side benefit offer new perspectives to the client. It must not be distracting or a way of offering advice. It challenges by inviting comparisons between the counsellor's and the client's emotions, behaviours and coping strategies.

Client: 'I feel so hurt and rejected since my husband divorced me. I really don't know what to do.'

Nurse: 'Listening to you say that makes me think back to my divorce; I felt a little like that, but mostly I was very angry. It eventually occurred to me that being angry wasn't very constructive. Do you see yourself in any of this?'

Unacceptable self-disclosure

Nurse: 'You should worry, if you had my overdraft, you really would be in trouble.'

or

Nurse: 'Yes, my husband left me last year, he was a nice man and I want to cry when I think about it.'

or

Nurse: 'What a coincidence, I'm...a...as well.'

The latter examples are not appropriate because, even if honest, they are too distracting, turning the counsellor into the client and reducing the proceedings to mutual sympathy and destroying the counsellor's credibility. After all, how can a client put trust in someone who is in a worse mess than themselves?

Information giving

Finally, the skill of giving information to clients is one with which most nurses are familiar. It is, however, important to give information tactfully, clearly and at the right time. For instance, John discloses that he is very distressed because he believes he has syphilis. He bases this belief on the fact that he has a painful sore on his penis. There are many possible responses but let us examine four typical ones.

1. 'Don't be silly, syphilitic sores are never painful, it can't be.' Confidently reassuring, but humiliating and breaks a golden rule by denying John's feelings.

2. 'Well, why don't you go to the doctor and get it treated?' Sensible advice, but shows no empathy and only selfish regard – i.e. I don't want to know, show a doctor.

3. 'Oh dear, how dreadful, I hope it's not. That would be difficult for you to explain to your wife.' Sympathy from the nurse's values and perceptions does little other than make the client more aware of how the nurse sees the problem and may not focus upon the concerns of the client.

4. 'You're obviously very upset about this John, but I'm wondering how much you know about syphilis. I believe it's not usual for sores to be painful. I sense that just worrying about it is not really helping.' This begins with an empathic response and offers information that may be useful to confront John's feelings and behaviour. The final challenge is a data-based hunch which motivates John to consider other opinions. Note that the nurse does not prescribe action but simply helps precipitate it.

Challenging skills rules

1. Only challenge when an empathic bond exists and the relationship could stand an unskilled challenge should things go wrong.

2. Challenging should be an invitation for the client to look at himself more closely, not an excuse for the nurse to attack or punish him.

3. Using challenges to shock, or as a disguise for prescribing, is not skilful and will usually succeed only in creating resentment.

4. Challenges are most effective when sandwiched between empathic responses, e.g. 'You're feeling puzzled and uncertain because you can't decide what to change in your lifestyle. On the other hand, you've said if you continue to smoke and drink you may not have time to change. – I see you're feeling anxious because of what I just said.'

5. If in doubt, use an empathic response not a challenge.

PROBLEM SOLVING

This section simply sets out, using the basic steps of the nursing process, how a counselling approach can be incorporated into the mental health nurse's practice. However, it must be acknowledged that this process is largely borrowed and adapted from Egan's problem management approach. Those readers seriously interested in pursuing counselling as a nursing option are strongly advised to read Egan's excellent (1994) book *The Skilled Helper*.

It is necessary initially to look at the route to effective problem solving and the individual steps in the process. We have identified four major stages and 23 necessary steps which may help the client find and reach his goals.

Assessment

The client needs to:

1. Know which are his real problems.

2. See his problems as his own, e.g. 'My problem is my wife' means the problem is not owned.

3. Have control of it personally, e.g. 'My death is not controllable, but the way I prepare for it is.'
4. Be motivated towards its solution.
5. Identify the main problem and auxiliary problems.
6. Express his problems in a specific form (rather than in vague terms).

Planning

The client needs to:

7. Identify the overall goal and where he is going.
8. Have an appreciation of steps towards the goal (subordinate goals).
9. Be committed to reaching the goal.
10. Feel it is his goal.
11. Express it as a worthwhile and realistic goal.
12. Identify what will help him and what will hinder him reaching his goal.
13. Have a timescale to work within, and know when it is achieved.
14. Identify the cost and consequences of achieving the goal, both to himself and to significant others. Also, what will be the result of *not* achieving the goal.

Implementation

The client needs to:

15. Identify resources and generate as many strategies as possible to help him reach his goal.
16. Understand the method of reaching the goal.
17. Succeed by achieving one step at a time.
18. Choose each step carefully, ensuring that it is reasonable.
19. Feel rewarded by each step.

Evaluation

The client needs to:

20. See what has been achieved.
21. Know what remains to be done.
22. Understand the changes that have taken place.
23. Be able to assess the overall results.

To achieve these objectives throughout the stages of problem solving will require all the nurse's counselling skills, but predominantly challenging skills will be invaluable.

It is suggested by Egan (1982) that one particular method of helping people make decisions and solve problems is to consider the problems and the goals as diametrically opposite. He suggests that goals and problems can be thought of as the two extremes of a force field (force-field analysis) and that the forces involved are facilitating and restraining forces. Connor, Dexter and Wash (1984) term this hindering and helping factors. Our amalgam of this simple but useful device is shown in Figure 2.2.

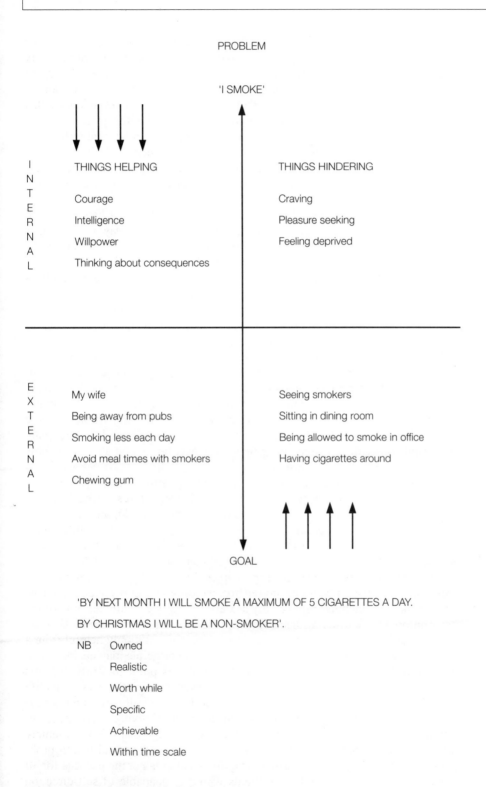

PROBLEM

'I SMOKE'

THINGS HELPING	THINGS HINDERING

INTERNAL

THINGS HELPING

Courage

Intelligence

Willpower

Thinking about consequences

THINGS HINDERING

Craving

Pleasure seeking

Feeling deprived

EXTERNAL

My wife

Being away from pubs

Smoking less each day

Avoid meal times with smokers

Chewing gum

Seeing smokers

Sitting in dining room

Being allowed to smoke in office

Having cigarettes around

GOAL

'BY NEXT MONTH I WILL SMOKE A MAXIMUM OF 5 CIGARETTES A DAY.

BY CHRISTMAS I WILL BE A NON-SMOKER'.

NB   Owned

Realistic

Worth while

Specific

Achievable

Within time scale

Figure 2.2   Helping and hindering factors

Egan suggests that if the helping (facilitating) factors are strengthened and the hindering (restraining) factors are weakened, the goal can be more easily reached. Essentially the idea is that the facilitating factors are a group of resources which, when fully used, may make up a solution. The restraining factors are a group of influences – people, places, things or behaviours – that are stumbling blocks and are counterproductive to reaching the goal.

It can be seen from Figure 2.2 that specific prompts can be used to help the client see these ideas more clearly. After dividing helpers and hinderers into internal and external resources, the client can be prompted with open questions: What emotions, thoughts, people, places, methods and objects will help or hinder him in achieving his goal?

This prompting will help the client generate ideas. The first lists of helpful and hindering factors are not censored, challenged or in any way influenced, as these are purely the client's 'brainstormed' ideas, which may be inappropriate, unrealistic or just plain silly. Nevertheless, the client should be allowed to choose freely from the list those which he feels are the most appropriate, effective and reasonable – as shown in the second list.

Egan's original idea holds great promise in helping the client explore his ideas and behaviours in an organized and structured way, and reveals obvious strategies for solving problems from the client's own value orientation.

It is then simply a matter of helping the client to see ways in which he may weaken the hindering things and strengthen the helping influences. For example, the first hindering factor was 'craving'. If the client is asked how many things he can think of that will weaken his craving and then selects the strategies that he thinks will work, they probably will. Conversely, if we take the first helping factor in the external section ('my wife') and ask him to explain what strategies will potentiate his wife's influence, he will be able to see how he can elicit his wife's aid most effectively.

By looking at these influences in a detailed and structured way, the client starts to appreciate what is going on in his life. He can at last see what has been holding him back from doing the things he has wanted to do, and finally find realistic strategies to succeed instead of continuing to fail. The skilled nurse may at this point be able to inform the client about how behaviours are reinforced, so that he can see how his undesired behaviours have previously been fixed by rewards (see 'Behavioural principles', p. 61). Maggie's example here would be 'I've been rewarding myself for avoiding facing my feelings – I've been drinking, which has relieved my anxieties [negative reinforcement] which has reinforced my drinking habit further, and snowballed into preventing me seeing what's really happening.' This type of insight is not only helpful from a historical perspective, but the understanding of the principle may enable her to avoid future traps. It is extremely important at this point to stress that this approach of trying to 'teach' the client about behavioural influences in his life is totally different from telling him what to do behaviourally, devising behavioural strategies or analysing him. Skilled information giving is required, not prescribing behaviours for individuals. We acknowledge that this is extremely difficult to do, especially with clients who have serious mental health problems, or clients with learning difficulties. Counselling is not the panacea for all ills, and for the small number of clients who are incapable of self-direction counselling may not be the most creative approach.

Steps 20–23 could be considered almost self-explanatory, but using appropriate challenging skills remains a priority. Simply because there has been an effect or a change does not mean it is cherished. An action programme devised by the client may not have succeeded, or may have simply uncovered more problems. Often, reaching the final stage simply means starting again from the beginning. It has been suggested that by far the commonest reasons for not effecting a solution are:

* The strategies devised by the client have not been followed.
* The problem was not the real problem.
* The goal was not achievable, realistic or worthwhile.
* The motivation for change was insufficient.

These areas are therefore most important to challenge in evaluation or much time can be expended following plans that are destined to fail. Far better to return to basics at this point than to pursue an unhelpful direction.

To refer back to the stages of problem solving, you may now be able to reflect on how challenging may be useful in each stage.

Assessment

The client needs to express specific, owned, real, controllable problems and subproblems, and be committed to their solutions, e.g. 'I smoke cigarettes' (main real problem) 'because I am under stress and I am bored' (subproblems) 'and I really wish I could stop.'

Planning

The client needs to express a specific, owned, realistic, worthwhile, stepped and measurable goal that he is determined to reach in a set period of time, e.g. 'I will give up smoking cigarettes at a rate of one cigarette a day and I will be a non-smoker by December 12th.'

Implementation

The client needs to examine the resources available to him, both internal and external, including people, places and things that will strengthen his strategies and help him to reach his goal. Conversely, he needs to examine the people, places and things that will hinder the process, and devise ways of weakening their effect, e.g. 'I am aware that to give up smoking I need to limit my craving, and spend less time at the pub. My wife will help me in the former, so I will spend as much time with her as possible. Being bored will increase my craving so I will endeavour to occupy myself with a new hobby. I spend more time at the pub when I really fancy a drink, so I will weaken this effect by having some cans of beer at home.'

Evaluation

The client needs to express: 'I am now a non-smoker.' 'I have succeeded in stopping smoking.' 'I like what I feel.' 'I like what I have become.' 'I am pleased.' 'Other things that have happened are...' 'I've only partly succeeded in...' 'I wish I could...' 'My next step is...'

Nurses commonly complain that clients they want to help cannot or will not be helped. It is our contention that this model of counselling skills, although by no means original, may in some way help the nurse to see new perspectives in helping. It is not our wish that the nurse should be straitjacketed by our ideas, but simply that they may offer an alternative approach for the care of some clients. The skilled nurse may well combine many skills she already possesses to potentiate what is presented here. We would commend this, as it is not our wish to discourage any initiative that will ultimately help your clients.

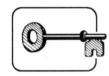

KEY CONCEPTS

1. 'People become engaged in counselling when a person, occupying regularly or temporarily the role of counsellor, offers and agrees explicitly to give time, attention and respect to another person or persons who will temporarily be in the role of the client.'
2. An effective counsellor must have an honest intention to help, a desire to promote growth within the client, and a reluctance to offer advice or judgement.
3. An understanding and a proficient ability to perform the skills of listening, paraphrasing, reflecting, questioning, clarifying, summarizing and challenging are essential.
4. It is our view that you must earn the right to counsel others, by acquiring the skills, owning the qualities and understanding yourself.
5. To be effective the counsellor has to dispense with her own values, beliefs, prejudices and stereotypes, in order to accept and try to understand the other person's values, ideals and beliefs, even if these are totally opposed to her own.
6. The qualities of empathy, warmth and genuineness are essential prerequisites for the client–counsellor relationship.
7. By being sensitive to your own and the client's non-verbal behaviours, you are likely to demonstrate to the client interest and warmth, thus increasing the likelihood of enhancing the relationship.
8. Exploration of the client's problems requires the counsellor to demonstrate understanding and the need to allow the client to express freely his thoughts, feelings and behaviours. The skills that help the client do this are paraphrasing, reflecting, clarifying and summarizing.
9. Sometimes the client finds it difficult to see his problems clearly because the realization and acceptance of the problems may provoke some anxiety. When this occurs, challenging skills are needed to move the client forward.
10. Once the client has identified and owned the problem, the counsellor may help him brainstorm useful ways in which he can set and achieve his goals.
11. Classification into helpers and hinderers is a useful way of looking at factors that will help or prevent the client achieving the goal.

12. By offering support and encouraging feedback, the counsellor can help the client evaluate the outcome of his attempt to change, thus offering an opportunity for further exploration.

FURTHER READING

Bond, T. (1993) *Standards and Ethics and Practice for Counselling in Action*, London, Sage.

Carkhuff, R. R. and Anthony, W. A. (1983) *The Skills of Helping*, Amherst, Mass., Human Resource Development Press.

Culley, S.(1990) *Integrative Counselling Skills in Action*, Sage, London.

Dryden, W. (1993) *Reflections on Counselling*, Whurr Publishers, London.

Egan, G. (1994) *The Skilled Helper: A Problem Management Approach to Helping*, 5th edn, Brooks/Cole Publishing, Pacific Groves, California.

Hardin, S.B. and Halasis, A.L. (1983) Non-verbal communication of patients and high and low empathy nurses (study). *Journal of Psychosocial Nursing and Mental Health Services*, **21**(1), 14–20.

Kalish, B. (1973) What is empathy? *American Journal of Nursing*, **73**(9).

Kennedy, E. (1977) *On Becoming a Counsellor: A Basic Guide for Non-Professional Counsellors*, Gill and Macmillan, Dublin.

Munroe, A., Manthei, B. and Small, J. (1989) *Counselling: The Skills of Problem Solving*, Routledge, London.

Nelson-Jones, R. (1993) *Practical Counselling and Helping Skills*, 3rd edn, Cassell, London.

Pratt, J. W. and Mason, A. (1981) *The Caring Touch*, H. M. and M Publishers, London.

Proctor, B. (1978) *Counselling Shop: An Introduction to the Theories and Techniques of Ten Approaches to Counselling*, Burnett Books, London.

Rogers, C. R. (1951) *Client-Centred Therapy*, Constable, London.

Rogers C. R. (1967) *On Becoming a Person: a Therapist's View of Psychotherapy*, Constable, London.

Stewart, W. (1992) *An A–Z of Counselling Theory and Practice*, Chapman & Hall, London.

Tschudin, V. (1991) *Counselling Skills for Nurses*, 3rd edn, Baillière Tindall, London.

3 Behavioural skills

BEHAVIOURISM AND ITS PLACE IN SOCIETY

First it may be necessary to say that although most nurses and allied professionals view behaviourism with a range of emotions from reverence to dread, it is in fact a basic component of our everyday lives. It is a school of thought which offers a distinctly different perspective and, when used thoughtfully, can be of immense help to the mental health nurse.

There should be no magical or mysterious power associated with behaviourism: only the uneducated or uninterested need to feel at a loss with it. It is hoped that you, upon reaching the end of the chapter, will be able to practise its simple principles, feel comfortable in its use, and assimilate it in your repertoire of skills.

The human being is essentially a complex creature, comprising skills, knowledge and emotions, each of which has been learned. It is in the way in which this learning has occurred that the behaviourist is interested.

All humans seek pleasure. This may not necessarily be in an overt form, but may take many diverse expressions. It may simply be in watching an interesting film, enjoying the praise of others or, more subtly, the satisfying feeling of taking a difficult task to a competent completion. Equally, however, a person avoids the unpleasant, or punishing, situation. These may include physiological occurrences, i.e. pain, discomfort, anxiety, or the more subtle situation giving rise to feelings of uselessness, hurt or failure.

From a very early stage of development, a child quickly learns that most behaviour will be followed by a predetermined consequence. For instance, crying will result in being picked up and soothed by a parent, and touching a naked flame is followed by pain. This direct method of learning may set up patterns of behaviour that will follow the individual throughout his life.

Even more intricate patterns of behaviour may be learned in this way. Take, for example, attitudes and thoughts: a schoolchild will quickly learn which attitudes and expressed thoughts will be rewarded – in a family where racial prejudice is evident, the child learns that statements such as 'I hate blacks' will be rewarded by a parent saying, 'I don't blame you, so do I.' If the first statement is accompanied by attention and a smile, it is far more likely to strengthen the attitude than if it was followed by a swift kick.

Within a family or social group, issues of prejudice or interest will be fostered by the already formed attitudes of the significant members of that group. This pattern is followed from the isolated family group to the larger institution of schools, and finally in the individual's working life.

It could be argued that if this is in fact the case, why do children grow up with attitudes and values different from those of their parents? Essentially very few significant variations do occur until circumstances separate the individual from the reward, or the reward loses its meaning, i.e. the approval of a parent is no longer highly prized and therefore it is no longer rewarding, or another view or attitude is being rewarded much more effectively. This can be seen to happen when an influential figure disagrees with previously set attitudes; most commonly these are teachers, friends and lovers.

At this point a few examples may help us to understand just how many of our behaviours may well have been learned in this fashion.

John (aged 11) was found naked one day in the garden shed playing 'mothers and fathers' with Julie (aged 9). His father severely rebuked him and beat him. When John subsequently experimented sexually with his friend Gordon, he was not punished. Should similar events continue to occur, this could lead John into adulthood with secure feelings in homosexual relationships and severe anxiety in heterosexual ones.

George found great social esteem from his friends because he was skilful at football, yet felt unrewarded by his 'B' grades in arithmetic; his arithmetic grades became worse and he spent more time practising his football skills. It is obvious from a very early stage that George is far more likely to become a sportsman than a mathematician.

These are simple illustrations and should not be taken as serious attempts to explain complex human behaviour, but none the less they do serve to show that rewards/punishments may influence behaviour. It could be argued that people's lives can be directed and prescribed from a very early stage by the amount of reward they receive. Conversely, they can be controlled by the degree of punishment to which they are subjected.

The previous examples could be said to be almost natural or coincidental influences, and this is true to a degree. However, what of the rules of society? Certain prescribed ways of behaving in various cultures are not only expected and taught, but contrived by statutes, i.e. the law dictates them.

The vast majority of people – termed 'law abiders' – conform to rules and obey. Generally this is to avoid punishment, but may well be because society rewards the law abider. The industrious and caring person is rewarded by the social group, not only by money but by elevation to the ranks of high esteem. Doctors and nurses, for instance, are generally highly respected and admired people. This social reward may explain why tiresome and irksome duties are still completed despite meagre monetary reward.

If all this can be accepted as being in essence true, it opens up many possibilities for the mental health nurse. It shows that if behaviours have been 'learned' in this way, then they can be 'unlearned'. Conversely, new behaviours can be learned and past behaviours removed. This in practice is the foundation of behaviourism as a therapeutic model. It is important that in all this we are not carried away in an enthusiasm to help, but as professionals we must never lose sight of the fact that we are dealing with people.

ETHICAL CONSIDERATIONS

There is no doubt in our minds that behavioural theory is one of the most potent forces the mental health nurse can employ. Whether this is for the benefit or to the detriment of the client depends largely on the knowledge and skill of the person running the programme.

The first issue that arises before any attempt is made at changing an individual's behaviour is one of consent. Behaviour can certainly be changed without an individual's consent, but such a fact raises obvious ethical considerations. In addition, in our experience the more consenting and consequently more motivated the client is, the more effective the treatment.

How can a programme begin without the client's consent? It seems reasonable that the two main circumstances are:

- When the behaviour is dangerous to the client, e.g. overdosing, head banging or similar physically hazardous behaviours.
- When the client is unable to give 'informed consent', i.e. he is unable to understand or appreciate the proposed choice and the concerned professionals agree that a change in behaviour will enhance the person's 'quality of life'.

Even if it is decided to go ahead with a behavioural programme, there remain several ethical or moral issues which will need to be carefully considered:

- Who decides what are desired and undesired behaviours in any given individual?
- Would it be right to change religious, cultural or social behaviours valued by the client?
- Should sexual or political attitudes be changed in clients when these are implicit in their values?
- Specifically, certain categories of client raise special problems. What right do we have to change the behaviours of those who are suffering from, for example, so-called 'personality disorders'; suicidal risk; institutionalization; anorexia nervosa or learning disability?
- What other considerations, if any, should be made when caring for children?

All these questions are honest ones which have to be answered by the individual team on an individual case basis. It would clearly be irresponsible of us to try to generalize in each category those which should or should not be treated by behavioural methods. On the other hand, general principles and guidelines can be suggested.

In the first instance, what is desired or undesired should not be decided by one person. When considering behaviour change, it should be evaluated objectively. The values and beliefs of the client should not be set aside simply because they are not held by the evaluator. For example, staying in bed until noon may not be very valuable to the therapist, but it may well be something prized and treasured by the client.

The nurse may be prejudiced against particular forms of sexual expression, e.g. homosexuality, masturbation or adultery. This should not mean that for the client they are not valuable, or do not add to his quality of life – they are not automatic areas for behaviour change.

This particularly sensitive area becomes more difficult when considering the client who is admitted compulsorily from the courts for something such as child sex abuse. Should his behaviour, however illegal, be changed without his consent? It would be our view that as the behaviour is not hazardous (within the institution), and as the client is usually able to give 'informed consent', then clearly he should not be compulsorily treated by behavioural means.

Occasionally a client may insist on or demand treatment. This equally may raise problems. Even if the treatment is thought to be inappropriate by the team, have they the right to withhold it? There must be room for flexibility and negotiation in all these areas, but in all cases careful and thoughtful consideration must be a precursor to treatment.

In areas of religion, culture and political beliefs, it would appear that most therapists agree that it would be unethical to interfere. However, there have recently been cases reported of religious and political 'brainwashing' which may require, or at least benefit from, some behavioural therapies. The question here is, do the two wrongs make a right? In the first instance the brainwashing broke the rule of consent, but would not treatment for the client's present state equally break the rule again?

People with personality disorders often have different values from the society in which they live. If this is causing problems for them in their everyday lives, or is continually bringing them into conflict with authority, then possibly behaviour therapy would be beneficial. However, it is our belief that consent is still required.

Suicidal and anorexic clients may be considered together. In both these cases it would seem clear that if intervention is not pursued, the individual may well die. If this is the case, it seems reasonable that any treatment that seeks to raise the potential for recovery is certainly worth careful thought. Once the person dies, he obviously loses his ability to choose and his ability to change his mind – and the preservation of this prerogative would seem to be one worthy of any effort expended, even perhaps without the client's consent. A case in point would be the deeply depressed person, for it could be argued that while in this state his judgement is seriously impaired, and therefore informed consent is not a realistic premise.

In certain circumstances, the institutionalized client and the person with a learning disability might fall into the category of those unable to give informed consent. However, they should be given every opportunity to discuss and plan with the mental health nurse any programme proposed, before its implementation. Some level of understanding is usually possible, and client involvement, no matter how limited, is both therapeutically empowering and ethically correct. The Code of Practice (HMSO, 1990) accompanying the Mental Health Act of 1983 should be seen as an essential source of reference in the planning of behavioural programmes for those considered unable to give informed consent.

The treatment of children is a special case that needs the full consultation and agreement of parents or guardians. Each case should be accurately monitored, preferably by an independent observer, to ensure that a child's behaviour is not changed out of context with his or her stage of development. Adult values and behaviour should not be imposed on a child, neither should his or her formative development be out of step with the social and cultural facets of the home and family. The child is, after all, going to return to the family and friends they left (if admitted) and the values and benefits held by peer groups should remain intact so that they can integrate back into the community on discharge.

Other ethical rules need to be established when using behaviour therapy. For instance, the use of punishment is extremely problematic. As a member of a caring profession, the nurse must be clear where she stands. It is our view that each individual will have her own values, and will place limitations on what she feels able to engage in – even in the best-planned behavioural theory. Each individual should decide, without pressure from any source, what she is prepared to do.

What types of punishment are acceptable? The Code of Practice (HMSO, 1990) clearly states that no programme should deprive a person of food, shelter, water, warmth, a comfortable environment, confidentiality or reasonable privacy. The suggestion, then, is that punishment has a limited part to play in behaviour programmes. Boundaries are very difficult to set, but again each individual should think carefully and see whether she can answer these questions in the positive:

- Would the programme be acceptable if I was the client?
- If the client was my relative or friend, would I easily agree?
- Is the programme potentially hazardous; has it been carefully considered and explained to my satisfaction?

If she can, most probably the programme is acceptable.

What is acceptable as rewards? Thought has to be given to how morally acceptable are such rewards as alcohol, drugs, sexual gratification and artificial social rewards. Each of these has built-in dangers and the individual should question how, when and why these are to be given and, more seriously, what the long-term effects are likely to be. The three areas previously examined for punishments remain applicable to rewards, and may be used as a guideline to assess suitability.

BEHAVIOURAL PRINCIPLES

Behaviour therapy is based broadly on the work of Pavlov, a psychologist experimenting in physiological responses in animals, and Skinner, who also worked with animals but generalized his work into human psychology.

Pavlov

Classical conditioning

The essential idea is that there are various stimuli in the environment that evoke reactions in response. If artificial stimuli are presented at the same time as the original, then there is a linking or association to such an extent that eventually the false or artificial stimuli will evoke the same reaction (Figure 3.1). In a more practical (mental health) setting, the person who has a fetish may well have been classically conditioned (Figure 3.2).

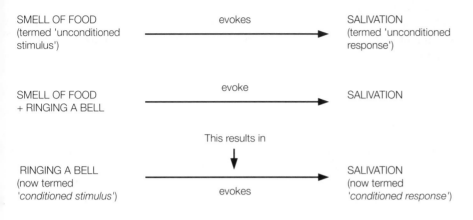

Figure 3.1 The classical conditioning process

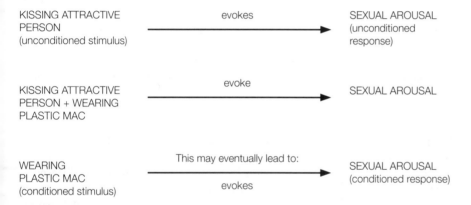

Figure 3.2 Plastic mac fetish

One increasingly rare type of treatment for people with alcohol problems uses the principles of classical conditioning in aversion therapy. Here an electric shock causes an unpleasant feeling. When drinking alcohol is linked with the shock, a gradual association is formed between alcohol and the unpleasant feeling (Figure 3.3).

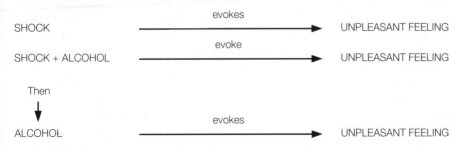

Figure 3.3 The classical conditioning process in aversion therapy

So, the work of Pavlov shows us that it is possible to create a response by linking a previously established stimulus-reaction together with a new one. From a practical mental health nursing point of view, this has quite a powerful potential.

The work of B. F. Skinner

Operant conditioning

The basic idea of operant conditioning centres on the observation that presenting something rewarding or appealing following a behaviour strengthens or increases that behaviour. Conversely, if a behaviour is followed by something of an unpleasant nature, that behaviour is weakened or reduced. Although the conditioning process can be demonstrated and proved scientifically in a laboratory using animals, its implications and ramifications when applied to human subjects are immense.

Human behaviour is so complex and its motivation so diverse that much intricate and specialized work has been done to enable the application of behavioural theory to the 'treatment' of human subjects. Much of the work of clinical psychologists and nurses or therapists in the field of mental illness is based on what has come to be known as the 'behavioural approach'. Hence in its simplest form we have 'behaviour modification' and in its more complex form 'behaviour therapy'.

BEHAVIOUR MODIFICATION AND BEHAVIOUR THERAPY

There appears to be some confusion in people's minds about the difference between these two expressions. Our understanding is quite simple: behaviour modification is generally accepted as referring to the principles of learning theory, and the various behaviour change strategies most widely used. These would include positive and negative reinforcement, extinction, modelling and shaping (see Poteet, 1978; Gentry, 1975). It could be argued that behaviour modification is concerned largely with Skinner's work, whereas behaviour therapy has a much broader definition.

We consider behaviour therapy as including any technique designed to change behaviour for the client's benefit. This would include much of Skinner's work and Pavlov's ideas, and perhaps even some of the therapies included within humanistic psychology theories. Behavioural counselling (Krumbolt and Thoresen, 1969) may be seen as a typical example of this. In addition, increasingly behaviour therapy recognises the cognitions which accompany behaviour and seeks to address both components in treatment programmes (see Murdoch and Barker 1991; Trower, Casey and Dryden, 1989). The difference between behaviour therapy, cognitive therapy and cognitive behaviour therapy can therefore be seen largely as a matter of therapeutic emphasis. Using behavioural principles in a rather more eclectic way to effect a behaviour change for the client's benefit would be our wider definition of behaviour therapy (see Wolfe and Lazarus, 1966; Barker, 1982).

To summarize, behaviour therapy is a general term which includes many therapies, and incorporates behaviour modification principles directed towards therapy. We take Barker's meaning of therapy here to mean 'an offer of help' (Barker, 1982, p. 11). Consequently we prefer the term behaviour therapy, as this implies a therapeutic design or intent, which behaviour modification may not.

Basic principles

The following is intended as a basic guide to the principles and techniques of behaviour change with which the nurse should be familiar. Focusing upon operant conditioning, behaviour change can be broadly separated into two main areas: increasing or strengthening, and decreasing or weakening.

Increasing and strengthening

This can be achieved in two ways – by positive reinforcement and by negative reinforcement.

Positive reinforcement

This occurs when a behaviour is followed by a response or event that the individual finds rewarding to such an extent that it will increase the likelihood of the behaviour being repeated. A positive reinforcer may be anything the person finds rewarding or pleasant and which tends to increase or strengthen a behaviour. A technical definition of a positive reinforcer is 'a pleasant stimulus presented to a subject following a response in order to strengthen that response' (Houston, Bee and Rimm, 1983). A positive reinforcer may be different for each individual – perhaps a chocolate for a child or a smile for an adult.

Examples:

- A little boy cuddled by his parent when he smiles is likely to produce an increase in smiling.
- A schoolchild praised for hard work is likely to work harder.
- If you are given £20 for predicting the winner of the 2.30 at Kempton Park, your 'predicting' betting behaviour is likely to increase.

Therefore, the positive reinforcers were:

- A cuddle
- Praise
- Money.

Negative reinforcement

This means increasing or strengthening a behaviour by removing an unpleasant occurrence or stimulus, following a response. So in colloquial terms it is in fact the 'relief' from the negative reinforcer (the stimulus) that rewards the preceding behaviour. A technical definition of negative reinforcer is: 'an unpleasant stimulus taken away from a subject following a response in order to strengthen that response' (Houston, Bee and Rimm, 1983).

Examples:

1. If a rat is placed in a box where the floor has a mild electric current, it discovers that jumping up removes the unpleasant stimulus and consequently its jumping-up behaviour increases. If the whole box is electrified and the rat discovers that pressing a lever inside the box removes the current, then the lever-pressing behaviour increases.
   Now to put this into human terms, which is far more complex:
2. When a baby cries its parent may find it unpleasant, but when the baby is picked up it stops crying. Here the parent is being rewarded by relief from the crying and subsequently her 'picking baby up' behaviour may well increase.
3. If an addict to diamorphine begins to experience withdrawal symptoms, nausea, sweating and stomach cramps, he will find this an unpleasant experience (aversive stimulus). He finds relief from this unpleasant experience by injecting himself intravenously with more diamorphine. Therefore the removal of these symptoms occurs when he increases injecting the drug. His behaviour is said to be negatively reinforced; by removing an unpleasant feeling, his preceding behaviour (injecting) has strengthened.
4. Persistent headaches may lead to increased aspirin taking.
5. Anxiety removed by diazepam may lead to increased ingestion of the drug.

In these examples the negative reinforcer was something aversive removed which subsequently increased a behaviour. The negative reinforcers were:

1. Electric current
2. Baby crying
3. Withdrawal symptoms
4. Headache
5. Anxiety.

The strengthened or reinforced behaviours were:

1. Jumping and lever pressing
2. Picking up baby
3. Increasing dose of diamorphine
4. Aspirin taking
5. Diazepam taking.

Decreasing or weakening behaviour

There are two ways of decreasing or weakening behaviour: punishment and extinction.

Punishment

In its technical sense this means the removal of something the individual finds pleasant, or the presentation of something the individual finds unpleasant. The use of either of these is designed to follow a behaviour and thus weaken or reduce its occurrence.

1. A schoolchild is eating his lunch, which he is obviously enjoying, but at the same time is 'messing about'. He is removed from his meal or his meal is removed from him until his 'messing about' stops. This is punishment by removal of a pleasant stimulus.
2. A motorist stopped by the traffic police for breaking the speed limit receives a spot fine. This is punishment by presenting an unpleasant stimulus.

It may be helpful at this point to consider the difference between punishment and negative reinforcement. A punishment is an aversive stimulus which follows a behaviour and is designed to stop that behaviour. A negative reinforcer is an aversive stimulus which, when removed, increases the behaviour which immediately preceded its removal. It can be seen, then, that punishment and negative reinforcers are both aversive stimuli – unpleasant. But punishment is applied to stop or weaken behaviour, whereas negative reinforcers are removed to increase or strengthen behaviour.

Extinction

The second method of weakening a behaviour is called extinction. Here the idea is to ensure that the undesired behaviour is not rewarded. No reinforcement is given or taken away: the behaviour is totally ignored. This applies the principle that if a behaviour is not rewarded, it ceases to occur.

One important aspect that should not be overlooked, however, is that when this procedure is followed there is almost inevitably a dramatic increase in the behaviour you are trying to reduce. This is technically referred to as 'extinction burst'. This is because the behaviour in the past has always a elicited a reward of some nature. Now there is no reward being given, the behaviour initially increases in a frantic attempt to gain the usual reward.

In practical terms, extinction, if it is carried through consistently, will work. However, there are several problems associated with this technique for mental health nurses:

- If the behaviour you are trying to reduce offers a hazard to the client, it is impossible, morally and perhaps legally, to ignore it. For example, if a person has previously been rewarded with attention when taking an overdose, or slashing his wrists, it remains impossible simply to ignore him.
- On a conventional ward or mental health unit there are many staff who perhaps would find ignoring a client's adverse behaviour difficult, if not impossible. This would mean in practice that extinction would not be complete. In fact, the behaviour would be spasmodically rewarded (intermittent reinforcement) and this would quite effectively maintain it.
- In the community setting the mental health nurse would find it almost impossible to control the client's environment to such an extent that extinction might be completed. The person's family, friends and acquaintances would be very likely to inadvertently disturb the consistent approach required.

A simple illustration of extinction and what has been referred to as intermittent reinforcement is the fruit machine. A person putting money into a fruit machine does so in the hope that he will be rewarded with a win. If he continued to put money in and had no success whatsoever, he would soon discontinue the practice – extinction would occur.

Generally, the individual does win reasonably often – initially. This produces positive reinforcement and leads to the person playing the machine more and more frequently. Each win is so powerfully rewarding that even if he receives little reward, he will continue to play. He will in fact continue to play even when the machine pays out very infrequently, as long as he is rewarded intermittently, and when long periods of non-payment occur his playing will increase frantically to achieve any kind of payout -extinction burst. At this point, non-payout will have to occur for some considerable time before he will stop playing the machine at all – extinction.

As can be observed from any social club or public bar, the fruit machine is extremely powerful; it appears to have no boundaries to its addictive power. Intellect, social, religious or cultural influences appear to have little effect on it, such is the power of positive intermittent reinforcement.

How then can these principles be applied in mental health nursing practice? How can extinction be useful?

In many ways behavioural principles should not be applied in singular form. The nurse must look to the general ideas and adapt and improvise them appropriately. As an example, let us see how, in the ward setting, an 'attention-seeking' client could be helped through the use of the principles we have looked at so far.

> Jim Middleton is a client originally admitted with bizarre behaviour, hallucinations and delusions. These symptoms have long since disappeared, but there now remain the residual effects of staying in residential care for twenty years. He does not take care of his personal hygiene, he refuses to eat with other people, and he constantly takes off his clothes and lies naked on the floor.
>
> First, it is important to observe his behaviour, to see what rewards he is receiving for his present state. It may be seen that:
>
> - Nurses help him dress, wash and shave.
> - He is allowed to eat alone in a comfortable chair, with the television or radio on.
> - When he undresses, a nurse intervenes and helps him to dress and return to his chair.
>
> The examples show that his behaviour is basically being reinforced by the nurses' attention, and by being treated differently from the other clients. Additionally, it may be that he is rewarded by the television, radio and sitting in an easy chair, and by the caring attitude, albeit chastising, of the nurses assisting him when he lies naked on the floor.
>
> Perhaps if we also look at the nurses' behaviour, it could be said that they too have behaved in such a way because they have been negatively reinforced. Having a person go without meals, lie on the floor

without clothes or live in an unhygienic condition may initiate feelings of anxiety, unpleasant feelings of unworthiness and inadequacy within them. The relief of these feelings by 'caring' for the client then reinforces their behaviour and allows them the positive reinforcement of satisfaction of a 'job well done'.

With a knowledge of the principles operating within the ward or mental health unit, the skilled nurse may be able to remedy this unhappy situation reasonably quickly. A simple programme for Jim, following due discussion with him and the care team, may be as follows.

Positive reinforcement. Jim would be rewarded with praise when he arose from bed – whatever state he was in. He would be left in bed until such time as he did arise.

At any time when his behaviour showed improvement, e.g. dressing, washing and shaving himself, he would be rewarded with either praise and attention or something more tangible, e.g. cigarettes or sweets. To avoid reinforcing undesired behaviour, his food would be served only at the table in the presence of other people, and again rewards would be offered for his acceptance of this situation.

Punishment (removal of pleasant rewards). Television, radio and his easy chair would be withheld from him whenever possible, without precipitating an aggressive incident, and used wherever possible as a reward for positive behaviour.

Extinction. Wherever possible, Jim's negative behaviour would be ignored. All social reinforcement, smiles, hellos and other acknowledgements of his presence would be unforthcoming while his behaviour was negative. However, when it is necessary to intervene, assistance should be given in the minimum socially reinforcing way, without smiling or social contact. Jim should only be helped to a stage where he is no longer a hazard to himself, and during the period where he is being ignored the nurse should continually observe for any behaviour that could be rewarded.

Negative reinforcement. Jim's hunger and need for social acknowledgement are powerful negative reinforcers, which would be removed at any period of positive behaviour.

The skilled nurse must be able to observe continually for factors Jim finds rewarding and use these to help reinforce desired behaviours. Although many problems may occurr within this programme, if the nurse can understand what has gone wrong and adjust the programme accordingly, then eventually the desired behaviour will emerge. By using the simple principle of not rewarding undesired behaviours and continuously rewarding those that are desired, the behaviour generally will improve.

Finally, two principles that are very important in behavioural work are shaping and modelling.

Shaping

Shaping is a technique that is analogous to sculpting clay. By gradual progression the clay takes shape into the final intended result, as does behaviour moulded by reinforcing responses that occur progressively nearer the final desired behaviour. The principles of shaping rely on rewarding any initial behaviour that even remotely resembles the final desired outcome. In order to continue receiving rewards, the behaviour must progress, so successive approximations are always rewarded. It should be noted, however, that the reward must be withdrawn once each further stage is reached, or it risks fixing the behaviour at that stage.

In Jim's case this would mean that once he had been encouraged to dress himself properly, he would be rewarded only intermittently for achieving this, and rewards would be concentrated on the next stage: washing and shaving.

Modelling

This is powerful when associated with shaping. Rather than waiting for the behaviour to occur spontaneously, the nurse may 'model' or demonstrate what she considers the desired behaviour to be, and reward the subject when he imitates it. Through rehearsal this method can be very effective, especially when a good rapport is in evidence and the subject is receiving some intrinsic reward for pleasing the nurse.

It is hoped that you now have an overall appreciation of some of the most important principles of behaviour change. The remainder of this chapter is concerned largely with examples of therapies which incorporate these principles in ways directed specifically towards helping the client. It is our hope that, with a better understanding of both principles and specific therapies on behavioural lines, the mental health nurse can add to her repertoire of skills to become a more effective helper.

The therapies selected are not intended to be an exhaustive description of all behaviour therapies available. There are many more less familiar and obscure ones that we do not feel able to describe. For this reason, suggested reading is given to fill any gaps and to provide direction should you be stimulated to research further.

The therapies described here have been selected on the basis that we believe they are currently the most likely to be practised, and it is probable that some nurses will become involved with them in the early parts of their careers. We believe they represent a fairly wide distribution of the behavioural skills that may be required of the mental health nurse in practice today.

TOKEN ECONOMY

Although token economy in its purest form is rarely used in contemporary mental health nursing practice, modified versions of this system of care are still used in some behaviour therapy programmes.

Token economy is essentially the use of artificial reinforcers which strengthen behaviours because they acquire the power of their exchange value, e.g. one token buys one cigarette. In much the same way as money is a reward and an incentive to most people in society, the token – usually a worthless piece of plastic – represents a saveable item that can be exchanged for anything the client may find rewarding.

In practical terms, ward or mental health units or hostels that use this system of behaviour modification have a shop which deals in tokens, where the token can be exchanged for anything in stock. Additionally, certain privileges may be paid for by tokens, such as a day off, an outing, leave, cinema, a late night out or a 'lie in' in the morning. Its usefulness becomes clear to the observant in that once the 'pleasure' link has been made between the symbol (token) and the purchase of a reward with it, the tokens become instant reinforcers of any behaviour the care team wishes to strengthen. The withholding or removal of tokens becomes a punishment and can be used to weaken any behaviour that is not desired.

Its simple management becomes a valuable asset to the mental health nurse, as she may build a programme that 'shapes' a client's behaviour by allocating 'targets' for him to reach. These targets are measured in tokens. For example, 'If you can save ten tokens by Saturday, you can go swimming instead of doing our normal chores.'

One major problem in helping with mental health problems using behavioural principles is what is referred to as satiation. This is when the reward offered becomes unrewarding. For example, a client is offered a cigarette for shaving himself when in fact he has a thousand cigarettes in his locker. It would be pointless using food as a reward when the person has just eaten a large and pleasant meal. The client is in a state of satisfaction, so offering rewards such as these will not strengthen his behaviour.

Avoiding satiation is necessary for token economy to be most beneficial. As the reward is artificially conditioned, the token will represent a reward that can be exchanged for anything the client truly wants or needs. It is unlikely in an organized system that the client will ever reach a point of satiation using tokens.

Table 3.1 shows an example of what a token economy scheme might be. The advantage of this is that the token reward can be adjusted when the client starts to find the task easier, and can then gradually be incorporated into his general behaviour with social rather than token reinforcement. An example of this would be: Jim refuses to get up. While he stays in bed he receives no reinforcement (no token); when he does get up he receives ten tokens. This is because he will get the most reward for what he finds most difficult. Subsequently Jim gets up more and more easily, so he is given three tokens and social encouragement for getting up, and seven for having a wash. This readjustment and sequencing can continue until the complete repertoire is built up and Jim's behaviour is positively fixed. This process is in fact a shaping programme, with a gradual reduction of reward as opposed to an abrupt end when a further stage is reached.

Table 3.1 An example of what a token economy scheme might be

Time	Behaviour	Reward token
08.00	Gets up	1
	Washed	1
	Showered	1
	Dressed	1
08.30	Eats breakfast using cutlery correctly	1
09.00	Helps clear tables	2
09.30	Goes to O/T	1
10.00	Participates in work	3
10.30	Helps give out coffee	2
11.00	Participates in work	2
11.30	Returns to ward and lays the tables	3
12.00	Socializes with other patients	1
13.00	Returns to work	1
14.00	Participates in gardening	Up to 10
16.00	Returns to ward	
17.00	Sets tables	
	Bath	Number of tokens
	Wash clothes	decided by nurse as
	Iron	appropriate
	Cook supper	

It can be seen, then, that token economy may be very useful in helping motivate the long-stay client, especially in his initial stages of rehabilitation, and has a potential, if skilfully used, to aid more complex social behaviours in the more advanced programme.

DESENSITIZATION

Desensitization is the behavioural treatment for people with phobias. A phobia will be expressed as some form of behaviour. Whether this is in the form of actions or thoughts, it is invariably shown in physiological terms, e.g. palpitations, sweating, pallor, nausea. For example, a person phobic towards rats will avoid places where he is likely to come in contact with them; he will think about them with dread, and should contact be unavoidable will certainly react physically to them, breaking out in a cold sweat, with increasing pulse and respiration.

Like all behavioural treatments, the use of desensitization should be carefully considered. A client with a phobia can sometimes be desensitized by a skilled nurse or therapist, but this does not mean to say that all the client's symptoms will disappear. The reasons for the development of the phobia may not have changed during therapy, and consequently other symptoms may arise and be just as debilitating. This phenomenon is referred to as 'symptom substitution'. To prevent this occurring, it is often desirable to begin other therapies simultaneously with desensitization. For example, a person who has developed a phobic reaction to leaving his house may have a deeper mental problem that will require treatment by psychotherapy or counselling, as well as a simple desensitization programme for the overt fear reaction to going out. If, then, a 'double-barrelled' treatment programme is started, the chances of symptom substitution developing are greatly reduced.

> Anthony developed a fear close to panic whenever he went outside his house. At first he forced himself to leave and go to work, but his anxieties did not subside and he found it impossible to concentrate once he had arrived at work. As he worked as an accountant and needed to concentrate for long periods, his superiors at work soon became unhappy with his performance, so he took sick leave and sought medical help. After a month of unsuccessful treatment with minor tranquillizers, it was decided to seek help from a behavioural approach.
>
> It was apparent at this stage that Anthony had a frank agoraphobia, and that in order for him to return quickly to work he would benefit from a desensitization programme. However, it was also clear that he was not suffering from a simple fear of the outside; his phobia had developed due to many complex factors involving unresolved personal conflicts.
>
> Before desensitization began, much time was spent with Anthony to uncover some of the psychological problems he was experiencing. For example, during discussions many things were discovered about him, the most significant being:
>
> * The cause of his parent's death the previous year had remained unresolved.
> * His wife, who had never worked before, had begun to talk about finding a job.
> * His teenage children were demanding more independence and making preparations to leave home.

It was clear to the nurse that urgent treatment must start by assisting Anthony's return to work, because while he was able to avoid the fear of going out this negatively reinforced his being housebound. It was also apparent that his last few days at work had been extremely unpleasant, which he had found punishing. While he was ill his wife would not consider finding a job, and similarly his children would not want to leave home; this he found rewarding.

A behavioural explanation of Anthony's phobia formation

As previously discussed in the section on behavioural principles, certain factors operated in Anthony's phobia formation, these being:

Punishment (serves to extinguish behaviours), e.g. going to work, followed by superiors complaining about his performance.

Result: weakens the desire to go to work.

Negative reinforcement (relief from an aversive stimulus strengthens preceding behaviour). Anthony's anxiety and unease when starting off for work were removed when he decided not to go.

Result: decision not to go to work is strengthened.

Positive reinforcement (rewarding situations).

While Anthony has this 'illness', his wife discontinues her plans to find a job (positively reinforcing his illness). Similarly, the children say they will stay at home until he gets better again (positive reinforcement for Anthony to remain ill).

The nurse's main job is clearly to desensitize the main focus of fear and continue counselling Anthony in order to help him uncover the underlying problems and deal with them.

From the above, it may well appear that if the reasons for the phobia's development are removed, all will be well, so counselling and psychotherapy may appear to be the better solution.

In fact, counselling was begun with Anthony two weeks before desensitization, but even if this had been completely successful the client would still be left with a learned behaviour. He has, in fact, been conditioned to respond physiologically to certain situations and circumstances, just as the simple rat phobic has learned to respond with fear to the sight of a rat. Similarly, Anthony, even when fully aware of the causes of his phobia through counselling, was still left with fear responses to leaving the house. Desensitization therapy was required to break down these responses and replace them with more appropriate behaviours.

The programme

First Anthony was asked to explain his fears, how he felt in various situations, and to place these in a hierarchy of fear (see Table 3.2). It may be helpful to study the table before reading on. Note the end column, which shows how the body is reacting. It is the body that acts as a reinforcer for Anthony's behaviour. When he relieves these symptoms, he negatively reinforces his behaviour.

Table 3.2 Anthony's hierarchy of fear

Situation	Feelings	Physiological responses
1. Knowing I'm staying at home	Calm	Normal
2. Looking out of the window	Uneasy	Pulse rate slightly raised
3. Going to the door	Anxious	Pulse rate up, B/P raised, palms perspire
4. Opening the door	Very anxious	Breathing becomes increased, overbreathing develops
5. Stepping outside	Feeling of panic	Breathing rate increases, sweating generalized, palpitations begin
6. At the gate	Faint, nausea	Symptoms increase, physical feelings of weakness, muscles refuse to work
7. At the bus stop	Uncontrolled panic, impulse to run	Indecision is enabling anxiety symptoms to continue, fainting is now a possibility due to extensive overbreathing
8. Arrival of bus	Complete confusion, panic building to terror	Physical symptoms of anxiety cannot be maintained further, all symptoms have reached a crescendo, adrenaline in the system will either be utilized in running or be broken down in the body.

Symptom (aversive stimuli)	Behaviour	Effect
Heart palpitations	Returns home	Feels calmer
		Strengthens his behaviour (by negative reinforcement)

This is called 'avoidance behaviour' and is the reason the phobia has been so well and truly fixed. If this pattern can be broken down, the conditioned behaviours can be replaced by more valuable ones.

The hierarchy helps the nurse because it allows her to understand exactly how the person is feeling, simply by asking him to pinpoint at any time where he is on a scale from one to eight. By explaining to the client what is happening, and reassuring him constantly, she can 'talk' the rating down and therefore break down this avoidance behaviour. To explain this a little more graphically, let us see exactly how the nurse begins.

First Anthony will be taught how to relax, using simple breathing exercises and muscle relaxation. For this he is asked to sit in a relaxed position and breathe deeply but slowly. Then, as he breathes in, he is asked to tense the muscles in his legs and arms and clench his fists; as he breathes out he says, 'I am feeling calmer' and simultaneously relaxes his tensed muscles. This technique takes only a few minutes to teach, but is invaluable in the process of desensitization, for several reasons:

- It provides an adequate supply of oxygen to the body and prevents over-breathing. This will affect the secondary physiological reactions that occur in panic attacks, such as confusion, palpitations, nausea and faintness.
- It relaxes the muscles so that blood flow is not restricted, and reduces the shakiness.
- Verbalizing 'I feel calmer' is reinforced when the body responds in a desirable way and allows the client to feel in control.

The nurse can now move on to take Anthony through his phobic journey, constantly asking him how he is feeling. He can now use relaxation appropriately to prevent him avoiding the situation until he is completely desensitized.

Finally, let us look at a brief dialogue between the nurse and Anthony at his garden gate:

Nurse: 'OK, Tony, you've made it to the gate, you're doing great, tell me how you feel now.'

Anthony: 'Awful, I want to go back in.'

Nurse: 'Well, awful doesn't tell me a lot; how do you rate it on your scale?'

Anthony: 'Around six.'

Nurse: 'Right. You're breathing too quickly, remember what we did before, breathe in and tense, breathe out and relax and repeat, 'I feel calmer'.'

Anthony: 'I feel calmer ... I feel calmer ... I feel calmer.'

Nurse: 'Carry on, you're doing fine, just a little slower.'

Anthony: 'I feel calmer ... I feel calmer.'

Nurse: 'Fine, how are you feeling now?'

Anthony: 'Much better, around three on the scale.'

Nurse: 'Good, that's great, we'll carry on for a few more minutes, then, when you're really relaxed, we'll finish for today and tomorrow we'll go a little further.'

This process is continued until all avoidance behaviour is broken down and Anthony feels quite relaxed at all stages of his journey. The nurse accompanies him until he is quite sure that he can succeed on his own. Failure at any one of the steps can be very traumatic, so the main aim is to make the steps meaningful but not insurmountable. Thus the client has additional reinforcement for the achievement but no negative reinforcement for avoiding the task.

If for some reason the nurse miscalculates the difficulty of the task and the client is unable to continue the exercise and, say, runs inside, this will create a potentially destructive situation. It can be offset to some extent by ensuring that the verbal reassurance given when back inside the house is directed not at how relieved he is feeling, but how well he has progressed. The reinforcement is therefore directed at his achievement of some goals, rather than his failure.

Alternative theoretical considerations

Within this approach to phobic clients we have focused strongly upon the operant learning theory of phobic formation, i.e. that the fear is rewarded by events following its avoidance. We have also intimated that rather complex mental processes may have contributed to this phobia formation. Additional theoretical considerations, which may help the nurse when evaluating the phobic client's behaviour, and in turn help the person understand how the fear was originally created, are given by Mowrer (1960). This theory combines a classical conditioning situation with subsequent operant reinforcement. For example:

Pain	*evokes*	Fear
Unconditioned stimulus		*Unconditioned response*
Pain + dog (dog bite)		Fear
Unconditioned stimulus		*Unconditioned response*
+ conditioned stimulus		*+ conditioned response*
Dog	*evokes*	Fear
Conditioned stimulus		*Conditioned response*

In Pavlovian terms, this explains why once you have been bitten by one dog you become afraid of all dogs. During his experiments with conditioning, Pavlov also discovered that this pairing phenomenon (i.e. the unconditioned with the conditioned stimulus and the unconditioned with the conditioned response) would not continue indefinitely. He showed that the conditioned response became weaker and gradually extinguished (extinction in classical conditioning terms) if the original unconditioned stimulus did not recur:

Sight of dog	*evokes*	Fear
Conditioned stimulus		*Conditioned response*
Second sight of dog	*evokes*	Reduced fear
Third sight of dog	*evokes*	Further reduced fear

Consequently, failure of the original pain to recur allows for the conditioned response (fear) to gradually reduce. Pavlov's trials showed individual differences between subjects in how long extinction took, and also that even after some time had elapsed and extinction was thought to be total, an isolated single response was possible.

If this is the case, how can phobias be maintained? It is evident that not every dog or even every tenth dog is likely to bite the conditioned person, so how is it that the conditioned response does not extinguish? Mowrer (1960) proposes that someone afraid of a dog will actively seek to avoid dogs, and that subsequently the negative reinforcement (relief of potential anxiety situations) maintains this avoidance behaviour. This is called the 'two factor theory'.

Another theory which may support the maintenance of phobic reaction is that of Ellis (1962). This theory suggests from a cognitive perspective that, once a fear exists, the individual may perpetuate it by 'self talk' which supports the fear. The subject says to himself, 'I must not go to the park, there will be dogs there, and they will bite me', or 'Dogs are dangerous', 'I'm scared of dogs', 'Dogs always bite me'. More significant perhaps is the possibility that when faced with a dog his thoughts may become the stimulus creating a fear response: 'Oh my God, there's a dog, it's going to bite me – I'll get rabies and die.' Running away from this situation may serve only to be a powerful negative reinforcement for subsequent avoidance of other dogs, and perpetuate the phobia.

Whichever theory is correct, and it is not unlikely that they all have relevant insights, it can be seen that desensitization may be beneficial in most cases. Gradual exposure to the focus of the phobia would serve to extinguish any conditioned response, using positive reinforcement, and reducing the efficacy of negative reinforcement in avoidance would helpfully reverse any learned behaviour pattern; and any cognitive reinforcement should be reversed by the evidence of experience ('The dog didn't bite me, dogs aren't dangerous, I've no reason to be scared of dogs.'). The latter idea of breaking down negative or unhealthy mental 'self talk' by the evidence of experience is well exemplified by the following therapy.

FLOODING

This procedure is based on the premise that the physiological responses of anxiety and panic cannot be maintained for prolonged periods, and that by being confronted by his fears the client will overcome them. In practice this is quite true. If it is impossible to avoid a phobic focus, the importance of the fear will dissipate relatively quickly. In other words, the client who is phobic to dogs may be confronted with a room full of them and be offered no escape. Similarly, the agoraphobic client may be taken into a town centre and made to stay until his fear is reduced.

However, it would be unusual for a client with a dog phobia or agoraphobia to be treated by flooding. Neither would appear to require such potentially traumatizing treatment, as both seem to respond to more gradual desensitization. The main advantage flooding has over desensitization is time, which may be a major consideration in some disorders such as examination or travel phobias. Provided the procedure and its likely effects are fully explained, and full consent is obtained, flooding may be a useful technique for such cases. However, some notes of caution would be wise. It should be remembered that, faced with no escape from a flooding situation, the client's state of arousal may be very high, which would certainly result in an increased blood pressure and heart rate. Failure to ensure that the client's health is able to maintain these cardiovascular changes would, in our opinion, be no less than professionally negligent. Should the person collapse or faint for any reason, irrespective of any possible physiological problems, flooding will have failed, as the client has achieved an escape. Finally, the nurse involved in the procedure should assure herself that the client will not suffer any psychological trauma as a result of this treatment.

POSITIVE CONDITIONING

Positive conditioning is a behavioural technique based on Pavlov's work, which extends the foundation work of desensitization. For example, if you have a client who is phobic to rats, it is possible to achieve by desensitization a state where he is no longer afraid of them, i.e. has a neutral attitude towards them. This is a desired result perhaps with rats, but what of the client who seeks help because she is having difficulty of a sexual nature? If, after desensitization the person is left with a neutral attitude to sexual behaviour, is this enough? Clearly the client is still not returned to full function. This is where positive conditioning can be used appropriately to take over where desensitization stops.

> Sally, a 22-year-old woman, was diagnosed as experiencing lack of libido and no subjective arousal responses. She had been in a steady sexual relationship for a year when finally, in desperation, she went to her GP for help.
>
> Sally had experienced pain during penetrative sex since her relationship had begun. This had at first inhibited her sexual arousal and led to her making excuses to her lover for not making love. On the occasions when penetrative sex had taken place, her anxiety and tension had led to an even more painful experience. Eventually Sally completely avoided all sexual contact, and the mere thought of sex precipitated an acute anxiety attack.

After several months of unsuccessful attempts to restore a fulfilling sexual relationship, Sally became increasingly depressed and was finally admitted to a mental health unit. After a period of assessment, the diagnosis was thought to be depression associated with sexual phobia. Sally agreed to a course of desensitization and responded very well to the treatment offered. She was taught how to relax and control her fear through breathing exercises. She was able to verbalize her anxieties and gradually conquer her fears of sexual activity. During her short stay in the unit she had three periods of weekend leave, and on the last of these occasions was successful in having penetrative sex with no pain or anxiety.

Although both Sally and her partner were delighted with the results of the therapy, Sally felt that after a few months she should be feeling more pleasure during sexual activity rather than the non-feelings she expressed. It was at a follow-up appointment that she related these feelings to the nurse/therapist, and in consultation with her doctor it was agreed to try to positively condition her towards a more pleasurable sexual experience.

The procedure

The theory of positive conditioning is simply to enable the person to associate feelings of pleasure from one specific situation and transfer them to another. In this case, this was combined with a programme of self-exploration and education to enable Sally to discover her sexuality as a pleasurable and sensual activity.

Sally was asked to choose some suitably relaxing music, which she found easy to listen to but not too distracting. The nurse asked Sally to relax and listen to the music, which at this point was playing at a very low volume, then to think of some pleasant experience she had in the past, and recall this to her. The subject of this 'pleasure experience' can be anything from a quiet conversation with someone she knew to lying on a beach in the sun. Sometimes, guided imagery can be used with the client in this experience.

Sally was then asked to intensify this feeling of pleasure in her thoughts, perhaps thinking of a particular experience that was even more pleasing. At this point the music was turned up slightly louder. Finally, Sally was asked to think of the most pleasing thing about this experience – intensifying the feelings of pleasure even further, and the music volume was increased accordingly.

This process was continued many times until the music itself could initiate these pleasurable feelings without Sally having to recollect the pleasant experiences. The process may take as little as one half-hour session, or as many as twenty, but it should be continued until the nurse is sure the association exists.

Once the association was made, Sally was encouraged to take her music to play at home during sessions where she explored and pampered her own body, associating her experience with the relaxed pleasure of the music. She was given a variety of exercises to do, ranging from luxurious bathing to massaging herself with oil, exploring her body and learning what touch she enjoyed and what she did not. In other words, she was able to get to know her own body intimately in an environment associated with relaxation and pleasure for her. She was then able to repeat the process introducing other artefacts such as favourite clothes, perfumes etc., thus making an association of pleasure with the articles and the music. Once this association was made, and Sally was confident in her sexuality being a source of pleasure, she was able to enter the final stage of the process.

Sally's partner had been acquainted with the procedure and was willing to cooperate with it. Both partners' understanding had been enhanced throughout the programme. Sally and her partner were then able to make love with all the conditioning articles, i.e. the music, the perfume, the clothes etc., so that sex was now not only anxiety-free for Sally but also actively enjoyable. Over the months, Sally was able to develop full sexual responses with her partner, with or without the accompaniments.

When a case history such as this is related, it often appears far-fetched or slightly ridiculous. However, for the sceptics among you, may we remind you that this technique is not limited to therapy. The so called 'great lovers' of the past have employed most of the techniques in this therapy, by attempting to associate themselves with good food, music, wine, setting the seduction scene in pleasure-arousing settings – soft lighting, soft furnishings, satin sheets etc. All these techniques are essentially Pavlovian:

Stimulus	*Response*
Food/perfume etc.	Pleasure
Food/perfume +	
Rudolf Valentino	Pleasure
Rudolf Valentino	Pleasure

The example of Sally's case was a special one, and will probably only be seen in outpatient clinics and special centres. The procedure is usually under the supervision of clinical psychologists or a consultant psychiatrist specifically involved in psychosexual treatments. However, the general principles of positive conditioning hold true in various mental health situations. It is up to the nurse to make herself familiar with these techniques and apply them within the resources available to her in appropriate situations. The principles involved probably explain how some of our own behavioural responses have been conditioned, and they are potentially very powerful if used effectively and ethically.

ASSERTION TRAINING

Assertion training is essentially taught through positive reinforcement, shaping and modelling. Many people who have been in long-stay care for a considerable time lack assertion skills, from the depressed person in the recovering stages to the institutionalized client of many years' standing.

Even some of the best residential care settings can have a detrimental effect on the individual's desire to be an independent person. Many clients have learned to be subservient, to be told what to do. It is for these people, and for many in the community, that assertion training can be a very helpful tool.

Ideally assertion training should be part of a course in social skills training, but certainly it is a necessary precursor for the timid, shy and inarticulate person before social skills training begins.

The purpose of assertion training is not to produce an aggressive, overbearing and truculent individual. It is simply to allow the individual to be more free to express his desires, feelings and thoughts in a clear and socially skilled way, without the accompanying anxiety that so many of us feel.

We wonder how many of you may have experienced the horrible feelings, the flushed features and sweating palms, when circumstances have prevailed where it has been necessary to complain? When it has really been important to state your case? How many times have you 'let things go' because it would be too traumatic or too much 'hassle' to say what you really feel?

It is, of course, your intellect that will determine in any given situation how to react, but additionally, how many times have your emotions ruled, restricted or inhibited your responses? Yet again, it can be seen how negative reinforcement by avoiding situations has in fact strengthened a reluctance to assert yourself. As with phobias, it can be seen that avoiding the focus is very rewarding, and breaking this down can only be achieved by positively rewarding the desired behaviour.

A few years ago, a colleague of one of the authors attended a behavioural course in assertion training. At the commencement of the course he was a rather polite, gentle and socially skilled individual. Roughly half-way through the course, during a dinner with the author, there appeared to be a total change in him. He was loud, rude and totally unskilled with waiters and the author to the extent that he was nearly left to finish his meal alone. He was, of course, suffering from an overexposure to therapy, which occurs quite frequently in short courses. It took him about a month gradually to assimilate his assertion skills into context on returning home. This graphic example serves to demonstrate that assertion training should be done slowly and surely, and preferably in conjunction with a social skills training course.

The procedure

It should be remembered that each programme should be tailor-made for each individual. This can be done by observation and discussion with the client. By noting situations that occur where a more assertive behaviour would be worthwhile and relating this to the person, it is possible to preorganize the individual for training and increase his motivation for change.

Individual or group exercises will enhance the desired outcomes at an early stage. Simple exercises modelled first by the nurse can be very useful as a basic step. Here are a few examples which, as can be seen, progress:

- *Eye contact exercise* A group of clients sit in a circle; each person in turn faces to his right and makes eye contact with the individual next to him, and states, 'I am (Joe Smith), what should I call you?' The person responds by returning eye contact and saying 'Hello Joe, my name is Fred Jones.' This continues in the circle, with the nurse giving social reinforcement for each pair.
- *Eye contact increasing volume* The above exercise is repeated but the volume of speech is subsequently increased with each round.
- *Touch eye contact + volume* The second exercise is repeated, this time with each client making physical contact with the other (usually appropriate contact is hand to shoulder).

Variations to these can be made, e.g. passing objects around the circle, stating loudly what the object is. Or clients can hold hands in a circle saying 'Charge', first in a quiet voice, progressing to loud, and finally standing on a chair, still holding hands, but with them raised in the air shouting 'Charge' at the tops of their voices.

The object of these exercises is gradually to allow the person to become less embarrassed in farcical situations and generally to disinhibit himself. The exercises should be made to fit the climate of the group. In each exercise the nurse's role is to model each step and reward the individual when successful.

Once this basic level is achieved, the nurse will design further more intricate exercises, tailored to the individual's needs. Following the 'Charge' exercise, for instance, a refusal exercise may follow. Each client politely requests something or some task from his partner, and the response should be: 'No, I don't wish to do that.' 'No, I don't wish to give you that.' 'I'm sorry, but I wish to keep that myself.' Once the nurse feels sure that each person is able to control his own wishes, and verbalize them confidently, more advanced and realistic exercises can be devised.

There are many practical applications of assertion skills training. Two practical and real programmes in which one of the authors was involved may be of interest.

Case 1

During psychotherapy Susan disclosed that one of her problems within her marriage was a lack of physical satisfaction during lovemaking. The problem stemmed mainly from her inability to discuss sexual matters frankly with her husband.

Using a modelling and rehearsal technique, employing an empty chair, she was able to use vocabulary that she had previously felt inhibited about. With constant reinforcement she soon became confident enough to disclose openly to the chair how she felt.

Before she was discharged this problem was discussed with her husband, who promised he would cooperate and help Susan explain how she felt with him as she had previously done in rehearsal. Susan's permission was, of course, sought before this, as it was an item of strict confidentiality.

Subsequently, Susan's sexual relationship with her husband improved and, along with this her confidence increased and some of her mental problems disappeared.

Case 2

Mike, a student nurse, complained that he was unable to communicate to his seniors certain reservations he had about policy and his role in the mental health unit. It was apparent that he would not be able to confront the charge nurse immediately in an open and honest way, nor would it be wise.

For him, then, a simple shaping programme was devised, with a student nurse colleague as the supportive therapist. Mike was to list the ideas and suggestions he wanted to make and the constructive criticism he thought would be helpful. At each opportunity that arose over a period of weeks, he and his colleague approached the charge nurse in private and discussed, in gradually increasing time periods, the less important to the most serious suggestions and criticisms. The student colleague was to make fewer and fewer contributions during the course of the programme, but was to continue the reassurance and support (see Table 3.3).

Table 3.3 A possible programme for increasing communication

Interview	Time	Topic	Student input
1	2 minutes	Wards reports	Verbal support for whole interview
2	5 minutes	Days off	Verbal support as appropriate
3	7 minutes	Patients' meals	Non-verbal support throughout interview
4	10 minutes	Personal clothing	Non-verbal support 1st half of the interview
5	12 minutes	Trips out for patients	Non-verbal support 2nd half of the interview
6	15 minutes	Drug administration	Simply in attendance
7	18 minutes	Doctor's rounds	Non-attendance but support afterwards
8	20 minutes	Holidays for patients	

By the end of the assignment Mike was surprised at how much he had been able to achieve with the charge nurse. Although he had not been able to change all the things he had hoped, he now felt more prepared to verbalize his ideas to other senior nurses in subsequent allocations.

It can be seen then that assertion training can be very effective, not only for the client but also for yourself if thought out well and with a little imagination, using behavioural principles applied intelligently.

SOCIAL SKILLS TRAINING

A knowledge of social skills training is extremely important for professionals working in the mental health field. Many people who have been in residential care for long periods, or acute clients who find relationship formation difficult, may benefit greatly from this training.

For many people in long-stay settings the need for social skill in any interaction has been removed, or its importance neglected. Clients tend to be given their daily requirements of food, warmth, entertainment and cigarettes without question, and certainly without a demand for 'please' and 'thank you'. These requirements have become the person's right without question or argument, and consequently the social graces have become redundant.

When one of the authors was last involved with social skills training with eight long-stay clients, most of whom had been in long-term residential care for over twenty years, he was quite startled to discover that none of them knew each other's names. Despite the fact that several slept in the same dormitory and sat together at mealtimes, none of them was aware of each other's existence. For them, life had become so monotonous, uninteresting and inflexible that a normal social interaction had been reduced to a blind meaningless togetherness, without acknowledgement or contact with their peers.

Some years ago, as a student nurse, one of us remembers his Principal Tutor defining mental illness as a 'breakdown of interpersonal relationships'. Without seeking causes, or anything more technical, we have always tended to agree with him. If this statement is true, and it is accepted that social skills are a cornerstone of interpersonal relationships, it can be seen that social skills training is essential in most manifestations of mental illness.

The procedure

Social skills training largely uses the principles of shaping and modelling. It is also hoped that when primary stages are reached, the intrinsic satisfaction and reward will self-perpetuate the learning or relearning process. Success will breed success or, as in this case, a smile will breed more smiles.

How can the average nurse begin in social skills training? What should she do? How can exercises be formulated? In fact, for the nurse, social skills training should be one of the most easily implemented schedules. The reasons for this are as follows:

- Most nurses are very socially skilled and present 'good' models for clients to follow.
- From examining their own social skills it is only a single step to generalize them into simple exercises for the client to engage in.
- The nurse is the most powerful person to reinforce social skills in the client, as they are in frequent contact.
- The nurse is present in very powerful reinforcement situations during the day, i.e. mealtimes, activities, cigarettes, recreation, hygiene and dressing.

It should be within all nurses' capabilities to list the components of their social skills, and by reinforcing them in their clients to teach a high degree of proficiency. A typical list may be:

Greetings: (non-verbal) smiles, nods, handshakes, waves; (verbal) 'Hi', 'Hello', 'Nice to see you', etc.

Names: rehearsal and memory of significant people in everyday contact.

Interest: remembering the significant interests of people around you. Mental notes of particular people's hobbies, pastimes – in order to make interesting conversation.

Conversation skills: appropriate listening, eye contact, encouragement and remarks. Appropriate responses at time intervals.

Hygiene: general and oral hygiene and an awareness of the effects of its absence.

Body space: appropriate space requirements for the rank, culture and type of relationship, i.e. acquaintance/friend/lover. This should also include appropriate use of touch.

Dress: differentiating types of dress customary for various situations and environments. This should include colour matching and choice of colours for congruence of occasion, e.g. black or dark for funerals, bright for weddings.

Eating: use and knowledge of conventional standards. Conversation during meals and ordering or preparation of meals.

Money: knowledge of currency, values and budgeting.

Social skills may be taught individually or in groups. Essentially, individually constructed exercises should be tailored to the stage of skills at which the client is currently operating. In long-stay wards or mental health units, everyone may need to begin at a very basic stage and progress via modelling exercises and shaping programmes.

An illustrative case

Four long-stay clients who had been in care on the same mental health unit agreed to work with a nurse purely on social skills, progressing to a daily living programme with a view to discharge together in a group home.

1. The clients were introduced to each other and rehearsed each other's names by throwing a cushion around in a circle and saying their own name and the name of the person catching it. The nurse was included in this, and this continued as a warm-up exercise daily in each formal session. Each person was asked to discuss with the others his particular interests or concerns, and then each client was asked to say what he could remember of each of his companions' interests. This also continued daily until each had a better understanding of the other, and then was repeated intermittently throughout the training.
2. Mealtimes were arranged so that the four clients were seated together. The nurse ate with them and made social contact throughout the meal, thus modelling a skilled interaction. Subsequently the nurse encouraged and praised similar imitative interactions on future occasions.

3. Gradual progression through the basic skills continued via two- and three-hour sessions of role playing, conversational skills, smiling, body posture and responding appropriately in various situations, e.g. a supermarket, public house, restaurant. When these had been achieved in role play, the sessions were extended into the real situations, with the nurse present giving support and encouragement.

4. The clients were asked at any time during the training to comment on each other's oral and personal hygiene, thus helping the others to become more aware of the detrimental effects this can have on social interactions. The nurse also contributed to this with comments, followed immediately by helping the person reach a solution, i.e. shower/bath/oral hygiene, and positively reinforcing the result.

5. Organized shopping expeditions for food and meal preparation were taken in turn by each client and followed by social reinforcement. People were encouraged to verbalize their praise of each other's abilities, and also to make constructive criticisms in a socially acceptable way.

6. Choice of personal clothing was linked with particular events and excursions, so that immediate social reinforcement was available appropriately in each situation.

7. Finally, before discharge, a trial period of four weeks on a set budget in a 'half-way house' was agreed, with the nurse supervising daily.

The outcome of this short course (approximately three months) was remarkable. The four clients were discharged and, with periodic support from the community mental health nurse and social worker, have been successfully reintegrated into the general community.

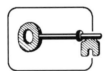

KEY CONCEPTS

1. Behaviourism has a significant role to play in people's everyday lives. Understanding behavioural science can be tremendously helpful to mental health nurses, and secure a better quality of life for the clients they seek to help. Skinner and Pavlov's experimental work has proved beyond reasonable doubt that behaviour is largely dependent on stimuli within our environment, responses to those stimuli and the consequences following those responses.

2. From the experimental work done by Skinner and others, behaviour modification principles can be extrapolated and applied to humans in real-life situations, e.g.
   • Weakening behaviour by extinction and punishment
   • Strengthening behaviour by positive and negative reinforcement
   • Developing behaviour by modelling and shaping.

3. Using a more eclectic approach, and incorporating the principles of both operant and classical conditioning, a wide range of treatment programmes can he created to help a person with mental health problems. This rather broader use of behavioural principles is termed behaviour therapy.

4. Before commencing any behavioural treatments, the nurse should consider the ethical and moral issues involved, i.e.

who   - is the client?
            - gave permission/consent?
            - decided what is desirable change?
what   - behaviours are being changed?
            - methods are to be employed?
why   - is it necessary?

Are all these questions being answered in an ethically supportable manner? How would you feel if you were the client?

CONCLUSION

This chapter seeks to explain some difficult concepts of behavioural science in a rather simplistic way. We hope that ending the chapter with some programmes may, by analogy, help focus some of the principles of behaviourism and aid the nurse to gain deeper insight. Since behavioural programmes were introduced into mental health nursing, much ingenuity and imagination have gone into making them work for clients. Many people who may have remained in residential care settings are now discharged and living effectively in the community owing to the help they received from behavioural strategies employed by conscientious, knowledgeable and caring nurses. It is our hope that this chapter may stimulate interest in and produce a greater potential source of help for mental health clients.

FURTHER READING

Barker, P. (1982) *Behaviour Therapy Nursing*, Croom Helm, London.

Barker, P. and Fraser, D. (1985) (eds) *The Nurse as Therapist: a Behavioural Model*, Croom Helm, London.

Eysenck, H.J. (1960) *Behaviour Therapy and the Neuroses*, Pergamon Press, London.

HMSO (1990) *Code of Practice. Mental Health Act 1983*, HMSO, London.

Marks, I. M. (1969) *Fears and Phobias*, Heinemann, London.

Martin, G. and Pear, J. (1992) *Behaviour Modification – What it is and How to do it*, 4th edn, Prentice-Hall, New Jersey.

Mathews, A. M. and Johnston, D. W. (1981) *Agoraphobia: Nature and Treatment*, Tavistock, London.

Murdoch, D. and Barker, P. (1991) *Basic Behaviour Therapy*, Blackwell Scientific, Oxford.

Richards, D. and McDonald, B. (1990) *Behavioural Psychotherapy: A Handbook for Nurses*, Heinemann, Oxford.

Schaefer, H. H. and Martin, P. L. (1969) *Behavioural Therapy*, McGraw-Hill, London.

Trower, P., Casey, A. and Dryden, W. (1988) *Cognitive–Behavioural Counselling in Action,* Sage, London.

Supervision $\boxed{4}$

Perhaps the first question that supervision raises is, Why does a mental health nurse need supervision? First, supervision is an integral necessity for any worker in the caring professions, to ensure the best-quality service for clients and best-quality developmental opportunities for workers. Secondly, our experience shows us that in both the voluntary and the statutory sectors the quality and availability of supervision for workers in high-stress situations is currently extremely variable; although there is evidence of good practice, there is equally evidence of supervision being organised on an ad hoc basis, which may leave workers and clients under-supported. Finally, we see supervision as a clear and purposeful activity for which managers, supervisors and supervisees may need to be trained in order to maximize its potential – it is more than either accountability or 'talking through'.

In addition to these main points it may be prudent to say more explicitly what is gained from supervision. A group of mental health workers in Grimsby we recently had the benefit of working with, make the point more graphically than either of us could. In discussion through a training exercise they came up with the following list of benefits for workers, clients and the organization if supervision is in place and is of a good standard:

Advantages of supervision

For the client	*For the practitioner*	*For the organization*
To have objective work done with them	To remain objective	To enable the practitioner to receive objective feedback.
Offers protection by ensuring shared resources.	To receive feedback.	Increases staff morale.
Inspires confidence.	Clarifies, informs and stimulates.	Promotes working within policies.
To achieve personal goals, not what the worker wants.	To remain client-centred.	To ensure good practice is maintained.

To receive the best possible from skilled practitioners.	To help define/achieve personal, client and organizational goals.	To identify areas that may require development.
	To ensure good practice.	Identifies training needs.
	To identify areas of practice that require development.	
	To identify areas of existing excellent practice.	

They also laid out what they believed were the requirements of effective supervision:

- Accurate communication: listening, feedback, consistency, information
- Clear realistic goal setting
- The ability to demonstrate empathy, respect and genuineness.
- Effective time management
- Use of objective perception
- The ability to encourage personal development.

It is from these perspectives that we offer the following client-centred model of supervision, a model devised for our own use and which we have found to be helpful. It is not intended as a device for constraining supervisors or supervisees into a straitjacket, or for reducing the flexibility or imagination of skilled workers – on the contrary, it may enhance the latter qualities. It is rather intended as a useful guide, offered for the reader to use, modify, benefit from or throw out. What we do hope to achieve at least is some added weight to the argument for adequate supervision for all workers in the caring professions.

We should at this point credit the major influences which lie at the root of our own development, and thus the model. In terms of our counselling practice, the greatest single influence has been Gerry Egan. In terms of case work, both statutory and voluntary, the systems approaches prevalent in the 1970s have left their mark. The unifying factor of each approach is in how they complement our belief that any complex process is made easier and more effective if it can be logically structured, while leaving scope for versatility and creativity. In terms of the supervision model, this reminds us that supervision is a purposeful activity, facilitated by communication skills and problem-solving techniques (see Egan, 1994), and with the ultimate goal of benefiting the client.

THE DEXTER AND RUSSELL CLIENT-CENTRED MODEL OF SUPERVISION

The model was first developed and used by Graham Dexter and Janice Russell in 1990. Since that time it has been used effectively by many organizations, mental health teams, voluntary agencies and individuals, mainly in the north of England (Figure 4.1).

The model consists of a six-stage circular process, dependent on skilled facilitation:

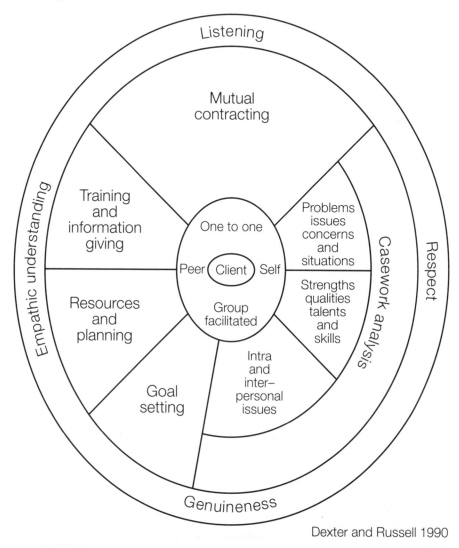

Dexter and Russell 1990

Figure 4.1   A client-centred model of supervision

1. Mutual contracting

2. Casework analysis
    - identifying current issues
    - identifying current strengths
    - identifying current inter-/intrapersonal dynamics.

3. Goal setting
4. Identifying resources
5. Information giving and training
6. Mutual contracting.

The skills within the process

The skills and values acknowledged in the outer perimeter operate from a counselling philosophy which underpins a belief that effective supervision is a facilitative process, hopefully enriching to all participants, rather than a mechanical procedure. Although the process itself is a simple one to follow, the communication skills required to empower it are specific and sophisticated, and become the fuel that drives the process.

In our view, this is because the major functions of the supervisor are twofold. One is to structure according to the mutual goals of supervision, which may need to incorporate agency expectations. The second, and equal in importance, is to recognize the need for supervisees to talk through any emotions, difficulties and anxieties. This is true of any 'people work' setting. Tschudin (1991), for example, suggests that this particular aspect of supervision is a valuable safeguard for nurses. Our own experience endorses this, in working with nurses, mental health workers, counsellors, social workers and voluntary agency workers. Tschudin links the process directly to Egan's counselling process. Although we see some relevance of that process here we would also stress that we would be wary of using counselling per se – indeed, we believe that supervisors should refrain from counselling supervisees.

The flexibility of the model

We suggest that this model may be equally effectively employed in one-to-one, facilitated groups, peer group or self-supervision. The advantage in any of these situations is that the purpose and logical sequence are not forgotten.

One-to-one supervision

This is often the most formal type of supervision, usually undertaken by a trained or experienced practitioner. The setting may vary considerably, and there are differences between, for example, consultative supervision and line management supervision. The differences need to be clearly recognized, and due attention given to the inherent power differentials and potential interest and conflicts in, for example, line management supervision, or in supervision directly linked to a training course, where feedback will be given to assessors. This is worthy of much more discussion, but for the purposes of this chapter the reader is directed to the importance of clear contracting (Stage 1 of the model).

Whatever the relationship of supervisor and supervisee, we would claim that while it may not be absolutely necessary to hold an identical value orientation, it is against the interests of both supervisee and client group to have a supervisor who is unable to understand and embrace the concepts of a non-judgemental approach, genuineness and empathy. Our own view in this is coloured, again, by experience, which falls in line on this occasion with Rogers' (1961, 1967) teachings relating supervision to the conditions of personal growth. At the very least, it must be agreed that good supervision cannot occur without the supervisee feeling safe to disclose the trickier aspects of their practice.

Facilitated group supervision

An alternative to one-to-one practitioner supervision is to use a combination of peer and practitioner supervision. In this arena it is possible to get the best of both worlds in terms of a more objective professional feedback, and in using the power of the shared resources of a peer group.

In group supervision the skills of facilitation are paramount. Egan (1973) suggests several functions of a facilitator that appear to be compatible with group supervision skills. These include modelling appropriate behaviour, being a resource for the group/client, and demonstrating a leadership role.

Peer supervision

Peer supervision is appropriate and effective in both one-to-one and group situations. It may be seen as an alternative to using a practitioner, or may be used to augment that process. It can be usefully employed on an intra- or interagency basis, tapping into and enhancing each other's resources – this may be particularly useful when there are practical and financial difficulties. This is not to suggest, however, that peer supervision is merely a substitute, rather to support an approach that asserts that there are always the resources for supervision.

One of the greatest benefits of peer supervision is the sharing of experiences, in terms of both personal and client-related issues. Peer debrief is essential for wellbeing and personal efficiency. The argument can be extended to suggest that the client's best interest is served when everything possible is being done to ensure the worker's ability to practise safely and efficiently.

Peer supervision provides an opportunity to share and debrief particular difficulties that occur in particular client groups. It also allows for the sharing of approaches, different styles of practice and techniques that may have been used to advantage, or which might have been disappointing. Such sharing is of benefit to the presenter and to those listening, and offers a medium for constructive feedback. In giving and receiving feedback, participants are also able to develop and enhance the skills of supervising and of being supervised. It is worth remembering here a point which recurs in our model, that while there is profit in sharing problems and anxieties, there is much to be gained from debriefing successes as well. It would be a great loss if learning were confined to the negative when development may be even more potentiated by studying the positive outcomes of sessions and interventions, and identifying the talents, resources and skills of the peer group.

Self-supervision

Self-supervision involves a reflective approach, an ability to self-check and self-assess which enhances quality of work without inhibition through self-consciousness. This involves a degree of self-awareness and an ability for self-analysis. Following a modular approach can aid clarity here, in being able to achieve some distancing. Within this, various techniques can be used as aids. Where possible, taping can be a useful practice, aiding interpersonal process recall. Where this is not possible, the immediate recording of sessions may provide food for thought. Identifying specific skills, attitudes or strategies which may help or hinder the process and charting them over time provides a useful backup to self-checking. Long-term notes may also be useful in reviewing work with a particular client group, to remind workers of contracts, of the purpose of the work, and to identify the positive and negative outcomes in terms of negotiated goals.

From here onwards we will present the model in terms of supervisor and supervisee. This is for clarity of presentation – the process is relevant to any of the above forms of supervision.

Mutual contracting

As stated, it is our view that the client is central and that their welfare is the supervisor's main responsibility. They therefore have an obligation to obtain the best deal for the client and to ensure that the supervisee is operating 'good practice', to the best of the supervisor's knowledge. Implicit in this fundamental premise is that they also have a responsibility to the supervisee to provide systematic supervision of a high quality and, where appropriate, e.g. in line management supervision, to ensure that the supervisee is not overloaded or agency-abused. Perhaps central to this process is the notion of a contract, which is mutually negotiated and which clarifies standards, expectations and what to do if it is felt that the client is not getting a fair deal. This is why mutual contracting is seen as the first stage of the supervision process.

Within a clear and specific contract, the supervisory relationship can negotiate and identify particular aspects of practice which require feedback. We would suggest that giving feedback, a term much bandied around, is not only central but is itself a specific skill, a view shared by Urbano (1984), who suggests that the most effective feedback is that given 'in a manner which is positive, immediate and agreed by the supervisee' (p.14). We would go further and say that feedback needs to be specific rather than general to be of optimum help. To achieve this end, it would seem that the contract should be flexible enough to allow for the development of the supervisory relationship and be frequently renegotiated to allow it to remain clear, specific and goal-orientated.

A typical contract may focus on:

- particular skills or approaches;
- individual goals of supervision;
- agency goals and expectations;
- personal/professional/practice debrief;

- timing for supervision;
- extent of confidentiality;
- the supervisor's responsibility to monitor the ethical context of the supervisee's practice;
- length of contract.

It may be helpful to look at some of these issues in slightly more depth.

Confidentiality

The complete confidential contract may not always be possible or desirable. Bohart and Todd (1988) cite the California Supreme Court Tarasoff decision, 1971, as a useful example of the need to have exceptions to complete confidentiality. In this case of a client who was intending to and eventually did kill their daughter, it was ruled that:

'Private privilege ends where public peril begins' (p.345). In our view, this relates also to supervision, while recognizing that there are many fine lines and grey areas surrounding the passover point. As a general guideline, the supervisee's client is also the supervisor's vicarious responsibility, and must remain the priority. In this context client endangerment may be substituted for public peril.

Less formidable examples of potential breach of confidentiality may also include the need for intra- and interagency liaison, or reporting to accreditation bodies, for example where the supervisee is enrolled in specific training programmes. However, confidentiality should only be breached in the interest of the client or the worker, and in any case only with the maximum opportunity for negotiation or consent. Confidentiality from the client's perspective has to be recognized and the relevant permissions obtained or limitations clarified. Perhaps the main point here is that the limits of confidentiality be openly recognized in any contracting.

Ethical considerations

The supervisor and the supervisee have to be equally clear on the ethical codes of conduct relevant to their working contract and to the supervisory contract. This entails having a clear understanding of what action may result should the supervisee disclose practice which is seen as unethical or prejudicial to the client's welfare. Although we are aware of the implications in terms of reducing potential disclosure, we feel it is vital that these issues are clearly negotiated and established at the first supervision session (see Information giving and training, p. 94).

Timing

The frequency and length of session need to be clearly identified. It is also useful if partitions can be drawn between particular aspects of the supervision, e.g. time spent on personal issues, training, casework discussion, analysis and administration. Any additional contract for informal or urgent telephone debriefing needs to be carefully considered and a policy determined. Concentration span for individuals will vary and be influenced by experience, mood, tiredness, environment and circumstantial distractions. It has been our experience that negotiating for these potential problems is beneficial.

Length of supervision

It may be useful to discuss the advisability of length of supervision at an early opportunity and contingencies developed for the possibility that the supervision contract be broken by either party. Also, a probationary period of supervision is often a good policy so that either party may withdraw if their personal goals or values are not being adequately served.

Supervisee's disclosure

The reciprocal skill that accompanies facilitation skills is the ability of the supervisee to disclose. Although it is the responsibility of the supervisor to establish a climate conducive to disclosure, the supervisee has to have the courage and ability to reveal difficulties, inadequacies and emotions where appropriate. Similarly, they will need to develop the skill of prioritization and, as mentioned in the section on peer supervision, that of analysis of positive interventions. These skills may vary according to experience, and the supervisor should keep this in mind when helping to focus the supervisee. Although the right to withhold disclosures remains the supervisee's, long-term inability to disclose or confront issues may, at its most extreme, result in forfeiture of the right to practise. Again, agency expectations, whether voluntary or statutory, need to be clearly spelt out here: where are the lines of accountability? Is supervision (which cannot operate without some disclosure) a part of the worker's contractual obligation?

Casework analysis

Identifying current issues

Current issues may be particular cases where the supervisee just feels stuck, where they need to review intervention for assessment purposes, or specific problems or concerns such as client dependence, overload, time management, administrative concerns or the appropriateness of any particular techniques or interventions. It is our belief that at this juncture it is not the supervisor's place to offer advice or guidance, but instead to employ the outer perimeter attitudes and skills in order to allow the supervisee to develop their own insights where possible. More directive intervention may be appropriate at a later stage in the process.

Identifying current strengths

If the supervisor has listened carefully to the supervisee's current issues, it should be possible to identify the skills, qualities and resources that they have available. The supervisor should be able to gently challenge clearer insights into what is potentially available within the resources of worker, agency and client, in order to move on within the process. Often supervisees need reminding at this point of the objective of their contract with the client, whether it is to enable a self-referred client to help themselves, or a statutory intervention within which they might have specific duties, whether willingly contracted with the client or not. Scenarios obviously differ greatly, but common to all will be issues such as time management, the use of particular techniques and commitment to progress and review. It is useful to be able to challenge supervisees to see themselves neat, with their deficiencies, weaknesses and mistakes alongside their strengths, talents, skills, personal qualities and resources. This implies a recognition of them as developing workers, and past experiences may be invoked in this process.

Identifying intra-/interpersonal issues

Within every case discussed will be elements of the interpersonal dynamic between worker and client, which may require debriefing. This can be as low key as 'I wonder why I like this client more than this one', to higher-profile feelings such as 'I hate seeing X, they really wind me up', or 'I feel sexually attracted to this client'. In other words, the interpersonal issues that require debriefing are the thoughts, feelings and behaviours that are stimulated between the two parties. It may be that there are some barriers, anxieties or difficulties that require identifying and working through before the relationship can progress. In some instances, particularly where the worker may be involved against the wishes of the client, it may be that hostility is encountered for which the worker needs support. Equally important may be the intrapersonal issues for the worker, e.g. 'What thoughts, feelings and behaviours are evoked for me through working with this client?' 'How do I feel when I contemplate this interview?' 'How do I feel when I come out?' These personal issues may not be directly related to the specific relationship with a particular client, but rooted in doubts about personal competence. It may even be the personal need to be helpful, the often overwhelming need to demonstrate skills, success or progress that is buzzing away in the worker's head, or frustration at the limitations of what the worker can realistically achieve.

It is vital that these issues are brought out into the open so that they can be dealt with sensitively and directly. How many of us can honestly say that such doubts, difficulties and frustrations have not occurred in our work? Knowing that this is the case, and that these are common and consistent themes, may be comforting for most workers, although such knowledge should not lead to complacency.

Goal setting

This stage of supervision is crucial and, in our experience, often underused in systematic supervision. There appear to be some vital questions that need to be addressed at this stage which make a significant contribution to effective supervision:

What are you trying to achieve with this client? If you are involved with the whole family, who is the client?

What do you believe the client is trying to achieve?

What are your preferred outcomes? Are any of them unethical, or contrary to either your own or the client's welfare?

Are your goals compatible with those of the organization you work for?

If you continue with what you are doing, will the interests of the client, yourself and the organization be best served?

If the answer to any of the above creates dissonance, how might this be resolved?

This is a generalized list of suggestions, certainly not intended to be either mandatory or exhaustive. The central point is that workers need to be in touch with their goals to aid effective work.

Resources and planning

Having explored the goals that the supervisee sees as important to the client and themselves, and which satisfy agency expectations where appropriate, it is now useful to initiate some investigation into what resources are required to enable those goals to be achieved. These might be of a personal or a practical nature, or perhaps involve the expertise of other workers. It may be that a plan is required to enable goals to be achieved. For example, the goal may be to proceed more quickly by using different approaches, but before this can be achieved further training or reading may be needed. Planning our own development is one possible outcome of contemplating how best to achieve goals, especially when investigation reveals a lack of immediate personal resources. Brainstorming can be a useful technique here for getting in touch with resources and planning strategies. Such reflections may also lead to the conclusion that the best interest of the client may be served by appropriate referral, rather than plodding on without profitable results.

Information giving and training

At some point within the process of supervision the supervisor will be called upon to venture an opinion or to offer ideas based upon their own professional experience and expertise. It is our view that this point is reached toward the end of supervision rather than the beginning. In the spirit of empowering, rather than inducing dependency, every opportunity should be given for the supervisee to develop their own insights and ideas through empathic response and insightful challenges on the part of the supervisor. However, it would be both wasteful and irresponsible for a supervisor to ignore obvious deficits in the supervisee's education or experience, especially if for want of some small input the client's situation could be significantly improved, or the supervisee's learning enhanced. The supervisor should be able to offer further insight and different techniques and approaches that will augment the competence of the worker. Such teaching should be limited to enabling development rather than overwhelming and thus disabling the supervisee.

One final note is clearly linked to ethical issues. It may be necessary on some occasions to be quite frank and say that if the supervisee continues with a particular technique or unethical practice, then 'x' will be the result. An extreme example of this may be where the worker is initiating or continuing a sexual relationship with the client, which would result in a breach of the code of conduct adhered to by the worker. The supervisor would need to explain the consequences of such behaviour, which would depend on the details of the situation and the agency/professional body code, but which may involve, for example, a report being filed with the appropriate ethical committee of the worker's professional body and/or agency, and discontinuation of supervision. This of course has implications for the supervision contract, and is where the process links back to mutual contracting.

Mutual (re)contracting

The original contract may have specified the supervision required by the supervisee, but this may change during the initial process where the supervisor has provided additional ideas of where feedback may be most needed or useful. Training needs, timing and frequency or type of supervision may now be more accurately assessed. Thus a renegotiated contract for the next session appears to us to be the most appropriate point to finish the process.

CONCLUSION

We began this chapter by stating that the model proposed is intended to be a useful tool, not a straitjacket. We would now add to this by saying that although the progress of the model is presented as linear and circular, this is only because it has developed that way. However, we note that when we have taught the model, and on occasion in our own use, there may be a need for the process to flow forward more quickly, or to flow backwards to previous stages. This is not only acceptable but commendable, as it demonstrates the model in use as a tool which enhances the supervision experience.

Finally, the model has a contribution to make in providing clear guidelines to the process of supervision which may offer a consistent approach, not only in consultative supervision but across a whole agency. This has obvious advantages for development and assessment processes, which will become more relevant with the introduction and intensification of NCVQ programmes across a variety of agencies. We believe that such advantages are for both supervisor and supervisee – the right to receive a high standard of supervision is equal to that of the right of an agency to expect a high standard of work from its employees. Ultimately, they aid the process of ensuring the best possible provision for clients.

FURTHER READING

Hawkins, P. and Shohet, R. (1989) *Supervision in the Helping Professions*, Open University Press, Milton Keynes.

Procter, B. (1988) *Supervision: a Working Alliance*, (Video Training Manual), Alexia Publications, St. Leonards-on-Sea.

Application of Skills

PART
2

Working with anxious people | 5

Matthew sat wringing his hands and rocking backwards and forwards with a strained facial expression.

'Hello, Matthew, is there anything I can do to help you at the moment?'

'I'm scared sick, I don't know what it is, but I just can't seem to think straight, everything is so difficult. My head aches, my heart is pounding, it is as if I've got some dreadful disease.'

Matthew has been complaining of a variety of bodily symptoms for some time, but underlying all these are his persistent feelings of fear resulting in a severe 'anxiety state'. This fear incapacitates Matthew to such an extent that he finds it difficult to do the simplest of tasks. The nature of his anxiety clouds his thinking to such an extent that he finds it difficult to pinpoint any specific area that causes it. This is generally known as 'free-floating anxiety'. However, anxiety can present in a multitude of ways, and may occur as a symptom in any psychiatric disorder. Another form of anxiety is where a specific fear can be isolated, which results in a 'phobic state'. Phobias such as fear of open spaces (agoraphobia) can be totally incapacitating and require very specific nursing interventions (see p. 68).

Anxiety occurs in an individual when he is confronted with some form of stress. It is a state whereby the body prepares itself for a 'fight or flight' reaction to the stressful situation. Its physiological origin (see Figure 5.1) gives rise to symptoms such as palpitations, increased respiration, diarrhoea, frequency of micturition, tension, headache, nausea and potentially many others. However, an appropriate level of anxiety can be very beneficial. For example, before a race, in examination preparation and other situations where the individual is put to the test, anxiety usually increases the motivation to do well, but once the anxiety goes beyond its useful level disaster can occur, i.e. examination or test failure. Examples of situations where anxiety is a major component of the individual's feeling state include examinations; interviews; important personal occasions such as marriage, the birth of a sibling, the loss of a loved one and funerals; competitive events; and personal danger. The body's response is geared towards helping the individual cope with these situations, but there are times when the physiological response remains when the stimulus situation appears to have gone. Recall how you felt before your interview; increase that feeling tenfold and imagine feeling like that for days and sometimes weeks on end; you will then be going some way towards understanding how it must feel to be suffering from an 'acute anxiety reaction'.

Some people are more anxious than others, which could be due to many factors: personality, family environment and influence, personal financial and occupational circumstances, education and ability to relax, for example. The ability to cope with anxiety stems from an awareness of what causes it and then a purposeful attempt to either avoid the cause or cope with the result. However, avoidance could lead to further anxiety when the stressful event is finally confronted, or just the thought of the event could be sufficient to set off an anxious reaction.

People have different ways of coping with anxious moments. These are often unconscious processes aimed at protecting themselves from the anxiety-provoking situation or thought. They are termed 'mental defence mechanisms' and were first described by Freud (1958). Using defence mechanisms initially serves a useful purpose in that it allows time for an individual to work through the anxiety situation, e.g. the student who fails the examination for the final time may say or think initially, 'Well, it is probably for the best anyway, I'm a more practical person and if I had passed I would have been stuck with the office responsibility which isn't really what I want.'

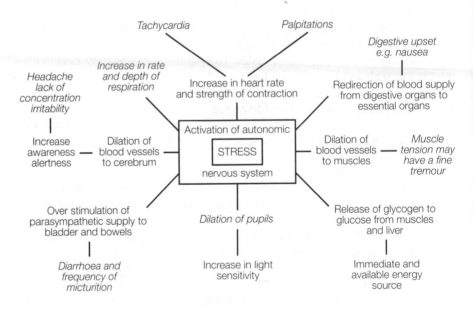

Other symptoms of anxiety are also due to alteration of sympathetic/parasympathetic action, adjusting blood supply and increasing function. These include: *increase in sweating, dry mouth, flushed face.*

Symptoms are shown in italic.

Figure 5.1   The physiological origin of anxiety

This 'rationalization' gives the person time, if they so wish, to work through to the actual thinking and acceptance of 'I have not got the intellectual or technical ability to pass this examination.' This form of thinking would initially have been anxiety provoking, so the unconscious use of the rationalization mechanism occurs. There are many other mechanisms that are used, depending upon the individual and the situation. Overuse of these, however, is not conducive to 'healthy' living, and many clients with anxiety states tend to rely rather heavily on them. It is therefore necessary for the nurse to understand these mechanisms and be aware of when they are being used excessively in order to appreciate the stressful areas in the client's life.

PROBLEMS AND NEEDS OF THE ANXIOUS CLIENT

The problems and consequent needs of the anxious client are mainly twofold: those presented as a direct result of the physiological response, and those related to the psychological effects of fear (see Tables 5.1 and 5.2). On assessment it is often necessary for the nurse to take reasonable control of the situation, conveying a calm air of confidence in order to avoid the client experiencing further anxieties related to 'Do they know what they are doing?' Clear explanations of 'what will happen next' are necessary in order to minimize the effects of the client's anxieties concerning the outcome of his admission. A steady tour of the environment and an early introduction to the client's personal space should help minimize his feelings of insecurity, at all times making clear the safety line of 'nurse availability'. It may be useful to concentrate on a one-to-one basis initially, until the client's confidence grows.

Psychological – well noted

Table 5.1   The physiological problems and needs of the anxious patient

Problem	Potential Problem	Need
Continual feelings of fear and dread	Panic attack	Calm, accepting presence of nurse. Clear safety limits explained
Insecurity	Uncertainty Loss of confidence	Highlight and reward any signs of progress. Give clear indications of any changes in treatment or care
Agitation	Exhaustion Social isolation	Enourage rest. Provide opportunity for privacy. Guide appropriateness of behaviour, i.e. protect from other patients' reactions to ceaseless agitation
Lack of concentration	Inability to complete simplest of tasks	Occupation given at appropriate level of patient's concentration. Regularly assessed and suitably changed to encourage distraction from personal worries
Frustration	Irritability, anger	Opportunity to vent and explore feelings, to be listened to and understood

Table 5.2 The physiological problems and needs of the anxious patient

Problem	Potential Problem	Need
Digestive upset, e.g. nausea	Anorexia, loss of weight	Monitoring of dietary intake and weight. Small, regular, non-irritating nutritional meals. Appropriate medication for indigestion
Frequency of micturition and diarrhoea	Incontinence, accidental soiling, dehydration	Easily accessible toilet facilities. Clothes that launder well and are practical. Extra fluids to compensate loss. Appropriate medication for severe diarrhoea
Excessive sweating	Body odour, discomfort, soreness	Frequent opportunity for bathing. Encourage self-care
Increased respiration and palpitations	Exacerbation of anxiety fears of physical cause/ disease	Clear and simple explanation of symptoms. Avoid dwelling upon patient's physical complaints. Focus upon feelings underlying the symptoms
Continual agitation, movement, restlessness	Irritability, frustration, aggression, exhaustion	Encourage rest and relaxation techniques at any opportune time

Priorities of care need to be quickly assessed and acted upon. In severe anxiety states it is likely that the nursing intervention will work in conjunction with the medical treatment. Anxiolytic medications, psychological testing, group therapy and relaxation techniques may all play a part in the care of the anxious client.

IMPLICATIONS FOR THE NURSE

When caring for the anxious client the nurse must remain calm and confident, acting in a sense as a model for the client. This is by no means an easy task, because the anxiety the client generates is often severe enough to cause anxiety in the nurse. A situation can occur where the client's expectations of the nurse to do something increase, the nurse's feelings of responsibility to do something increase, and at the same time the nurse realizes how powerless she is to help, thus creating a 'mutual anxiety-provoking' relationship. The danger then is that the nurse's anxiety reflects further on to the client, thereby increasing the client's anxiety. An extension of this could be when a client detects his anxiety being reciprocated and becomes increasingly frustrated to the extent of directed aggression towards the nurse. The tendency for the nurse to withdraw with feelings of rejection is considerable, and may influence the nurse to the extent that she may avoid the client in the future. It therefore becomes clear that while interacting with anxious individuals, it is important for the nurse to be aware of her own anxiety levels and to understand the possible causes within any interactions. The causes are often concerned with the nurse's self-doubt or lack of confidence (see Table 5.3), the effects of which are minimized if she is prepared for this and given some idea of the strategies she could use when anxiety levels increase in a nurse–client interaction. These strategies are concerned with relying on genuineness, i.e. being honest with yourself about self-doubt and personal limitations. This will help in the perception of intended interactions with realistic expectations, thus reducing what often becomes 'personal pressure' of having to do something well and in concrete terms. During interactions the strategy used is the practical application of skills, and the more effective these are the less likelihood there is of 'personal distracters' causing anxiety in the nurse.

Table 5.3   Some causes of 'nurse anxiety' during interactions with patients

Personal	Environmental	Patient
Am I helping?	Have I got time?	He is becoming more
What am I doing?	Should I be doing	frustrated.
Will I be able to help?	something else?	He is becoming very
Am I saying the right	What about the other	emotional.
things?	patients?	What if he turns his
What shall I say next?	I must go soon.	frustration towards me?
	How do I end this?	Can I cope with all this?

PRINCIPLES AND SKILLS REQUIRED

The skills required to help anxious clients are mainly those associated with encouraging them to explore their feelings in order to identify in more concrete terms the areas in their lives that contribute to the anxious state. Referring back to Matthew's statement when he was asked by the nurse if there was anything she could do to help:

'I'm scared sick, I don't know what it is, but I just can't seem to think straight, everything is so difficult. My head aches, my heart is pounding, it is as if I've got some dreadful disease.'

Nurse: 'You feel frightened because you are not sure what's happening, you have all these symptoms and you suspect there may be something physically wrong with you.'

This response demonstrates the use of paraphrasing and reflecting in order to convey empathy to the client, but also allowing him to hear again what he has just said, thus giving more time to focus on what he actually feels. The tentativeness in the nurse's response at this stage is important in order to allow the client to correct or focus in further on the nurse's response.

Matthew: 'Yes, it makes me wonder sometimes if there is something physically wrong, but at the same time, I know it is to do with my thinking, my feelings, the worry about home, relationships and work.'

Nurse: 'So you realize that the way you are at the moment is to do with your thinking, feelings and worries about home, relationships and work. I'm wondering which of those is the crucial issue for you at the moment?'

One of the skills when interacting with anxious clients is to distract them from dwelling too long on their bodily symptoms, as this is likely to increase their fears, yet at the same time the nurse must acknowledge and show understanding of the client's feelings. The response above is a 'clarifying' skill, in that it is an extension of a paraphrase asking the client to sort out priorities, which may mean the client responding to something that is the most crucial issue, or something that the client feels comfortable to talk about at this stage. Either way, it is helping him to explore his situation with the aim of identifying feelings and problems.

Matthew: 'Well, I suppose a lot of it is to do with home and my wife. She's changed so much over the last few years, she has so many new interests it's as if she's a different person.'

Nurse: 'How does this change in your wife make you feel?'

The open question is used here for two main reasons: one is to gain more information, and the other is to help the client focus upon his own feelings in the present rather than his wife's behaviour in the past. This is important, for it enables the client to continue talking about himself, whereas the details about the past and others, although relevant and possibly serving a purpose in some cases, may cloud the issue of the 'client's feelings now' in this type of situation.

Matthew: 'I just know that I'm becoming less important to her, that one day she's going to go off with someone who's on her level that she can share more interests with. I just can't keep up with her.'

It is often the case that because of the high level of anxiety within the client, even when asked directly how he feels, he may still come back with more detail concerning his feelings but not identifying them. When this occurs, it is important that the nurse uses an empathic response to ensure that understanding has taken place and that the client has a chance to pinpoint his feelings:

Nurse: 'Are you saying you're feeling inferior in some way to your wife and this makes you feel insecure within the relationship?'

The stronger the feeling words used the more tentatively the nurse should say them, as they can sometimes be received with some surprise and, if said dogmatically, the client may become defensive and refuse to explore the possibility of owning the feelings put to him.

The skills described so far are the listening skills from the counselling model (see p. 33). To expect to use advanced skills in a severely anxious client is unrealistic, as much working through of the client's feelings is required before problem solving should be considered. This 'working through' is facilitated by the nurse if the skills above are used in conjunction with observational skills. Sensitivity to the client's non-verbal behaviour will help the nurse appreciate the general state of the client: restlessness, pacing, rocking, wringing of hands, nail-biting and many others are indicative of anxiety. Also, being acutely aware of more subtle changes during interactions, e.g. looking away, resorting to closed posture, change in tone of voice, will help identify possible areas of particular difficulty in the client's life. This does not necessarily mean that it would be right for the nurse to focus on these areas, as this would depend upon many factors, e.g. how secure the client feels within the nurse–client relationship and the ability of the nurse to cope with the possible consequences. At the very least, any appreciation of the client's anxiety situations will enhance the empathy that the nurse achieves.

Another area of skill that is very useful for the care of the anxious client is related to facilitating relaxation and teaching methods of self-relaxation. There are many different methods of relaxation, but one that is commonly used involves the physical relaxation of the body by systematically tensing and relaxing groups of muscles. This involves following instructions either from a teacher or a tape. The skills needed to perform this are: appreciation of the appropriate environment, i.e. a quiet, comfortable, dimly lit room; the use of a tone of voice that is soft, clear and free from obvious distractions such as stutters, lisps or strong accents; and a sensitivity to timing, ensuring that while the nurse is taking the person through the experience she allows sufficient time to carry out the individual exercises. This is one advantage over the tape recorder; another is that the nurse can be sensitive to a particular area of the body that is visibly more tense than anywhere else, and spend a little more time helping the client to relax that part. Once the client has learned the principles of physical relaxation, the nurse can help him to apply those principles to himself at times of stress, in order to minimize the effects of anxiety.

SUMMARY

Anxiety is a part of all of us and can be useful in increasing our motivation to do certain things. However, when anxiety becomes the predominant emotion in our lives its usefulness turns to destruction, fear and helplessness. Its physiological and psychological nature requires the nurse to have a clear understanding of its origin and effect, and the subsequent problems and needs. When caring for the anxious client, the nurse must be in touch with her own feelings and be aware of her own anxiety levels, so as not to compromise the attention she gives to the client. The skills required to help the client explore his anxious world are the listening skills of paraphrasing, reflecting, questioning and clarifying. These are used to help gain empathy with the client, while at the same time supporting him through confused and sometimes painful emotions.

KEY CONCEPTS

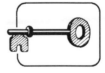

1. Anxiety can present in a multitude of ways and may occur as a symptom in any psychiatric disorder.
2. It is a state whereby the body prepares itself for a 'fight or flight' reaction.
3. Its physiological origin is due to the overactivity of the sympathetic and part of the parasympathetic nervous systems.
4. Mental defence mechanisms are unconscious processes aimed at protecting the 'self' from anxiety.
5. The problems and needs of the anxious client are those presented as a direct result of the physiological response and those related to the psychological effects of fear.
6. When caring for the anxious client, the nurse must remain calm and confident.

7. The nursing skills required are those of effective listening to gain empathy and help exploration of the client's emotions.
8. Other skills are related to observation, sensitivity and the use of non-verbal communication, and the facilitation and teaching of relaxation.

FURTHER READING

Goliszek, A. (1993) *60 Second Stress Management: the Quickest Way to Relax and Ease Anxiety*, Bantam, London.

Goodwin, D. (1983) *Phobias, the Facts*, Oxford University Press, Oxford.

Hallam, R. (1992) *Counselling for Anxiety Problems*, Sage, London.

Madders, J. (1980) *Stress and Relaxation*, Martin Dunitz, London.

Melville, J. (1980) *First Aid in Mental Health*, Allen and Unwin, London.

Powell, T. J. and Enright, S. J. (1990) *Anxiety and Stress Management*, Routledge, London.

Priest, R. (1980) *Anxiety and Depression*, Martin Dunitz, London.

Working with depressed people 6

Andrew: 'I've had enough. I'm such a big fat useless slob. I just can't get anything right. I'm totally useless.'

Nurse: 'Totally useless?'

Andrew: 'Yes, I can't do my job properly. I can't keep relationships. I cock up everything I do and then I run home like a big kid...I had a house once but I couldn't hack it. I sold up after three months, lost a load of money and ran home to my mother. I go out to the pub, act like the life and soul of the party and pretend everything's OK. You know, have a laugh and a joke, but it's all a sham, an act. I'm just a figure of fun, bit of a joke really. Everyone expects me to be like that all the time...but when I get home I start blubbering like a baby, weeping and wailing all over the place. Who'd want a pathetic man like that?'

Nurse: 'Pathetic?'

Andrew: 'Yeah! Useless, a failure, total mess. I can't see an end to it. It seems to go on for ever. Me cocking things up, upsetting people, blowing it.'

The picture illustrated above is one of a man with severe depression. His thought processes are all negative, about himself and the world around him. He is miserable, preoccupied and wrapped up in self-criticism, berating himself constantly. He appears to have lost his sense of purpose, is confused, dejected and has a hopeless and powerless vision of his future. This continuum of depression (see Figure 6.1), however, is not necessarily experienced by all. Individuals may never proceed to the depths of hopelessness described; others may not experience sadness, but find themselves suddenly in the grips of despair.

There are many theories relating to the causation of depression (Barker, 1992), varying from the psychoanalytical theory of loss of a love object (Freud, 1917) to the neurophysiological theory that relates the alterations of feeling states to chemical disturbances, to the cognitive theory which implicates the thinking style of the sufferer (Beck, 1980). It is our opinion that it is unlikely that a single theory could adequately cover the aetiology of depression; it is probably a combination of factors that play a part in each individual. However, when dealing with someone with depression the cause becomes academic, for each individual is unique, as is their experience. Consequently any attempt to generalize and find a common denominator should have little effect, if any, on the nurse's attitude and skills.

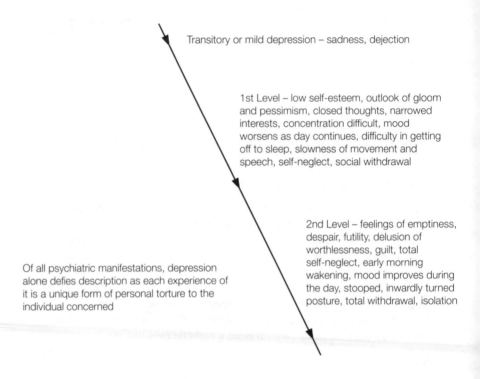

Transitory or mild depression – sadness, dejection

1st Level – low self-esteem, outlook of gloom and pessimism, closed thoughts, narrowed interests, concentration difficult, mood worsens as day continues, difficulty in getting off to sleep, slowness of movement and speech, self-neglect, social withdrawal

2nd Level – feelings of emptiness, despair, futility, delusion of worthlessness, guilt, total self-neglect, early morning wakening, mood improves during the day, stooped, inwardly turned posture, total withdrawal, isolation

Of all psychiatric manifestations, depression alone defies description as each experience of it is a unique form of personal torture to the individual concerned

Figure 6.1 A continuum of depression

The individual manifestations of depression are many and varied, and an outline of the most common features associated with feelings, thoughts, behaviours, communication and sleep will help to clarify this point (Tables 6.1–6.4).

Table 6.1 Depressive feelings

1st Level	2nd Level
Achievement of pleasure and satisfaction negligible. Feels helpless. Generally pessimistic. May show clear evidence of crying. Experiences feelings of heaviness and emptiness. Anxiety may be present mildly or intensely.	Often 'expressionless', as if without feeling. Experiences feelings of 'nothingness', 'bottomless', despair and futility, worthlessness and hopelessness.

Table 6.2   Depressive thoughts

1st Level	2nd Level
Thought process slow. Concentration becomes difficult. Interests increasingly diminish. Becomes unsure and indecisive. Ruminative thoughts interfere with problem solving, dwelling upon the lack of future prospects and a meaningless existence.	Orientation to reality becomes increasingly difficult. Delusional thinking may be present, often confirming negative feelings. Delusional content may be associated with guilt, poverty, 'nothingness' (nihilistic) and bodily functions.

Table 6.3   Depressive behaviour

1st Level	2nd Level
General slowness of movement. Every task takes a great effort. Very little effort to invest in self-care. Weakness and fatigue. May overeat or more often become anorexic and lose weight. Marked decrease in sexual interest. Agitation may result in persistent movement. Tendency to withdraw from others leading to isolation.	Becomes almost motionless or indulges in agitated purposeless movement. No evidence of self-care. Posture often slumped, head and eyes down and generally curled inwards. If left, would never move out of bed. Every task becomes a major ordeal.

Table 6.4   Communication observed in depression

1st Level	2nd Level
Slow speech, often with long gaps between sentences, often delivered in a montonous manner. May forget the original train of thought due to poor concentration span. Posture and facial expressions are often reliable aspects of non-verbal communication.	Often mute, or monosyllabic. Little acknowledgement of others present. Very subtle changes in non-verbal communication.

Depressive reactions can occur at any age and in either sex. Individuals may communicate their feelings differently. People tend to be at risk from depression at times of crisis or during some developmental period of their life, e.g.:

- Loss of a loved one or separation anxiety
- Having a baby   Puerperal depression
- Entering the change of life   Menopausal or climacteric depression
- Retirement   Depression of old age

Of course it is not just the process of change that gives rise to the depression, as many physical, psychological and social components will play their part, resulting in what can be referred to as a 'complexity of painful despair'. The following was written by someone regarding this aspect of depression.

'I think I'll just sit here – but I've got so much I should do, it doesn't matter. If I do start something I'll only do it wrong. Oh God why should there be so much pressure? I can feel them all wanting so much, almost like a physical pressure on me dragging me down. So I'll sit here – just sit. I refuse, no-one can make me do anything – but they'll try. I'll fail again. They all expect so much, and I'm just not able. I try so hard but I'm just not up to it. If only they could see, but they just keep smiling and saying it's all right. But I know it's not, just look at me, I'm a mess, I'll never feel better. How will I ever face them after they've seen me like this? I can't let them – but what can I do? Why should I do anything? If I sit here I'll die eventually then I won't have to do anything ever again. I'll study that carpet until I die, it's better this way, I can never fail again. I don't even have to do anything, I couldn't even do what I've rehearsed so many times. I even bought a tow rope, tested the garage beams but I couldn't even do that. I thought about the kids at the last moment – if I'd done it, then it'd be over now. The kids would cry, but at least they'd respect me for doing something right. Now all they see is this sorrowful pitiful mess they call their father. If I am their father. I wonder if I even did that right. Who would blame her for taking a lover, married to a mess like me? If only I could get it together just enough to get it over with, but it's just too much effort. I'll just stay here and look at this carpet till I die – please God if you'll just help me to do this. I even need help just to sit here and die. God – that's a laugh, he should worry about me. My God what a mess I am just sitting here feeling sorry for me. I don't deserve to live when I can't even feel sorry for the people I've hurt. Please please someone help me die.'

This transcript illustrates that suicide is always an option for depressed people and is often thought of as the only way out of what is perceived as a desperate situation. **It must be made clear that any depressed individual may attempt to end his life by suicide**. It has been said that those individuals who have very little energy or drive, or who lack clarity of thought due to severe depression, as in this case, are unlikely to succeed in killing themselves, but the nurse cannot ignore the possibility that they may find sufficient resources to fall through a window, walk in front of a car or wander off towards the river. When nursing clients who are depressed, it is safer to consider them all as potentially suicidal. Clients are most 'at risk' when their physical and psychological state has outwardly improved but the feelings of desperation still remain. At this time the patient may resolve never to experience the same depths again, and in order to ensure that it does not happen, decides to 'end it all'. Other risk periods related to depression are summarized in Figure 6.2.

It is not only people who suffer from depression who attempt suicide. Others are also at risk, e.g. those who are continually tormented by disordered perceptions and wish to rid themselves of the torment, or as a direct response to hallucinations or delusions. Some people may not intend to kill themselves but use the attempt as a 'cry for help' with problems that overwhelm them. All attempts at suicide are serious and raise many issues that require exploration by the nurse.

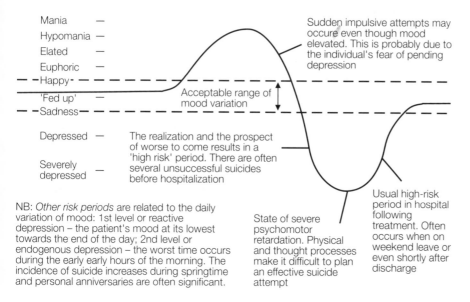

Mania —
Hypomania —
Elated —
Euphoric —
– –Happy· – – – – – – –
'Fed up' —
– –Sadness– – – – – – –

Acceptable range of mood variation

Sudden impulsive attempts may occure even though mood elevated. This is probably due to the individual's fear of pending depression

Depressed —

The realization and the prospect of worse to come results in a 'high risk' period. There are often several unsuccessful suicides before hospitalization

Severely depressed —

NB: *Other risk periods* are related to the daily variation of mood: 1st level or reactive depression – the patient's mood at its lowest towards the end of the day; 2nd level or endogenous depression – the worst time occurs during the early early hours of the morning. The incidence of suicide increases during springtime and personal anniversaries are often significant.

State of severe psychomotor retardation. Physical and thought processes make it difficult to plan an effective suicide attempt

Usual high-risk period in hospital following treatment. Often occurs when on weekend leave or even shortly after discharge

Figure 6.2 Mood variation curve showing the 'high risk' times for potential suicides

IMPLICATIONS FOR THE NURSE

Imagine yourself walking across a bridge; in the distance you see a figure sitting precariously on the edge of the bridge, looking down on the busy road beneath. To fall would mean almost certain death. As you approach you recognize that she is an ex-client who was discharged a few weeks ago. She had been treated for depression, but was considered fit to leave by all concerned. As you walk, you recall the conversations you had with her, particularly the one that related to her wanting to commit suicide, arguing that it was her right to do so and giving what appeared to be quite logical reasons for this. When you are almost at arm's length from her she turns and recognizes you. She shouts, 'Leave me alone, this is something I must do.' By putting out your arm and grabbing her, it is likely that you could stop her at no risk to yourself. Attempt to answer the following questions:

- What would you do?
- Would you stop her?
- Would you let her jump?
- How would you feel if she jumped without your attempting to stop her?
- Have you the right to interfere with someone else's decision about their own life?
- Why is she about to kill herself in a place where she may be discovered and prevented from doing so?
- How can you be sure her thinking is logical and without distortion?
- How can you be sure she will not blame you for the rest of her life for saving her?
- How can you be sure she will not thank you for saving her when her depression lifts?

These are questions about your human response to someone's despair. It is important for the nurse to explore these issues and questions in order to prepare for the situation occurring, thus increasing the likelihood of effective intervention taking place during a crisis. When the nurse is clear in her mind what she thinks, the issues are prevented from being distractions during the 'crisis intervention'.

However, there are also professional boundary issues for the nurse working within residential care as part of the multidisciplinary team caring for a group of clients. She has a responsibility to preserve life and prevent suicide attempts and, to a large extent, the institutional response will either reinforce this set of beliefs or directly contradict and outweigh the individual's human beliefs.

It is often the case that the institution will increase the level of observation of the depressed patient to minimize the risk of suicide, in seeming contradiction to the principles of client autonomy, freedom and choice. These issues need to be discussed and debated on the basis of what is best for the client, rather than to fit the nurse's principles and theories.

Caring for a client in the community carries with it a degree of risk. Assessment of suicide risk, often by direct questioning - 'Has it ever been so bad that you've felt like harming yourself?' – is often an essential first step. The nurse who is reticent about asking the client about suicidal intent is not only doing the client a disservice (he or she will often be only too relieved to either acknowledge these feelings or to strongly deny them) but also doing herself a disservice, since assessment is now based more on observations than on hunches (admittedly these are occasionally right) and hard data and frank discussion.

The question may lead to a discussion of ways and means or merely indicate that the client is worried that 'If it gets much worse, I'm frightened I might start considering it'. In either case a clearer picture is formed of the risk involved. Clients may be encouraged to look at all the factors which have prevented them taking this course of action, or to review better times as the first step in reinstilling hope.

Development of a support network for the client is also crucial as the level of support around is often as important an indicator of suicidal risk as is expressed intent. A useful question might be: 'If I were not around who else could help you with your current difficulties?' Heightening support for the client as well as providing support for relatives and others concerned helps to maximize support for the client and minimize isolation for the nurse.

Important questions for the community nurse to ask of herself might include:

- Can I help this person?
- When would I need to refer the client on?
- How would I recognize that time?
- Where am I getting my support?
- Where is he getting his support?
- What has helped this person previously?
- What has not helped?
- What is our contract?
- When will we know when this person is 'better'?

Supervision for the nurse (see Chapter 4) and a knowledge of how and when to refer clients would seem to be crucial.

Another potential distracter that could interfere with the therapeutic process is the expressed depression from the client affecting the feelings of the nurse. It is possible to find yourself sad, low, irritable and often helpless during an interaction with someone who is depressed. It is necessary for the nurse to realize this possibility, as it could result in her avoiding the depressed client and thereby reinforcing his feelings of rejection. By being aware of this potential distracter, and sensitive to the way it is communicated, i.e. mainly by non-verbal cues, the nurse should be able to avoid interference from it and use the added awareness to 'tune' into the client's problems and needs.

PROBLEMS AND NEEDS OF THE DEPRESSED CLIENT

The problems and needs of the depressed client are varied and many. We intend to outline these only in general terms in order for the student to perceive the total picture of complexity, thus appreciating the scale of the problem. As with any intention to embark upon caring for an individual, a thorough assessment must be made and priorities of care set. These will vary, depending upon the severity of the depression. Perhaps the most obvious priority is to ensure the client's safety and minimize the risk of suicide; some of the principles involved here are outlined in Figure 6.3.

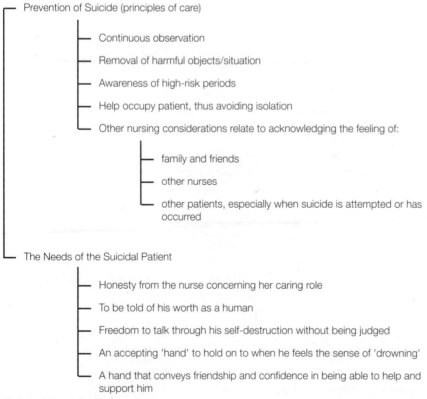

Prevention of Suicide (principles of care)

— Continuous observation

— Removal of harmful objects/situation

— Awareness of high-risk periods

— Help occupy patient, thus avoiding isolation

— Other nursing considerations relate to acknowledging the feeling of:

  — family and friends

  — other nurses

  — other patients, especially when suicide is attempted or has occurred

The Needs of the Suicidal Patient

— Honesty from the nurse concerning her caring role

— To be told of his worth as a human

— Freedom to talk through his self-destruction without being judged

— An accepting 'hand' to hold on to when he feels the sense of 'drowning'

— A hand that conveys friendship and confidence in being able to help and support him

Figure 6.3   Suicide prevention

Basically, physical problems, which may include anything from neglecting personal hygiene and not shopping for food through to not eating or drinking, may be dealt with on a continuum from problem-solving with the client (inviting the client to set goals and actions to achieve those goals), to prompting, cajoling and, in the most severe case, 'doing for' the client.

We do not wish to underplay the part played in caring for teeth, personal hygiene, diet and sleep within the institution and acknowledge that the nurse has a crucial part to play in performing those activities for the client which he is incapable of performing himself (see Figure 6.4). However, in many cases the work that is done with clients is aimed at preventing this degree of stupor, or at helping the client to recover from that point.

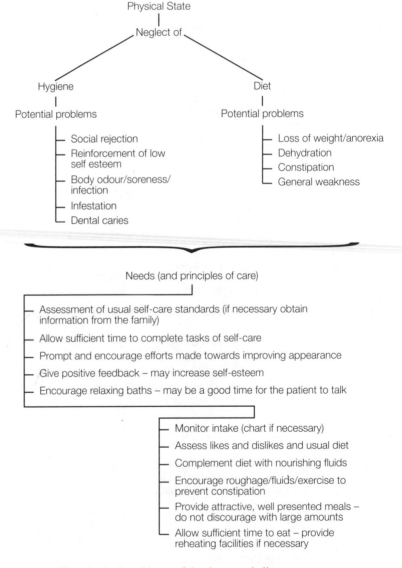

Figure 6.4   The physical problems of the depressed client

The psychological problems of someone who is depressed are uniquely entwined around their personality, environment, circumstances and relationships. There are, however, some clear common problem areas that can be experienced in varying degrees and combinations. Not all depressed people experience them all, but most experience some of them (see Figure 6.5). This simplified diagram shows how problems overlap and often reinforce the feelings expressed. The needs related to these problems are concerned with allowing the client to talk through and express his feelings to someone skilful enough to facilitate this.

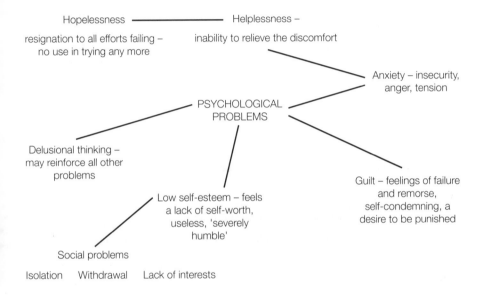

Figure 6.5   The psychological problems of the depressed client

PRINCIPLES AND SKILLS REQUIRED

Sensitivity and awareness skills

Severely depressed people have limited resources to use in self- care. They may neglect their most basic needs to such a degree that many, if left alone, would just sit, oblivious to their own physical discomfort and environment. When this state exists to any degree, the nurse must be sensitive and anticipate the needs of the client, for example:

* He may sit in a draught and not state that he is cold.
* He may sit in his own urine and not admit to being sore.
* He may be severely dehydrated and not ask for drink.
* He may be crying out for love and acceptance yet deny himself tears.

Accepting that the client may be unable or unwilling to communicate his own needs, the nurse must rely on her observational skills in order to perceive accurately what is going on for that particular client. The observations made should give sufficient information for the nurse to be able to approach the client with appropriate sensitivity. It is important for the nurse to be aware of her own feelings and mood state, for it is a common enough mistake to believe that superficiality and over- cheerfulness may somehow help the client who is depressed to change his mood. This does not happen, and this insensitive approach can quite often have the reverse effect, making the client withdraw even further. This process of mood influence can work both ways, for the client's depression may affect the nurse, as mentioned earlier. This is why, particularly with clients who do not readily respond or comply, the nurse must always be prepared to look inwards and self-evaluate in order to ensure that the approach and care that she gives are tailored towards the client's needs and not her own. The following are examples of some questions that would help the nurse to explore for herself a less than satisfactory nurse–client interaction:

Did I have a preconceived idea of what the outcome of the interaction would be?

Did I enter the relationship with some negative feelings that may have been communicated non-verbally?

Am I more concerned with the way I am feeling at the moment and this is distracting me from understanding the client's feelings?

Are my expectations of the client and/or myself too high?

Am I bringing my own frustrations into the interaction?

Am I displacing my frustrations on to the client?

Is there something about the client that reminds me of someone else with whom I did not have a good relationship?

Do I see something negative in the client that I see in myself?

Am I being honest with myself and am I really interested in this client?

This series of questions demands a degree of self-challenge, which is an aspect of self-awareness and should be part of a continuous process of self-evaluation, to guard against rising barriers which prevent the formation of relationships based on honesty, trust, genuineness and understanding.

Non-verbal skills

The client may often respond only when 'contact' has been made, through eye contact, touch and tone of voice, all of which are essential in order to break through the 'wall' of depression. When the aim in this sort of interaction is to gain a response, this approach is necessary to prevent total isolation in those who have withdrawn. Efforts to make contact with clients who are severely depressed should be aimed at gaining a response that will minimize the tendency to withdraw, reinforce reality such as the time and the nature of the environment, and increase the chance of further communication.

Sometimes just being with someone experiencing depression may be enough to show them that you care, and also to make contact. Sitting with the client, acknowledging his presence and being aware of subtle changes in his breathing, eye movements and posture may give him a sense of belonging and acceptance, which such clients often lack. This awareness of posture may consciously or unconsciously aid the nurse to 'mirror' by making subtle adjustments to her own breathing, leg positions, head and body movements and arm positions. Such mirroring is very powerful and is a physical way of communicating 'I'm interested in you, I want to invest some time with you, and I'm prepared to accept you and your present state by understanding your life as much as I can.' So, by using your own body language and being sensitive to the client's it is possible to communicate, thus going towards helping him satisfy his need to be accepted and valued.

Verbal skills

The principles underlying the use of verbal skills when talking with individuals who are depressed are that they must be allowed to verbalize and explore their feelings without reinforcing their negative thinking (Beck, 1980). We believe that the state of 'depression' is in many respects similar to the state of 'bereavement' (see p. 196), and is particularly relevant when the importance of helping the client work through his feelings is considered. It is generally accepted that unless someone who is bereaved works through most of the stages of bereavement, prolonged grieving and depression may result. It is our experience that the longer someone who is depressed is left to dwell upon the 'complexities of his despair', the longer he will take to recover. The skills that seem particularly pertinent here are the listening skills of paraphrasing and reflecting, conveying to the client basic understanding and allowing him to hear his own words and rationale, so that he can further explore his own world in an atmosphere of genuineness, warmth and empathy. This relationship between the nurse and the client must be one where the client can feel safe enough to explore many emotive issues that he may not have expressed to anyone before. His innermost conflicts may be verbalized, as he places trust and confidence in the nurse who is listening. She must respond to this trust by conveying acceptance and understanding, thus facilitating further exploration. The nurse must be prepared to accept verbalization of some very strong emotions, particularly anger, which is directed inwards towards the client, his significant others or even members of the nursing staff. Anger is quite a common component of depression and one emotion that tends to be controlled, causing much inner frustration and preventing further exploration of other thoughts and feelings.

By using observation and sensitivity skills, tension, agitation and frustration can be detected. Emotional release can be encouraged by highlighting and communicating these observations to the client, while at the same time giving him permission to be angry. For example, while listening to Alice the nurse noticed her voice becoming less relaxed; she started fidgeting and her face began to look tense:

Nurse: 'Alice, I've noticed when you started to talk about your mother you seemed to become tense, I'm wondering if there is a connection?'

Alice continues to talk about her mother in an angry frame, but still holds back on releasing any particular emotion.

Nurse: 'You seem to be holding back your feelings, as if you're saying to yourself, 'I shouldn't be talking about my mother like this'.

The theme of anger and guilt continued until Alice found herself freely expressing anger without guilt, which helped her explore further her relationship with her mother.

Actively listening to someone who is depressed and encouraging them to vent their feelings in an atmosphere of trust will help them to work through their despair as an important part of the overall care and attention they need.

Understanding and 'being with' the client is often enough. However, in many cases it is often the first step and, in the case of Andrew, although he believed himself to be understood, he still considered that he could not be helped. Thus, it is important to enable Andrew to address tasks he has been avoiding which, once tackled, will give him a sense of success and achievement. These may be very 'simple' tasks, such as getting out of bed at 9 a.m. instead of hiding there all day, or taking the dog for a walk. None the less, simple structured activities give the client a sense of control and direction, may help take his mind off painful thoughts and will make him feel less tired and lethargic (in spite of his initial belief that he will become more tired). On subsequent visits these tasks can be reviewed and the client may want to begin new activities or pick up old ones which have recently dropped off as he succumbed to the effects of his depression.

In later conversations with Andrew he states: 'I used to bike to work every day, go swimming once a week and do a bit of gardening, but I'm so exhausted I just sit all day and do nothing. The day seems like it's 48 hours long and I just can't get moving.'

He seems to be seeing everything in concrete, all-or-nothing terms – 'I could do it all before and now I can't do anything'. The implication is that he believes he will never be able to do anything ever again. He also demonstrated similar patterns of thinking in the earlier transcript, particularly awfulizing everything (seeing the worst in every situation) and overgeneralizing (one failure indicating failure in everything.)

At this point, getting him to identify what he *is* doing rather than what he believes he *can't*, and reviewing the things he has previously seen as valuable about himself, might be productive. It is also helpful to enable him to obtain a more balanced view of himself by asking him to review the evidence regarding his total failures.

Addressing negative thinking is a challenge to both the client and the nurse. Doing it too early may leave the client with the belief that you have not fully understood his situation, and may sound 'Pollyana-ish' and unduly optimistic. Doing it clumsily may leave the client feeling bludgeoned. The following are brief examples of the types of responses which might encourage the client to begin to adopt a more balanced view:

Client: 'I can't do my job'

Nurse: 'Which aspects are you doing?'

Client: 'Nobody loves me.'

Nurse: 'Could you list them?'

Client: 'I'm a total failure.'

Nurse: 'Total?'

See Gilbert (1992) and Trower, Casey and Dryden (1989) for a more thorough description of this approach.

CONCLUSION

Depression is a potentially life-threatening state of 'being'. You must never underestimate the personal pain an individual may be going through. You will need all your personal resources to withstand the barriers of silence, monosyllabic utterances and futility expressed by the severely depressed. Using your sensitivity, warmth and understanding, it will be possible to enter into the client's world. In doing so you must be strong enough to withstand the enveloping nature of the client's mood and stand back to respond with empathy. This will help you lead the client out to look forward to some future where he can value his life.

KEY CONCEPTS

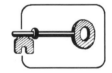

1. The manifestations of depression vary in severity from sadness and dejection to despair and futility.
2. The main areas of depressive symptoms focus around:
   • depressive feelings
   • depressive thoughts
   • depressive behaviour
   • communication.
3. People are particularly at risk from depression during developmental stages of life, or when experiencing some personal crisis such as the loss of a loved one.
4. Any depressed person may attempt to end his life by suicide.
5. It is essential for the nurse to be aware of the 'high- risk' factors in the potentially suicidal.
6. The implications for the nurse involve exploring personal ethics and being self-aware during interactions with depressed clients.
7. The problems and needs of the depressed clients revolve around:
   • physical needs
   • prevention of suicide
   • psychological and social needs.

8. The skills required are aimed at encouraging the client to explore his own feelings and work through his despair without reinforcing his negative thinking. They include:
   - sensitivity and awareness
   - non-verbal skills
   - verbal skills of listening, i.e. paraphrasing, reflecting, questioning, clarifying and challenging
   - sensitive cognitive challenge.

FURTHER READING

Barker, P. (1992) *Severe Depression*, Chapman & Hall, London.

Beck, A.T. (1973) *Diagnosis and Management of Depression*, University of Pennsylvania, Philadelphia.

Beck, A. T. (1974) *The Prediction of Suicide*, Charles Publishing, Bowie, Maryland.

Beck, A. T. (1980) *The Cognitive Therapy of Depression*, John Wiley, Chichester.

Freden, L. (1982) *Psychosocial Aspects of Depression: No Way Out*, John Wiley, Chichester.

Gilbert, P. (1992) *Counselling for Depression*, Sage, London.

Hauck, P. (1983) *Depression*, Sheldon Press, London.

Mitchell, A.R.K. (1974) *The Nature of Depression*, NAMHO, Penguin Books, Harmondsworth.

Morgan, H. (1979) *Getting Death Wishes? The Understanding of Deliberate Self Harm*, John Wiley, Chichester.

OHE (1981) *Suicide and Deliberate Self Harm*, Office of Health Economics, London.

Rowe, D. (1983) *Depression: the Way Out of Your Prison*, Routledge and Kegan Paul, London.

Helping the depressed client. *Nursing Times*, 26 October 1983, pp. 62–3.

Stengel, E. (1964) *Suicide and Attempted Suicide*, Penguin Books, Harmondsworth.

Trower, P., Casey, A. and Dryden, W. (1989) *Cognitive Behavioural Counselling in Action*, Sage, London.

Working with people experiencing delusions

7

Mary was recently admitted believing herself to be perfectly well. She insists that she is a victim of a Soviet plot to destroy her. Her brain is receiving transmissions from Russia which are gradually interfering with her thinking. Her next-door neighbours are spies. She knows this because it was they who informed the doctor that she was unwell. At one time she trusted her GP but that was probably her big mistake, for he is undoubtedly the head of the local spy ring, and by admitting her to a mental health unit he has prevented anyone believing her story.

Mary's belief is typical of the deluded client receiving treatment in mental health units all over the world. The great tragedy is that whatever is done for Mary, until such time as her ideas become more logical she earnestly believes them. Any attempt to treat her may simply be incorporated into her delusional system as another plot and make her more resistive.

Delusions are said to be false beliefs which cannot be shaken by reason or argument, and not in keeping with the person's cultural or religious background. They may take many shapes and forms, but we can list the more common.

Paranoid

These are primary delusions, i.e. having an initial theme and usually taking the form of suspicion of plots or malice towards the client.

Systematized

From a primary delusion new ideas or experiences are incorporated and weave a complex linking network of delusional ideas.

Nihilistic

Usually these are found in depressive and withdrawn individuals believing themselves to be without organs or parts of their bodies, e.g. 'I have no stomach'; 'I have swallowed my tongue'.

Unworthiness

Again associated with depressive illness: 'I'm not worth your time, I deserve to die'.

Grandiose

These delusions are often seen in organic dementia types, especially in neurosyphilis. Here the client believes himself to be omnipotent or vastly wealthy. Some clients invent past lives for themselves, e.g. 'I was a Stuka pilot/tank commander/Prime Minister/the Queen's hairdresser'. These become even more difficult to deal with when linked to hallucinations that support them, e.g. when the doctor arrives he is perceived as Prince Philip, General Rommel, the Prime Minister etc.

Ideas of reference

Here the client believes that words, gestures, television announcements or any innocent communications have a hidden and special significance to them, e.g. when the nurse sits opposite the client and looks at her watch, he may say or think that this is a coded message directed at a hidden observer to signal some malicious act towards him.

PROBLEMS AND NEEDS OF THE DELUDED CLIENT

The client has difficulty discerning reality from fantasy but no amount of persuasion seems to help. He may be very distressed that no one believes him and is at a loss to understand why. He may search desperately for an ally, for someone to place his trust in, but a great anxiety surrounds him as he has every reason to be suspicious. After all, he is well, and perhaps being held against his will, and the people he feels he should trust -the doctors and nurses – seem to be in total disbelief.

The deluded client may have physical problems due to lack of nutrition. The grandiose client could not eat such a basic diet - 'Bring me some caviar' – the paranoid client believes it to be poisoned and the nihilistic type cannot chew or swallow it, and anyway, without a stomach what is the point? The taking of medication becomes equally difficult for similar reasons.

IMPLICATIONS FOR THE NURSE

Using Mary from the introduction, several principles and skills can be illustrated to show how nurses can best help the deluded client.

Non-verbal communication

This will be the first exchange of information between Mary and the nurse, and as such will largely influence the positiveness of the eventual outcome. It is important to approach Mary openly and directly, giving no hint of surreptitiousness, and certainly without any posture or facial expression that could be misinterpreted as threatening. Perhaps one approach may be to speak to several other clients in the vicinity before speaking to her, using a consistent approach to each client so that Mary does not suspect she may be a specific target. We have found that making positive eye contact is very important with deluded clients, as this reinforces an honesty and a desire to be open. Tone of voice should be firm rather than hesitant, as well as being clear and loud enough to leave no room for misinterpretation. Adopt a posture that is non-threatening. We would suggest sitting next to Mary at the same height, or slightly lower, so that she may feel in control of the interaction. It is very likely that Mary's potential for misinterpretation is extremely high, so a minimal use of possibly ambiguous non-verbal signals should be used. For instance, touch can easily be interpreted as threatening, so although its powerfulness for reassurance may be useful, it should be avoided initially until a safe rapport is established.

Listening and attending skills

Here listening and showing Mary that you are listening (attending skills) is imperative. The skill of reflecting is probably most important. Whether you are able to believe what is being said is largely irrelevant; to show her you care enough about her to listen is essential.

It is often argued that delusions should not be reinforced, i.e. agreed with, nor should they be argued against. Therefore, by employing the skill of reflecting the skilled nurse should be able to build up an empathic understanding and concentrate on Mary's feelings rather than the thoughts and ideas that form the delusion, thus responding to the emotion and not the context.

Client (distressed): 'Nobody believes me when I tell them I'm being interfered with by these dreadful Russians. You believe me, don't you?'

Nurse (carefully, thoughtfully and slowly): 'I can see that you feel very distressed by your beliefs and that's what I'm concerned about. I would like to be able to help you feel less anxious.'

Client: 'I would feel calmer if someone believed me, then I'd feel safe.'

Nurse (ensuring maximum eye contact): 'I can see you feel very frustrated that no one believes you, and that makes you feel in danger. I hope you will believe me when I say I only want to help you and I'll do everything I can to make you feel safer.'

We believe that this approach would be typical of a skilled response. Note that the nurse is not dishonest: she does not agree with Mary, nor does she argue with her. She carefully concentrates on how the client feels, without discussing and thereby risking reinforcing the delusions. This may help Mary to feel better understood and that the nurse is honest and deserving of trust. This approach may help Mary confront the feelings attached to her ideas and deal with them more effectively. When she is able to deal with her feelings of anxiety, her behaviour may change and her ideas may accordingly become less disturbing.

Once an atmosphere of trust is established, intervening in the client's ideation is more likely to be effective. By listening to Mary, other interests, concerns and problems may well emerge. The nurse who is able to establish an empathic relationship with Mary will have more channels available to distract her into when her thoughts turn back to her delusional ideas. The skilled nurse will be aware that Mary has problems in her relationship with her mother, that she likes to play badminton, or that she is interested in music, cooking and art. These are the areas into which Mary's conversation is profitably directed. For instance, look at these two different interactions:

Mary: 'I'm not really sure, but I think Dr Jones is working for the Russians.'

Nurse: 'I can see you are starting to feel anxious again, Mary, perhaps it would be a good time to:

- write to your mother;
- see if we can get a game of badminton in the hall;
- go out to the shops and fetch something for your tea;
- listen to some soothing music.'

Mary: 'I'm not really sure, but I think Dr Jones is working for the Russians.'

Nurse: 'Let's watch TV.'

The difference is, of course, obvious in its depth, skill and appropriateness. Distraction is a useful skill, even in the second response, but it only becomes powerful to potentiate the client's recovery when it is an integral part of the empathic relationship.

Similarly, the use of encouragement and persuasion is only skilful once a safe rapport has been established. If they are used initially in order to make Mary do something, they will create resentment. They may even be responsible for the nurse being incorporated into the delusional system. This inappropriate use of encouragement and persuasion may be as damaging as arguing with the delusional ideas.

The skilled nurse will know when the rapport of trust has been established sufficiently to stand the use of encouragement and persuasion to eat meals and take medication. The nurse's judgement is critical in this area, and should be respected by other members of the caring team. In our experience, nothing is more damaging to a relationship of trust than a premature use of persuasion.

Devices such as eating with the client and encouraging the client to prepare her own meals may be useful, but should be used carefully and with thought. After having tasted her food for her, consider what she will think when you refuse to taste her medicine also:

Nurse: 'Mary, here's your medicine.'

Mary: 'I'm not ill, why do I have it – it may be poisoned – will you taste it like you did my dinner?'

Nurse: 'I know you believe you're not ill, but I think you are very anxious, I can see that now in your face. This medicine will help you feel calmer. If I was anxious like you, I would need some, but as I'm not, it would only make me sleep.'

Mary: 'I'm only anxious because you're making me drink poison.'

Nurse: 'I can see you are very anxious, I won't make you drink it, but it isn't poison and I think it would help you feel calmer. I'll ask you again later.'

The nurse here may or may not get through to the client but the relationship remains intact, with more possibility of success next time.

Many experienced nurses reading this may feel that it is rather idealistic and that it may be expedient to give intramuscular medication in this case – the hope being that the medication, when effective, will succeed where the relationship failed. We do not rule out compulsion as an expedient; as we have said, these clients are extremely difficult. We do, however, suggest that the slower route is safer and more lasting if it is possible to implement, and should be given every opportunity first.

Implications for the nurse in the community

Building up trust and rapport can be difficult, yet it is crucial. The challenge to the nurse may be as profound as gaining access to the client's home and gradually developing a wary relationship, or not colluding with the client's delusional ideas about others in an attempt to maintain the one relationship which is still working.

At a simpler level, not assuming that the client's statement is delusional is also necessary. One client claimed that a man in a nearby city had a black box which was transmitting invisible rays into his body to drive out his stress and tension. Upon further investigation it became apparent that his mother was paying large sums of money for precisely this form of 'alternative' medicine to alleviate his distress.

Equally, it is not uncommon that one partner, engaged in extramarital activities, can go to extreme lengths to convince the other partner that their suspicions are unfounded and a sign of illness, in a desperate attempt to cover up.

Finally, Macphail (1988) argues convincingly that it is possible to confront a client from within his delusional system, in this instance claiming to believe you are Jesus Christ when the client believes he is God. While we do not necessarily recommend this approach to the novice or for use with clients with whom the nurse has not established some rapport and tried alternative approaches, it has certain merits. Not least is the fact that it can create sufficient dissonance to lead to an agreement by both parties to 'talk sensibly'.

SUMMARY

There are many forms of delusional thinking, and we have offered but a few of the most prevalent within this chapter: grandiose, nihilistic, ideas of reference and feelings of unworthiness, systematized and paranoid delusions. All these, but particularly the latter two, may lead to severe difficulties in forming and maintaining a rapport. This is especially true if the nurse becomes incorporated into the system as a suspect. This lack of trust in the client will almost certainly produce management problems when attempting to implement care, which is often manifested as problems arising in the administration of medication, diet, hygiene and the client's sleep disturbance.

We have suggested that it is possible that the frustration this creates within the nurse may result in interaction difficulties. The nurse may become reluctant to approach or spend time with the client, particularly after she has been subjected to hostility by the client.

In order to be of some help to these unfortunate clients, it may follow that some very practical skills and principles are needed. We suggest the following:

1. Do not argue or agree with delusions.
2. Maximize the potential empathic relationship by using:
   - clear non-verbal communication;
   - an open honest approach;
   - skilled listening;
   - reflecting the feelings of the client and sharing your understanding of his emotions, while limiting responses to the content.
3. Use distraction to limit delusional thinking.
4. Use encouragement, praise or any other rewarding responses to reinforce 'normal' or 'non-delusional' behaviour.
5. If possible, without jeopardizing rapport, use persuasion to increase the client's occupation or activity in productive areas, i.e. resocialization, work, projects, recreation.

CONCLUSION

Initial interactions are extremely important when dealing with people suffering delusions. It is vital to gain their trust and to understand them by establishing an empathic relationship. In this way the nurse uses herself as a therapeutic agent to help the client recover. Restoring these clients to health may largely depend on good physical care and appropriate medication, which will not be accepted until some valuable and trusting relationship is established. The nurse is therefore the central focus of effective treatment and her skilled interaction is imperative.

FURTHER READING

Berkavitz, R. and Heinl, P. (1984) The management of schizophrenic clients: the nurse's view. *Journal of Advanced Nursing*, 9(1), 23–33.

Buckley, M. (1983) Nursing care study. Tormented by delusions (treatment and care of chronic schizophrenic clients). *Nursing Mirror*, 1, 43–6.

Frost, M. (1974) *Nursing Care of the Schizophrenic Client*, Kimpton, London.

Hill. L. B. (1973) *Psychotherapeutic Intervention in Schizophrenia*, Chicago University Press, Chicago.

Working with people experiencing hallucinations

8

Thomas was sitting in the corner of the ward staring at the floor. Occasionally he would lift his head, look to the side and smile. The nurse approached and sat down beside him.

Nurse: 'Hello, Thomas.'

There was no response. It was as if the nurse did not exist.

Nurse: 'Hello, Thomas, how are you?'

Slowly Thomas turned and stared. It was as though he could see right through the nurse. He suddenly opened his mouth wide, took a deep breath and groaned as if expressing some agonizing pain.

'This place I am in is warm and dark. I can see the depths of colour moving around my feet. The mist is all around, everyone seems to be moving slowly. Someone is laughing up there, it is very funny.'

'Stop looking up there, Thomas, listen to me. Don't listen to him, Thomas, he's only out to hurt you. Who's this coming to laugh at you?'

Nurse: 'Hello, Thomas.'

'Open your mouth and swallow his pain. Let out the hatred from your bowels.'

Nurse: 'Hello, Thomas, how are you?'

The above is a description of one event from two different perspectives. The first is how the nurse attempts to communicate with a client who appears to be preoccupied about something. The second description attempts to convey the experience from a client who is being distracted by hallucinations. It can be seen that two completely different worlds can exist, and in such a situation a bridge must be formed between them to allow effective communication to take place. To do this, an appreciation of how a hallucinatory experience can affect an individual is needed.

'A hallucination occurs when an individual experiences a sensory stimulus without any apparent external cause for that stimulus.' It must be clearly distinguished from an 'illusion', which is when a 'misinterpretation of a sensory stimulus' occurs. The following examples should clarify this.

A person may experience 'illusions' when delirious. For example, he may see shadows, or the shape of a curtain as an intruder, or misinterpret a nurse's identity. In contrast to this, however, a client could experience hallucinations without any external stimulus:

- He may hear voices or other sounds during silence (auditory);
- See lights, colours and/or faces while staring at the floor (visual);
- May smell rotting vegetation or burning rubber when no one else can (olfactory);
- May sense the taste of faeces in his mouth while eating what seems an ordinary meal (gustaciary);
- He may feel the sense of things crawling in his hair or under his skin (tactile).

Any one or a combination of the five senses can be experienced in an hallucinatory form. The auditory and visual are the most common forms of hallucinations.

PROBLEMS AND NEEDS OF THE HALLUCINATED CLIENT

When caring for someone who is experiencing hallucinations, it becomes apparent that the problems and subsequent needs all relate to the client's conflict of two worlds – one which involves very real and personal sensations with a compelling nature, the other a rather vague and somewhat impersonal world of everything going on around him. The actual effect of this can vary, depending upon the intensity and nature of the hallucination: the problems and needs of a client who is hearing continual auditory stimulation will differ from one who occasionally sees bright lights flashing in front of him. This emphasizes the fact that every client is an individual and that every experience is unique to him. So, although we describe skills and principles, it is the application of these in the context of knowing the client that makes them effective. The fact that caring for one hallucinated client may differ greatly from caring for another is made clear in Figure 8.1. It can be seen, then, that the problems vary from lack of adequate diet and personal hygiene to self-injury, with different feeling states depending on the nature and reaction of the client, e.g. anxiety, depression, confusion and frustration. The needs will be specific to each problem, but generally speaking we can summarize as shown in Table 8.1

IMPLICATIONS FOR THE NURSE

The question arises whether you should approach a client who is showing evidence of hallucinating but who seems quite happy in his own world and does not seem to be hurting himself or others. Here, knowledge of the client is

Table 8.1 Contrasting hallucinatory experiences and effects

Partial loss of reality	Problem	Need
Continual loss of reality	Self-neglect	Nutrition Safety Hygiene Sufficient sense of reality to maintain or improve quality of life
Loss of reality – with distress	Self-harm Isolation Depression	Defined limits Acceptance Reassurance
Loss of reality – interfering, annoying, embarrassing	Confusion Frustration	Sensitivity, listening, reassurance
Loss of reality – directed outwards	Dangerous, disruptive behaviour Effect on self and others	Clear identifiable nursing action with explanation.

crucial. It may be that, for example, if Thomas were left on his own he would go further and further into his hallucinatory world and might eventually act upon it to the detriment of himself or others. So, attempting to communicate and distract Thomas from his world now may prevent future difficulties. Conversely, if it is unlikely that he will deteriorate as a result of the hallucination, it may be that with minimum persuasion or interference he can function effectively. This really emphasizes the point that you do not need to direct your attention to all clients who are hallucinating, only to those who might deteriorate if left to their own devices or, as shown in Figure 8.1 overleaf, where the needs become evident because of a particular experience.

The significant issues for the nurse relate to the fact that she cannot validate what is happening to the client. For example, she cannot see or hear what he sees and hears, which may be very frustrating for her, so it is important that she is aware of her feelings and avoids arguing with or denying the reality of the client's perceptions.

PRINCIPLES AND SKILLS REQUIRED

Appropriate use and sensitivity of non-verbal communication

Sensitivity to non-verbal communication is an essential aspect of the skills required, in order to detect the more subtle signs that show a client may be hallucinating. The client may laugh, talk to himself, smile, grimace or distort his face inappropriately, or he may turn his head to one side as if to listen, all probably out of the context of usual interactions. The client's use of gestures, body movements and tone of voice may give the nurse vital information as to the nature or theme of the hallucination, thus increasing the chance of her responding appropriately. The verbal response is often enhanced by using

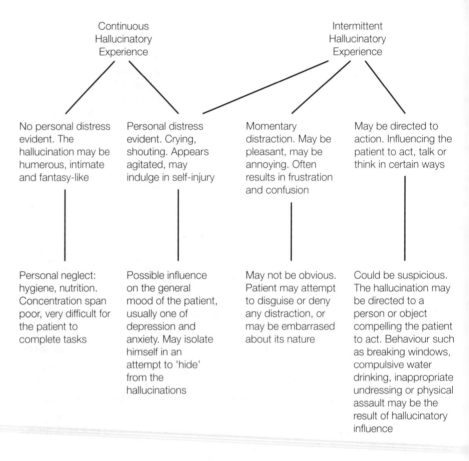

Figure 8.1 The possible effects of hallucinatory experience

appropriate touch, posture, eye contact and tone of voice. It often requires the effect of all these used at the right time in order to bridge the gap from the client's world to that of the existing environment.

> Thomas began shouting, then jumped out of his chair and started banging on the window.
>
> 'Leave me alone, leave me alone!' he screamed and started crying.
>
> The nurse approached Thomas, stood close, placed her arm firmly around his shoulders, turning Thomas towards her, and looked straight at him.
>
> 'Thomas, it's all right, I'm here and I won't let anything happen to you. You're safe with me, come away from the window and we'll have a chat.'
>
> The nurse led Thomas away, still holding him and talking in a firm positive manner, communicating to him that she was in control.

The likelihood of the above situation turning out successfully will depend largely upon the degree of trust that exists between the nurse and the client. If the nurse is to interfere or enter the world of a client's hallucination, then the development of trust is vital in increasing the likelihood of positive outcomes.

This is an ongoing process whereby the attitudes and qualities of the nurse are communicated to the client at all times, alongside the confident use of skills, showing that in the event of the client losing control there is someone capable of taking hold of the situation safely. This usually involves reinforcing reality. The client's world is often frightening, but also compelling for that client. It often occupies the whole person, sometimes to the extent that all reality is lost, as in Thomas's case, where the internal visions and voices were indiscernible from the external ones. It is the use of reality that can often bring back and maintain the client away from the distractions of his hallucinations. The nurse, by acknowledging the client's feelings and at the same time denying that she shares his perceptions, is reinforcing the reality of the feelings experienced, e.g.:

Nurse: 'I do not hear the voices you hear, Thomas, but am I right in thinking that you feel confused and may be frustrated?'

The same principle of reinforcing reality can be shown by:

* Use of appropriate touch;
* Questioning about the client's current interests;
* Asking about the client's recent activities and how he feels about them;
* Encouraging the client to do something that requires connecting his thoughts directly with actions, e.g. going for a walk, joining in an activity, making something constructive;
* Use of appropriate tones of voice, i.e. firm and calm when limit setting is required, but also loud enough to interrupt auditory hallucinations, especially when they are predominant.

So, by knowing the client and his likely response the nurse can utilize the skills of questioning and reflecting to attempt to bring him out of a world foreign to her and often frightening to him.

It has been suggested that the use of portable cassette players has proved to be beneficial with clients who are hearing voices; listening to preferred music mutes the voices and limits the distress caused by them. Obviously this is not a permanent solution and may go hand-in-hand with periods of discussion in a quiet, non-stimulating environment, which may help to reorientate the client to the 'real' world.

Finally, never underestimate how real a hallucination can be to the client, never argue with the client about its validity and always accept the individual without judgement or analysis. In this way the person lost in a world of strange perceptions may be found.

SUMMARY

The client may experience disordered perceptions concerning one or a combination of the five senses, resulting in auditory, visual, tactile, olfactory or gustaciary hallucinations. These may occur in varying degrees of intensity, giving rise to a multitude of needs and problems, some of which may be related to: nutrition; hygiene; safety; self-esteem; isolation; depression; anxiety; confusion; frustration; suspicion; and dangerous behaviour.

It is important to note that although to the nurse hallucinations may appear strange, alien or even intriguing, it is actually their effect on the client's mood and behaviour that determines the type of nursing interventions and not solely the type of hallucinatory experience. The nurse should never underestimate the reality of the disordered perception to the client, and should also be aware of her own feelings, especially when the client requires control to be communicated to him in a crisis situation.

The skills required are:

- Sensitivity' to non-verbal communication:
- Detection of hallucinatory experiences;
- Awareness of client's feelings and theme of hallucinations;
- Appropriate use of non-verbal communication, i.e. touch; tone of voice; posture; eye contact; reinforcement of reality; and development of trust.

FURTHER READING

Berkavitz, R. and Heinl, P. (1984) The management of schizophrenic clients: the nurse's view. *Journal of Advanced Nursing*, 9(1), 23–33.

Falloon, I. R. and Talbot, R. E. (1981) Persistent auditory hallucinations: coping mechanisms and implications for management. *Psychological Medicine*, 11, 329–39.

Hiler, P. (1984) Schizophrenia: an inside story. *New Society*, 68, 439–40.

Slade, P. D. (1974) The external control of auditory hallucinations: an information theory analysis. *British Journal of Social and Clinical Psychology*, 13, 73–9.

West, L. J. (ed) (1962) A general theory of hallucinations and dreams, in *Hallucinations*, Grune and Stratton, New York, pp. 275–91.

World Health Organization (1977) *International Pilot Study of Schizophrenia*, WHO, Geneva.

Working with overactive people

9

'I'll see you on the dark side of the moon light becomes you it goes with your. Bugs Bunny is on I'll have to watch it, botch it can't do it well. Imagine all the people living life that way. What do you think of it eh?'

'I've written to the Queen, I've written to the Prime Minister, they haven't answered yet, I bet they won't so I'll phone. What do you think?'

Alice paces around the room pointing out the phone, gesticulating and absently picking up and putting down items while talking. The cup of tea which she'd managed to make for herself when offering one to the community mental health nurse (CMHN) remains untouched in spite of frequent prompts to have a drink.

'My husband moans at me, says I'm high. Silly devil, I'm not Everest double glazing, although we could do with some, get it chirpy, chirpy cheap, cheap. What do you think?'

The symptoms portrayed here – pressure of speech, flight of ideas, overactivity – are indicative of someone experiencing hypomania bordering on mania, the latter being a rarer and more serious situation, sometimes culminating in a delirious episode. Hypomania is an affective disorder with an insidious onset. It begins with mild elation or euphoria, a general feeling of wellbeing, and progresses to general overactivity and grandiosity. It can occur in isolation but is more commonly associated with severe mood swings indicative of manic–depressive psychoses. A complete picture of someone experiencing a hypomanic state would include:

- A feeling of wellbeing, denies that he may be ill;
- Easily provoked, may be impulsively aggressive;
- Mood can quickly change from laughing to crying (lability);
- Pressure of speech and flight of ideas, comprising a continuous and rapid change of topics, often includes rhyming and punning, as in Alice's case;
- Grandiose delusions may be present; if so, a history of gross overspending is usually common;

- Neglect of or inappropriate self-care. Dress and personal hygiene may be generally neglected, or dress may be overexpressive and not in the client's usual style. Aspects of clothing or additions may have special meaning;
- General increase in physical activity, always on the move, doing three or four things at once, continuously interfering in other people's business;
- Disturbed sleep pattern, will often fight rest until close to exhaustion;
- Sexually disinhibited, may describe indiscreetly and in expressive detail personal sexual exploits, or engage in sexual acts foreign to his usual judgement;
- Extremely distractible, focusing upon anything novel for short periods, often misidentifying and misinterpreting certain stimuli.

From the above description it is clear that this particular individual's situation has the potential for many serious problems. It is essential that the nurse is aware of the client's needs, for it is likely that he is not.

PROBLEMS AND NEEDS OF THE OVERACTIVE CLIENT

Assessing someone experiencing hypomania will require a quick establishment of priorities. These are usually related to the client's physical problems and needs, e.g.:

Problem: The client will fight sleep, deny the need to rest and may be at risk from physical exhaustion.

Needs: The nurse must be aware of the client's general physical state in order to appreciate his limitations. General encouragement from the nurse is required to allow the client to rest. Include the client in activities that involve him sitting down, and do not discourage times when he is resting, even during the day.

Problem: The client will neglect his diet, will claim he has no time to eat.

Need: His intake should be monitored and, if necessary, recorded. Rather than insist on him sitting down for meals, provide nutritious snacks and complemented fluids to enable him to include them in his demanding schedule.

Problem: May neglect his self-care, i.e. hygiene and appropriate clothing.

Need: Provision of opportunity to concentrate on himself, with the skills of the nurse to encourage, suggest and persuade.

The psychological problems are more likely to be varied, depending upon the individual, but generally speaking they may be related to underlying conflicts and anxieties that are often neglected by others because of the front of 'wellbeing' and elation. A psychological problem arising from the client's actual behaviour may be one of social neglect, i.e. other individuals avoiding or shunning the client because of his demanding behaviour. The client is vulnerable to feeling frustrated, insecure and not being accepted. Therefore the needs of security, belongingness and self-esteem should be considered in any nursing care plan.

The social problems and needs concern themselves with the client's occupation and interactions with others. Social problems arise out of the client's inappropriate behaviour and faulty judgement, giving rise to potentially embarrassing situations. The client will have to interact in the same environment as he improves, with the same people, which will involve him gaining insight into his previous behaviour. It is therefore essential that the nurse attempts to protect the client from unnecessary embarrassment. This fact must be considered when assessing the client's interests and abilities in order to plan suitable activities. The following considerations may be useful:

- The client's interests, hobbies, occupation;
- His concentration span and level of distractibility;
- His physical limitations;
- His need to express his energy in some physical way.
- Music and painting are often useful activities as they involve large motor movement and are sufficiently expressive to enable the client to release emotions and frustrations in a positive way.

PROBLEMS AND NEEDS OF THE OVERACTIVE CLIENT IN THE COMMUNITY

Assessment will involve decisions about whether the client can be managed in the community or whether admission into a mental health unit for assessment and treatment is indicated. This is not always easy due to the client's general feeling of wellbeing and denial that anything is wrong. Consequently, compliance with treatment or advice is often difficult to enlist.

In the case of Alice, the CMHN may increase the frequency of the visits to keep a check both on her physical state (she is not eating and drinking) and on her behaviour (she may begin to put herself at risk by her restless and potentially socially embarrassing (to her) behaviour).

The CMHN also spends time with Alice's husband giving him support and time to express his feelings and also exploring ways of helping Alice better. Her husband has already 'banned' Alice from getting out of bed before 4.30 a.m. to stop her disturbing his sleep; he cannot make her sleep, but it has effectively slowed her down and limited the disturbance. He is also aware of her tendency to spend vast amounts of money when 'high', and he now gives her an allowance and channels her energies into buying Christmas presents for the grandchildren (even though it's June), so that at least the money is not wasted and she still gets the pleasure of spending. These strategies were discussed with the nurse and no doubt other strategies will need to be created in the future.

IMPLICATIONS FOR THE NURSE

Nursing an overactive client makes exhausting demands on the nurse. She will be expected to be patient and tolerant in her interactions with the client, which becomes extremely difficult if she is tired. It is therefore necessary for her to be able to evaluate her own capabilities and limitations. All members of the nursing team must be sensitive to this and allow for realistic expectations from all concerned. In practice this means finding a balance between one nurse spending a lot of time with the client, getting to know him very well and possibly becoming exhausted, and several nurses working in rotation for a realistic time span, thus enabling them to use their skills effectively. Even so, patience and tolerance will be tested. It is important not to rise to the personal insults and argumentative tones of the client, as this would result in further stimulation, which may end in the nurse being assaulted. The principle of reducing environmental stimuli for the overactive client has implications for nursing management. Realistically, very little can be done to control everything in the client's environment, but at certain times, especially on admission and early on in the illness where distractibility is at its highest, it would be beneficial to all concerned if the client could be kept away from the busy and intensive areas of any caring unit. Planned admission is therefore preferred, although due to problems of insight compulsory detention is an option. In this case there are potential hazards to the relationship between nurse and patient.

Implications for the nurse in the community

Caring for an overactive client can tax the nurse's creativity as well as raise questions about the need for admission, which should be fully discussed with the client, relatives and GP.

In the case of Alice, working with her husband has paid dividends, and in her local community shop assistants will check whether she really wants the items she is buying and have learned to tolerate frequently returned goods.

In other cases training the client to spot any changes in mental state and attempt to take early preventive action can be productive. One client, observing that his GP had told him that he lacked insight into his condition, had learned to listen to what his friends said about his behaviour and to seek early medical help rather than await a full cycle of overactive behaviour.

PRINCIPLES AND SKILLS REQUIRED

In order to implement the principles already mentioned, certain skills must be specifically applied, one of these being sensitivity to non-verbal communication. This is necessary in order to reflect observable emotions through the distraction of the verbal content. Is it possible to make sense of the opening paragraph illustrating Alice's flight of ideas? Looking at the content, very little sense can be made, but listening to how she says it and observing her non-verbal communication may give clues to how she is feeling behind the barrage of words. As she was talking tears sprang into Alice's eyes and her shoulders sagged.

Nurse: 'I guess you're feeling upset Alice, although I'm not totally sure why that is or what it is about.'

Here the nurse uses her sensitivity to the non-verbal communication and the skill of reflection and clarification in order to gain some understanding of the client. She also attempts to convey this understanding, which is important to establish rapport. We are not saying that the nurse should ignore the content, just its fine detail, as the overall theme of the content may also be helpful in detecting how the client is feeling or what need he is trying to communicate.

What possible feelings or direction of content may be useful to explore with this patient's communication, which is said rather sternly?

'If she thinks as I thinks and stinks I would knock twice before entering the pathway of punishment, no way is she cash and grabbing my little bird's nest before going in and doing hell.'

There seem to be two, maybe three, consistent elements to this content. They are:

- Directed to someone – 'she';
- Entering or going into somewhere;
- Possible fear about being harmed by that person on entering.
- Now if we were to say that this client stated this while pacing outside the interviewing room, waiting to see the doctor, then it may be appropriate to reflect: 'Am I right in thinking you're anxious about seeing the doctor this morning?'

Suggestion and persuasion

Often a tactful approach is more successful than an authoritarian one in facilitating the client in certain directions. In Alice's case the nurse has learned that frequent gentle reminders to have a drink are ultimately more productive than demanding and leading to a possible argument.

It is worth noting that the stronger the relationship is the stronger the level of suggestion and persuasion may be. Consequently, Alice's husband is able to ban her from getting up early because she knows he has her best interests at heart. This indicates that the time spent in developing rapport, listening to the client empathically and developing a mutual and trusting relationship is time well spent.

Pacing

In many cases mirroring the client's words or behaviours and reflecting feelings are ways of developing this trust and can convey deep understanding. With the overactive client these skills are essential, but equally pacing can be of enormous value. By this we mean initially responding at the same pace and in the same frame of reference as the client, but gradually slowing down one's own pace of speech and its volume with the intention that the client mirrors you and slows down to a more acceptable rate. This can have the effect of liberating the client from her pressure of speech, enabling her to relax sufficiently to communicate freely and, in some cases, address the real causes of concern.

It is not uncommon to find that the overactive client is actually depressed and that the overactivity has become a screen, or denial or even flight from issues of deep concern.

CONCLUSION

When caring for someone who has very little time to share with you, then the contact you do make becomes very valuable. The client will think he is always one step ahead and make out that he is coping extremely well. You must appreciate that under this perception of energy someone is fighting for survival, and indeed may be experiencing conflicts that only he is vaguely aware of. During this time of extreme activity, his basic needs must be met. As his mood drops, you need to be sensitive to the implications this may have for him. These may involve the client experiencing embarrassment, guilt, remorse, insecurity and, in the extreme, he may swing very quickly to depression. So, you will have to be prepared for all eventualities, and rather than the client being one step ahead of you, it becomes the reverse.

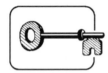

KEY CONCEPTS

1. The client may be overactive, disinhibited, distractible and easily provoked. He may express flights of ideas and grandiosity. Self-neglect and exhaustion are real dangers.
2. The overactive client needs sleep, nutrition, hygiene, security and to feel needed.
3. Other important areas of assessment include interests, hobbies, concentration span, physical limitations and the need to express energy.
4. The implications for the nurse involve having realistic expectations and insight into her own limitations; also, using a team effort rather than a singular one.
5. A team effort involves working closely with friends, family, relatives and carers.
6. The skills required are:
   - Being sensitive to non-verbal communication, particularly tone of voice and gestures;
   - Reflecting any theme that may be present in the content;
   - Using suggestion and persuasion rather than an authoritarian approach;
   - Pacing as a way of helping the client to slow down;
   - Managing the environment, i.e. protection and reducing stimuli.

FURTHER READING

Buckwalter, K.C. and Kerfoot, K.M. (1982) Emergency department nursing care of the manic patient. *Journal of Emergency Nursing*, **8**(5), 239–42.

Corker, E. (1983) Nursing care study. Manic depression. *Nursing Mirror*, **157**, 43–5.

Working with clients experiencing obsessions and compulsions | 10

I must always wash my hands before putting the clothes into the spin dryer. If I can't remember whether I have done so or not, I think to myself 'It doesn't matter, I'll hang them out to dry anyway', but it will go on and on in my mind until the clothes are dry and I have to wash them again, this time ensuring I wash my hands first.'

Mrs Armstrong evidently washes all her clothes three times, each time after drying.

'I must clean something before I touch it, then after I've touched it I must wash my hands. Sometimes I don't realize I'm doing it, but then I know if I didn't do it, I would never rest. I spend most of my day cleaning clothes and the house. My husband has been very tolerant up to now; he used to try and help by cleaning parts of the house for me, but that was no good, I had to do it myself, I had to make sure it was right.'

The above account illustrates how one woman's life has become increasingly dominated by obsessive–compulsive behaviour. An **obsession** is a repetitive, intrusive thought, image or impulse which cannot be easily dismissed. It is distressing and often leads to a **compulsion**, the urge to act in a way that the mind knows to be irrational but which can only be resisted with the greatest effort. In Mrs Armstrong's case the obsession is the persistent thought of having to ensure something is clean and uncontaminated by her touch, and the compulsion is the actual act of cleaning and washing, in a precise order. If that order is disturbed her personal 'rules' are that the ritual has to be started all over again. Compulsive rituals, whether the overt behaviours of washing, cleaning and checking, or more covert strategies such as repeating a 'bad' thought twenty times, serve to reduce or neutralize the anxiety caused by the original obsessive thought. When clients seek help because of washing or cleaning excessively they are likely to have developed this behaviour to reduce their fear of 'contaminants', such as dirt, germs, blood or disease, harming themselves or others. Compulsive checkers, including the client who risked losing his job due to time spent repeatedly checking that every light, electrical and gas appliance was switched off before leaving the house, typically believe they are responsible for averting illness, death or disaster by their actions. Despite having insight into the irrationality of their thoughts sufferers can feel helpless to change as only the compulsive behaviour brings relief from the anxiety of the obsessive thought. In addition, over time the absence of any actual harm befalling themselves or others seems to indicate that the compulsive behaviour provides a successful protection that it would be increasingly dangerous to omit.

The obsessional person's rituals often involve the significant people in his world by repeatedly requesting reassurance, eliciting their participation in rituals or their conformity to rules such as orderliness. It is quite usual for someone with obsessive–compulsive behaviour to develop an accompanying depression. This may be a reaction to being involved in and responsible for domestic chaos, yet feeling helpless to alleviate the resulting strain on potentially supportive relationships. This frustrating picture usually results in a cry for help from the whole family, in which case all should be involved in the care of the individual concerned. Client and family are likely to ask questions such as: 'What causes it?'; 'Why should it happen?'; and 'Is it to do with us?'

It is often the case that the nurse will have to use her skills to explain to the family the nature of the behaviour and the possible reasons for its development. One theory is that obsessive–compulsive states are a result of unresolved conflicts and anxieties unconsciously pushed back and taken over by various defence mechanisms. It is also likely that the underlying conflicts are concerned with the 'significant others'. The obsessional character develops out of the need to obtain approval by being excessively tidy and controlled. A child will react to standards set by the parents, and sometimes these conflict with normal developmental tasks. This may lead to the child being very frustrated, which could contribute to the development of obsessive–compulsive behaviour when faced with difficult life events as an adult. Whatever the reason for its occurrence, the family is usually very much involved, therefore they have an important role in helping the individual understand and overcome their difficulties.

PROBLEMS AND NEEDS OF THE OBSESSIVE–COMPULSIVE CLIENT

When the nurse is asked to enter the world of the obsessive– compulsive client and their significant others, they often encounter fear, frustration, shame and isolation. Clients may expect rejection or ridicule for obsessional thoughts which they themselves find distressing and unacceptable. Addressing this reluctance in an empathic manner can facilitate the client's disclosure of socially embarrassing fears, of contamination from faeces or urine for example, or horrifying intrusive images of causing harm to others. The nurse's willingness to explore likely causes and meanings of distressing thoughts and seemingly incomprehensible rituals continues this communication of acceptance to the client. Additional messages, that such difficulties are not uncommon and that the nurse is offering help with the problem, as others have been helped in the past, can reduce isolation and instil hope.

Where assessment indicates that obsessions and compulsions are features of an underlying depression, psychosis or history of abuse, the client should be offered treatment for the primary problem, with the involvement of other members of the multidisciplinary team as appropriate. Obsessive–compulsive features can be addressed as part of this work. Most of us have experienced brief episodes of repetitive thoughts or behaviour, perhaps with a 'superstitious' belief that something bad will happen if we do not complete a ritual. We might decide that stepping on a crack in the pavement is unlucky but can overcome the ungainly result by deliberately standing on a crack until any initial anxiety subsides, i.e. applying the principle of exposure from behavioural treatment approaches. The absence of any unfortunate consequence following deliberate or accidental contact allows cognitive reappraisal to take place, and we can safely change our behaviour in the knowledge that our fears are unjustified. Obsessional thoughts, however, are more intrusive and distressing, and the anticipated consequences of failing to complete compulsions are so catastrophic that such effective methods cannot be risked. Instead of deliberate exposure the sufferer begins to avoid situations or behaviours that trigger obsessional thoughts. The van driver who planned routes to avoid pedestrian crossings, which triggered an obsessional impulse not to stop, found he had started a pattern of self-imposed restrictions that eventually left him unable to sit behind the wheel. In addition to the limitations of avoidance, distressing obsessional thoughts and demanding compulsive rituals, many clients with severe states are at risk from self-neglect, mainly in the areas of sleep and nutrition. Because of the time-consuming compulsive behaviours these areas are given low priority by the client. Their needs are obvious but, as in the case of hand-washers who continue to scrub sore and injured hands, the physical pain experienced is minimal compared to the psychological pain of doubt, uncertainty and torment they would have experienced if prevented from carrying out their rituals. Under these circumstances, or when depression and shame have put the client at risk from self-harm, the benefits of admission should be discussed. If admission does follow, the increased potential for contamination or disruption to routines can cause a period of continual high levels of anxiety and the possibility of severe panic attacks if the rituals are thwarted. The need of the client in this situation is therefore, for the first 48 hours or so, to be able to re-establish some form of security in his own personal routine in order for the anxiety to drop to tolerable levels. As the client is open to ridicule by others, it may be that as well as modelling an accepting approach, the nurse will need to explain tactfully to other clients the need for acceptance throughout the ward. Teaching the client relaxation methods to manage acute anxiety symptoms is a useful preparation for response prevention therapy, where the client is encouraged to face his fear, gradually increasing time with the anxieties until the tendency to carry out a particular ritual diminishes.

IMPLICATIONS FOR THE NURSE

Communicating acceptance can be very difficult with clients who seem not to respond to their own logic and insight. It can be very frustrating, not only for the client, but also for the nurse, when change does not easily follow from clear agreement that the highly unlikely consequences of stopping compulsive behaviour are outweighed by disruption to the lives of the client and significant others. This may develop at times into a feeling of helplessness on the nurse's part, which can grow into anger. It is important that the nurse is aware of this possibility in order to prevent these emotions compromising the delivery of care. Reflecting on practice and supervision will aid self-awareness; being patient, understanding and helping the client set small achievable goals will help both parties to achieve realistic expectations. Acceptance is not conditional on the client always achieving such planned goals, however, and a critical or subtly punitive response will reinforce the client's sense of failure and may lead them to terminate the sessions. Viewing homework tasks, for example, as 'experiments' where even a seeming failure can provide valuable information to refine the next attempt, allows all participants to maintain a collaborative, positive approach. Finally, there are times when we see things in others that we see in ourselves. Obsessive elements in anyone's personality can be helpful, especially in certain occupations where precision, accuracy and detail are essential. The organized and conscientious mind is a useful asset to any team leader. It is when the organization and responsibility become dominated by torment, doubt and uncertainty that they cease to be useful.

PRINCIPLES AND SKILLS REQUIRED

Initially the skills required for the obsessional client will be those of assessment and rapport building common to other client groups. The client's home often provides a sense of security lacking in ward or interview room settings, which reduces the likelihood of the client's anxiety level inhibiting assessment. The nurse can then use her skills of listening, non-verbal sensitivity and questioning to gather information from the client which will be significant for the planning of future care. At the same time, by understanding and giving empathic responses, she is developing the therapeutic bond of the nurse–client relationship. In addition to providing a baseline for evaluating future progress, assessment of the obsessional client provides information and insight which allows the individual, perhaps for the first time, to understand the links between triggering factors, obsessional thoughts, avoidance and anxiety-reducing compulsive rituals. Some clients may never have considered the significance of childhood or later life events in the formation of their particular difficulties; others may have been so successful in employing defensive rituals at the merest hint of discomfort that they have 'forgotten' the original anxiety-provoking thought until prompted by the question: 'What do you think would happen if you were unable to carry out that behaviour?'

The nature of the obsession and the form of the compulsive behaviour are established and clarified by working through specific examples of the problem in terms of associated cognitions, affect physiological changes and behaviour. Summaries punctuate the assessment process and it is this skill, allied to information-giving about the nature of the problem, that begins to translate the distress, shame and isolation of the client into a more objective mutual understanding which can form the basis for change. With the client's permission their significant others can be included in the assessment to provide additional information, to benefit from a new understanding of the problem and to discuss their contribution to the treatment plan. In Mrs Armstrong's case, assessment showed that her obsessional thoughts were related to contamination by germs, disease and cancer. She remembered having become concerned about germs after a number of episodes of cystitis. Although successfully treated, she began to wonder if she or objects around the house harboured the beginnings of a disease that could harm her and her family. However unlikely, the threat was so frightening she could not risk ignoring it. The only way she could lessen the dominance of these thoughts was to complete a comprehensive cleansing ritual.

Her obsessional washing was mainly of herself following her obsessive thoughts; around the house, particularly the bathroom and toilet; and her own and her children's clothing.

Mrs Armstrong's wish not to take what seemed like unnecessary chances resulted in a further problem area, i.e. **avoidance**:

- of gatherings such as crowds, queues or parties where she might inadvertently touch strangers;
- of public toilets;
- and reading, viewing or talking about any topic that was even remotely to do with illness.

Information from the family about Mrs Armstrong's increasing reluctance to touch her children and repeated requests for reassurance that something was clean completes the picture of disruption the client and her family have been experiencing. In addition to using her listening skills, the nurse could also use questionnaires designed particularly for rating an individual's anxiety levels, extent of obsessions or even mood. It must be remembered that it is not uncommon for a client tormented by obsessions and rituals to be severely depressed to the extent that suicide could be an option. The anxiety rating scale could be in the shape of a 'fear inventory', whereby a hierarchy of anxiety-provoking situations is established ranging from the least provoking, e.g. being prevented from washing her clothes the third time, to the most provoking, e.g. not washing following a particularly frightening obsessional thought of her children suffering a terrible illness. This hierarchy will become useful in setting realistic goals, depending on the treatment approach used. At present, many of the principles of care involve allowing clients to discuss or demonstrate their behaviour in an atmosphere of acceptance, thus helping them to lower their anxiety sufficiently to facilitate the exploration of causes and effects. As outlined above, the skills of effective treatment involve assisting the client to face the anxiety associated with the obsessional thought, image or impulse without the use of avoidance or compulsive rituals until it is apparent that the feared consequence does not occur and anxiety subsides. To allow the client to make an informed choice a proposed treatment plan should be drawn up with him, describing short- and long-term goals.

Cognitive and behavioural methods to assist successful exposure and response prevention should be outlined and the client informed of the need for practice between sessions, perhaps with the involvement of significant others, and the likelihood of increased anxiety at first. The nurse will need to offer the client the opportunity to raise any concerns about the plan, then, if the client agrees, contract for duration and frequency of sessions, with a joint evaluation of progress after a certain number of meetings depending on the severity of the problem. Approaches that have proved to be very effective in assisting obsessive–compulsive clients to overcome their difficulties involve one or a combination of the following techniques.

Graded exposure *in vivo*

A hierarchy of anxiety-producing situations is constructed. The client agrees to confront these situations, beginning with the least anxiety-producing and working towards the greatest.

Flooding

The client agrees to confront a most feared situation until the overwhelming anxiety begins to reduce naturally.

Response prevention

The client is encouraged to face a particular fear, e.g. using the toilet without ritually washing his hands and the toilet immediately afterwards to 'switch off' his obsessional thoughts. The length of time between using the toilet and washing allows cognitive reappraisal to take place and anxiety to diminish.

Modelling

This involves the nurse showing the client the appropriate behaviour and reinforces the fact that no harm has occurred.

Contract therapy

A mutual agreement between the parties concerned is made so that it is very clear and explicit. It establishes a bond or an obligation in such a way that the actions of one party demand the conduct of the other according to the terms of the contract. These techniques are all dependent upon the agreement and commitment of the client. The appropriate skills here are those related to being able to explain and to educate the client about the nature and benefit of the methods involved. Before embarking upon these, however, the client may require the additional technique provided by relaxation training. The ability to relax physically may mean the differences between success and failure, especially with techniques that involve gradually increasing anxiety levels. A client's reluctance to commit himself to these regimes is understandable, and it may be appropriate to challenge the client skilfully, e.g.: 'You have said you want to stop these rituals, and that you can see the benefit of these techniques, yet you still don't feel able to commit yourself to them. I'm wondering if there is anything else getting in the way?'

This response points out some discrepancies between what the client says and what he does, and gives him a chance to explore further his feelings and behaviour. Another challenge to someone who has already committed themselves to a particular therapy could be: 'Although you decided to only check the house once before going out you are now telling me that one more check will make all the difference. What evidence do you have to support that?' By allowing that the client may be right in his assertion, the nurse avoids an argumentative confrontation and maintains a collaborative search for the truth. If the client replies honestly in a review of the evidence for and against another check, they are likely to remind themselves that, for example, that the cooker cannot switch itself on again or that one more check has in the past led to many more. The dangers of unskilled challenging must be carefully considered, especially with people who have insight and are frustrated by the helplessness of not being able to act out their own logic. There is no therapeutic benefit from challenging the discrepancy between 'I know it's wrong, silly or irrational' and the continuation of their behaviour with obsessive–compulsive clients, as this is the consequence of their conflicts and not its origin.

When working with individuals with obsessive–compulsive problems contact with the family is usually necessary and beneficial. Keeping them informed, especially partners, of the principles of care and progress will enhance the likelihood of support and understanding. Where relatives have seen their desire to help lead to increasing demands being made on them for reassurance or participation in rituals, the nurse will need to give guidance and perhaps permission to gently refuse to comply. If admission has been required the community mental health nurse can be involved at an early stage, to help plan a specific programme of care to be continued in the home and to facilitate family sessions preparing the way for the client's discharge. The greater the awareness of the plan and the support offered, the greater the client's chances of success in the battle against his own 'constraints'.

SUMMARY

The individual whose life is governed by ritual and who then becomes uncertain whether that ritual is enough is expressing internal anxieties and conflict in his own way. The nurse, in caring for this individual, must aid him in conquering his personal loss of control and at the same time help him express his anxieties. A major obstacle to this is that one enhances the other, i.e. attempting to control or limit his compulsion increases his anxiety, yet expressing his anxieties and exploring areas of conflict is likely to increase the occurrence of his compulsion. It is therefore essential to devise a balanced programme based upon individual needs and problems and the resources available to cater for them. The overall skills required, however, are those needed initially to facilitate exploration to a level essential for accurate assessment, i.e. exploratory counselling skills, and later to help the client express personal conflict areas; teaching skills to aid the client through his therapies; behavioural and cognitive skills, depending upon the treatment approach taken; challenging skills for the reluctant client; and finally, 'family skills', i.e. those skills required to enable a family to work together, communicate and support each other throughout this crisis.

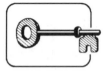

KEY CONCEPTS

1. An obsession is a repetitive, intrusive thought, image or impulse which cannot be easily dismissed. It is distressing and often leads to a compulsion, the urge to act in a way that the mind knows to be irrational but which can only be resisted with the greatest effort and difficulty.
2. Obsessions often relate to fear of 'contaminants', illness, disaster or being responsible for causing harm to others; compulsions and avoidance can be understood as ways of reducing anxiety associated with these fears.
3. Because of the time-consuming nature of many rituals, clients are often at risk from self-neglect of their physical needs, e.g. nutrition and rest.
4. It is important for the nurse to be aware of her own feelings of helplessness, lest these turn to frustration and anger, possibly compromising the care that she gives.
5. It is not uncommon for a client tormented by obsessions and rituals to be severely depressed to the extent that suicide could be an option.
6. Many of the principles of care involve allowing the client to express his behaviour in an atmosphere of acceptance, thus helping him to lower his anxieties sufficiently to facilitate exploration of underlying conflicts and potential for change.
7. Certain behavioural and cognitive methods have been found to be very useful and effective. These are mainly graded exposure in vivo; flooding; response prevention; modelling and contract therapy.
8. Keeping the family informed of the principles of care and involved in the treatment process may enhance the likelihood of a successful outcome for the client.

FURTHER READING

Marks, I. M. (1981) *Fears, Phobias and Rituals, Panic, Anxiety and Their Disorders*, Oxford University Press, New York.

Marks, I. M. (1992) *Living With Fear*, McGraw Hill, Maidenhead.

Melville, J. (1977) *Phobias and Obsessions: Their Understanding and Treatment*, Allen and Unwin, London.

Rapoport, J. (1990) *The Boy Who Couldn't Stop Washing – The Experience and Treatment of Obsessive Compulsive Disorder*, Collins, London.

Rowe, D. (1987) *Beyond Fear*, Fontana, London.

Salkovskis, P. M. and Kirk, J. (1989) Obsessional disorders, in *Cognitive Behaviour Therapy for Psychiatric Problems – a Practical Guide*, (eds K. Hawton, P. M. Salkovskis, J. Kirk and D. M. Clark), Oxford Medical Publications, Oxford.

Working with people who orchestrate | 11

Clients we previously called manipulative may now be described less detrimentally as 'orchestrative'. Searching for a word that describes certain collective descriptive behaviours without instantly stigmatizing the person was, we confess, difficult. 'Manipulative' tends to be a pejorative word which we would seek to avoid. The client who manages with proficient skill to orchestrate both his environment and the people around him should not be judged in a negative sense. This is, after all, his attempt to get the best for himself, although it often takes a maladaptive form. However, it is not inconsistent with behaviour which all human beings adopt in adverse situations, and which some more socially skilled people (notably politicians and entertainers) engage in from habit or for personal profit.

> Jane has been in the mental health unit for six months; it is her 25th admission. She will probably be discharged soon, but there is little hope she will remain in the community. Jane comes into the unit usually following an overdose of aspirins, or having slashed at her wrists. This has become a regular occurrence and generally follows some unpleasant incident in her life. She has many boy 'friends', but no close friends. Her parents say they cannot cope with her and no longer visit. She has a long list of offences, mostly minor, and is well known to the local police; she is 22. Jane's whole life appears to have been like a racetrack circuit – going from one dangerous bend to the next, the straights, like her relationships with people, being very short. The bends in Jane's circuit are perhaps only minor events for us, like keeping a job, friendship, resisting temptation to steal or to tell lies, even just getting up in the morning; for Jane they represent major hurdles almost impossible to negotiate. Even while in the unit, Jane seems unable to stop telling lies and goes from one member of staff to another with requests until she receives a favourable answer. When she does not get her own way she causes terrible scenes, makes suicidal gestures, breaks windows and furniture. Attacking clients both verbally and physically is her way of responding to frustration or boredom.

Jane's medical diagnosis would probably be personality disordered, sociopath, maladjusted, inadequate or just a plain psychopath. Whatever the diagnosis, the case history is probably a recognizable one. A very high percentage of people like Jane end up in residential care, mental health units or special care units, with nurses not quite sure what to do with them.

Jane's case is by no means unique, but is seen in various guises. Some drug- or alcohol-dependent clients have similar backgrounds and problems to Jane; their overt symptoms of dependence are simply their individual ways of portraying their unhappiness. Excessively aggressive people, sexual abusers, baby batterers, prostitutes and recidivists may have in their ranks people not dissimilar to Jane. Indeed, all people like Jane have one factor in common – they have great difficulty in forming meaningful relationships with other human beings. They have learned ways of behaving which are not endearing to others, and seem incapable of changing.

It is our belief that many of their problems are inherent in their absence of values, due perhaps to a failure of learning in their early psychological development. Some of the elements most noticeable in Jane's character are as follows:

1. An inability to love or to recognize love, warmth and friendship when it is offered.
2. An inability to make thoughtful decisions to be independent and free.
3. An underlying insecurity which breeds mistrust and anxiety.
4. Feelings of inadequacy – being different and unable to change.
5. An overwhelming frustration that life is not fair, that people do not care about her.

This being the case, perhaps rather than condemning the 'Janes' we nurse, we should try to understand them and help them to fulfil their needs. It is our belief that Jane can be helped with skilled nursing. The orchestrative person, like any other person, has potential for growth. We believe skilled nursing may be the facilitator for that growth.

The deficits highlighted in Jane's character suggest the needs that nurses may help her fulfil. For instance, if Jane is shown a consistent warm and caring approach, does she not have a better chance of developing these qualities herself? If the nurse is able to listen and try to understand her, will she not be more eager to try to understand herself? If Jane is offered some trust, will she not subsequently be able to grow to trust others? If she is offered a stable and committed relationship, will she not be more stable and committed in return? The answer to these questions is undoubtedly, in the short term, no. Jane will take advantage of your trust and manipulate your weakness, for that is how she perceives it. She will laugh at you, pour scorn on your genuineness, continue to be deceitful and lie and cheat whenever the opportunity arises. Indeed, why should we be so arrogant as to believe we can change in a few weeks a process that has taken 22 years to develop? It does not seem likely. We do, however, suggest that it will work. Your warmth, genuineness and empathy, if used skilfully and consistently, will overcome even the most difficult of manipulators if it is continuous and is given time.

IMPLICATIONS FOR THE NURSE

When nursing the orchestrative client the nurse must be prepared for a long campaign. It is not one that can be won in weeks, and may take years. During this time you will have to have the patience of a saint to put up with all the disappointments and frustrations you will encounter. Jane will consistently let you down when you have faith and trust in her; she will misrepresent you, betray you and tell lies about you. When she realizes you still accept her, do not resent her and remain warm towards her, things will probably get worse. At this point she may abuse you, threaten you, even physically attack you. If, despite this, your approach is immovably consistent, then, and perhaps only then, she may eventually learn to trust you. It is important to remember that in her disordered perception she has always been let down, no-one has ever been reliable, no-one has ever accepted her totally before. It is almost as if her entire previous behaviour has been an elaborate and marathon test of your honesty.

During this process, it has to be said that unless the nurse is a paragon of virtue, many crises will have occurred. Conflicts of loyalty, strains on emotion and just plain physical tiredness may have interfered with this therapeutic process. When Jane has stolen or bullied other clients, or had tantrums to seek attention, you may have given up. We believe the reason these clients have such a poor prognosis is that they require such intensive and continuous nursing that few establishments or individuals can fund it financially or emotionally.

PRINCIPLES AND SKILLS REQUIRED

Communication

At all times accurate and consistent communication must be maintained between client, nurse and other staff involved. It is important that the nurse is totally honest with the client at all times. If possible, the ward or mental health unit should have planned policies for dealing with antisocial or undesirable behaviour, and these should be understood by both parties, e.g.:

Jane: 'But why can't I have my weekend leave this weekend?'

Nurse: 'We discussed this when you first came into the unit, and you knew if you were found stealing clients' cigarettes you would not be allowed home for weekend leave. You stole Brian's cigarettes on Wednesday, so you can't go home this weekend.'

Jane: 'It's not fair, I don't get enough money to buy cigarettes, and I feel so frustrated here at weekends, I'll probably end up smashing something. You don't really care about me.'

Nurse: 'I understand you are very upset about not going home, but you're wrong about me not caring. I care very much. It would be easier to let you go, but it wouldn't do you any good in the long run. We have a deal and we have to stick to it. If you break something this weekend, I'll be upset and disappointed, but I hope you think about it seriously before you do, as I'm not sure it will help anything. Wouldn't it be better to discuss your frustration and deal with it more realistically?'

It can be seen from this exchange that the nurse shows she is totally honest, she is firm in her decision and is not interested in the 'implied blackmail'. She takes the opportunity to say how she feels – that she does care – and also suggests a possibly more appropriate behaviour. It should be emphasized that there is no attempt to judge Jane's statements; the nurse simply listens, understands and responds in a calm, consistent and caring way.

Dealing with undesirable behaviour

The ground rules have to be set early in the relationship. Although it is difficult to generalize, these suggested guidelines may be helpful.

Aggression

Wherever and whenever possible attention-seeking behaviour is best ignored, and the behaviour discussed later, e.g.: 'I noticed how aggressive you were this morning – when you act like that I will ignore you. I think you were just trying to get my attention, and I'm sure there are more positive ways of doing that than with aggression.'

Self-mutilation/suicidal gestures

Suggest to the client that this behaviour is unacceptable but that you will not intercede unless life-threatening situations occur. Explain that you do not intend to take responsibility for his life, as that robs him of his independence. Explore more acceptable ways of dealing with problems.

Telling lies/stealing

Discuss the situation with the client, being careful to listen and not to judge. Present the evidence as it appears and discuss this openly. When you have decided, say honestly how you feel, take any action you think is appropriate, or which is according to ward or unit policy, and state that this is the way it will always be dealt with in the future. It is important that, even though sanctions may be operated against her at this point, your accepting attitude does not change, e.g.:

Jane: 'So you don't believe me, and now I can't go on the trip tomorrow.'

Nurse: 'Look, Jane, I believe you did steal Harry's soap, and yes, that means you can't go on the trip, but I am trying to understand why you behave like this, and I really want to help.'

It may be seen from this that although the nurse may have judged Jane to be guilty of the act, she did not judge her as a person, and continued to offer help in a caring way.

Antisocial behaviour

Swearing, spitting and overt and offensive sexual behaviour are not uncommon in these clients. Largely ignoring this appears to be the most effective way of dealing with it, but intervention may be necessary when other clients are caused distress. Once a trusting and respecting relationship is attained, the nurse should be able to model appropriate behaviour for the client to learn more skilled social interactions.

Disloyalty and selfishness

These traits are commonly seen, and can only be dealt with by a total acceptance of them and disclosure of the nurse's feelings when appropriate, e.g.:

Nurse: 'I think I understand that you needed to complain to Dr Jones about my behaviour, because it seemed to you I was being unfair and asking a lot of you – I don't feel resentful about it, but perhaps a little disappointed you think so little of me.'

This becomes more difficult, however, later in the relationship when trust has been built and yet disloyalty still occurs. Nevertheless, no profit is gained by hostility and confrontation.

Once a rapport is struck between the nurse and the client, the nurse becomes a teacher. Her effectiveness in teaching will depend largely on the respect, trust and integrity she engenders.

In all interactions the nurse should attempt a positiveness so that she is perceived as honest, reliable, stable, warm and caring. We believe that if this is maintained for any length of time, more positive outcomes are both possible and probable.

SUMMARY

In this chapter we have tried to show that the orchestrative client suffers from an emotional deficit which has been potentiated by learned maladaptive behaviour. In order to help, the nurse has to be aware of the client's needs, which are closely involved with the underlying condition that the client suffers. To reverse the maladaptive behaviour and repair the emotional deficit, the client needs to be accepted and to be shown honest regard. New learning has to begin, as the client needs to learn acceptable behaviour patterns and to be more trusting, warm and honest.

It has been suggested that the client may seek attention by suicidal gestures, aggression and antisocial behaviour. Indeed, the nurse should expect dishonesty, disloyalty and selfishness. Although this paints a rather gloomy picture, and the nurse may be frustrated, disappointed, irritated and at times feel completely defeated, if the client is to be helped she must battle on. Her main allies are good communication with the client and her colleagues, a consistent approach, and her underlying qualities of honesty and warmth. If these qualities can be taught, modelled and suggested to the client, the task, although awesome, may be considered more realistic. Considerable patience is required to listen to and try to understand the client, especially when the nurse feels like giving up.

Finally, it would be wrong of us to suggest that successful outcomes will always result from this approach, but we do commend it to you as a caring approach that will at least enhance your self-respect and professional standards, when perhaps it is tempting to give up.

Working with people experiencing dependency $\boxed{12}$

Frank is 43 years old, thin and emaciated. He looks much older than his years, as he is completely grey, rather stooped in posture, with wizened skin and decaying teeth. He started drinking alcohol in his early teens and, as most young people do, considered it to be socially acceptable and a rather adult thing to do. He went to university, where his drinking habit was sustained, and achieved a degree in engineering. In his early twenties he married a school-teacher and had a happy domestic life. He had two children, whom he loved very much, and life generally seemed to be progressing pleasantly.

As his career and the subsequent pressure of his ambitions developed he began to drink rather more heavily. He would pop out at lunchtime, and stop for a drink on his way home. The significance of this did not really occur to Frank at this time, and his habit simply evolved. It was not long before he began keeping a bottle in his desk drawer 'for after a hard day', and his visits to the pub at lunchtimes and evenings became longer. Having a drink before important meetings became normal practice, only shortly before it became normal to have a drink after an important meeting.

It was probably around this time that his boss reprimanded him for the first time and his wife began to insist he spends more time at home with her and the children. Frank responded to these criticisms by getting absolutely drunk. He came home, hit his wife and shouted at the children. He had never behaved like this before. The next day Frank was shocked when confronted with his own behaviour, and swore it wouldn't happen again.

Frank managed to stop drinking completely for nearly a month after this incident. However, the pattern began to repeat itself the next month, when Frank told himself that it was the pressures at work and his wife's lack of understanding that had precipitated the incident, and that it had very little to do with drink. In fact, drink was the support he was getting. No-one really understood how he felt; hardly anyone knew he had a problem. This cycle continued, getting worse and worse.

Six months later, Frank was drinking all the time, consuming a full bottle of whisky a day with very little effect. His work deteriorated, as did his relationship with his wife. Six months later he lost his job. His wife tried to help and remained with him for another three years. The final blow for his wife was the realization that she was working only to support his drinking, and on discovering that he had remortgaged the house to its maximum and had spent several thousand pounds of this money on his habit, she left.

After his wife left, Frank gradually sold the furniture to buy drink, and spent all his social security money designated for mortgage repayments similarly. When the building society foreclosed he was left penniless and homeless. His first appearance in court was for stealing money from a parking meter. His second was for assault in an attempt to steal from an elderly woman. His third appearance led to his first admission to the psychiatric unit and now, five years later, he is up to his 30th admission. The pattern of his admissions has been similar over these five years. Admitted in a dreadful state, he is given good nursing care and 'dried out'. Subsequently he remains sober for some weeks. He enters group therapy determined to shed his problem, becomes depressed with his insight and discharges himself. He usually remains stable for several weeks, then gets hopelessly drunk for several days and is readmitted to the unit.

Frank has become dependent upon alcohol which, like many other drugs, is capable of causing both physical and psychological dependence. For our purpose in this book we make no distinction between dependence upon diamorphine, cocaine, alcohol or, for that matter, tranquillizers. Although these may have significant differences in physiological disorders or abnormalities, there is, we believe, a common component of psychological dependency. For example, there is no difference in principle between the socially acceptable cigarette smoker who finds it impossible to give up his drug and the young adolescent who inhales toxic fumes from glue to effect a 'high'. They are, of course, completely different subjects, but there is some common ground in that both are in some way dissatisfied with their strategies for dealing with their lives. Both demonstrate a need for outside agents to influence their internal emotional state. These dependencies, whether linked to physiological craving and bodily disorders or to a more immediately destructive form of suicidal wish, would both benefit from skilled intervention in order to achieve a healthy state. In the case of the alcohol or drug-dependent person, averting a premature death is the more serious objective.

Effective treatment begins with an understanding of Frank as a human being. Clearly, his physical dependence was built up over years of excessive drinking, but what originally motivated him to begin and continue to consume alcohol? A most popular contemporary theory is that we model our behaviour on others. For example, observing our parents and our peers consume alcohol or drugs will inevitably reinforce the idea that it is permissible. Conversely, rebellious adolescents may act in diametrically opposed directions to their parents, simply to show independence and control over them. No research we are aware of has conclusively shown that alcohol-dependent parents create alcohol dependent offspring or, for that matter, total abstainers, so clearly these influences must be only one factor and not the end of the story.

Another current theory is that dependent clients have peculiar personality traits. However, although Frank may be a typical 'personality type' seen today, there did not appear to be any significant features in his early years to single him out as being at particular risk of becoming alcohol dependent. Neither is there some particular IQ range which suggests he is more at risk. Any evidence collected so far suggests that becoming dependent on drugs or alcohol seems to be a cultural phenomenon having no respect for class, age, intelligence or personality type. Neither would it appear that physiological factors are significant in the development of dependency, in as much as women are just as much at risk as men; nor, as far as we are currently aware, are fat, thin, tall or short people particularly susceptible.

From this short resumé, of what can only be described as 'non-facts' we may take some comfort in thinking that dependency is not predictable, but by the same logic, although less comfortably, neither is it inevitable for any individual. Many people still believe that it is their own weakness of character, that they have some qualities attributable to others in less quantity, and that perhaps they do not deserve our help. They appear to be a section of the client population which is almost universally unpopular, evoking very little optimism or sympathy. Many people would maintain that they do not even require our help. Our feelings are most adamant on this subject – we believe that if a certain set of circumstances is applied to a certain type of person at the optimum time, at the most critical pressure, 'x' is the result. If 'x' turns out to be an alcohol dependent person, a person with sexual problems or a potential suicide, all are equally entitled to our help. To withhold our help and our skills detracts from our own value. To allow our prejudices and preferences to interfere with our care casts doubts on our professional integrity. Despite our previous experience and our jaundiced views concerning the 'success' rate of such clients, we must attempt to consider each readmission or rereferral as another fresh start – to reassess, replan and reimplement our care. To take any other course tends to predetermine the result. If it is debilitating for us to view potential success pessimistically, think of the detrimental effect it will have on the client. Unless we are able to inject hope into his perception of himself, he is bound to fail again. A 31st attempt to succeed is far more positive an outlook than his 30th failure.

PROBLEMS AND NEEDS OF THE DEPENDENT CLIENT

Alcoholics Anonymous considers the fundamental breakthrough in the rehabilitation of an alcohol-dependent person to be the point when he finally admits he has a problem, i.e. when he finally admits that he is alcohol dependent. Following this through logically (and we have no reason to dispute this theory), it appears that the dependent person is protecting himself with the mechanism of denial and that he is very able to project and rationalize his situation and misery. Indeed, this largely supports our own experience of the dependent client. In our experience the most remarkable rehabilitation has occurred when sudden insight has inspired the individual from a position which could only be described as the depths of degradation. The client appears to have reached rock bottom, has no self-respect, and his emotions and thoughts are left naked and open for all to see. The choice appears to be change and life, or to die in this sorry state. It is perhaps at this juncture that, if help is not forthcoming, if someone is not able to show they care, or if we are not alert to the potential for change, the client may be completely failed.

The client who is motivated to change will meet many obstacles, and he will almost certainly have to contend with the unbeliever. After all, who in their right mind would employ a self-confessed 'alcoholic'? Who would offer him a home and trust him in their house? Who would believe, on seeing a history such as Frank's, that such a person could change, would not steal, lie and cheat to obtain a drink? Certainly not someone who had known him.

The client needs someone to trust him, to have faith in him, to care enough to encourage him. His uphill battle for sobriety will not be made easier by people doubting him. How can he be expected to have faith in himself when others do not? Every aspect of his environment, of people's experience and his own thoughts tells him he will not succeed, but he knows he must. Even his own physical condition casts doubt on his ability to survive. How could such a frail, run-down body hold down a job? His thinking, memory and problem-solving ability have also been diminished by his habit. All the assets he had within himself have been taken from him by his drinking.

Frank's past life is of no consequence or credit to himself or others – he has proved to be unreliable, dishonest and aggressive, and only time can extinguish this stigma. He needs, more than ever before, some attainable goals and some distant dreams. He will need strength to work tirelessly towards remaining sober until the end of the day and the next, and the next, and he will need perseverance ultimately to be able to hold up his head again in society and to see his children in a climate of mutual respect. Starting all over again with a clean slate is almost impossible, indeed undesirable, for he needs to remember how easily his resolve can be lost, and how awful his previous existence really was.

IMPLICATIONS FOR THE NURSE

To nurse Frank skilfully, the nurse must have a fundamental belief that, should he want to change, he is capable of it. If the nurse has any doubt, this will inevitably be reflected in the attitudes she conveys towards him. To believe that Frank does not want to change is human; to believe he cannot is debilitating. The second most important prerequisite for effective treatment is for the nurse to believe she can help Frank if asked to do so. Casting aside all evidence and statistics that spell failure for dependent clients, and with an objective knowledge that most attempts at rehabilitation will fail, she must undertake each successive attempt at rehabilitating Frank as if it were the first, and consequently the most likely to succeed.

The skilled nurse will be able to appreciate that at times Frank will be ungrateful, so she must not seek gratitude. She must know that he will test her trust and support, so she must be trustworthy and supportive. She should know that he requires honesty, so she should reward him with the truth in a way he will not feel is punishing.

We believe dependent clients can only be treated voluntarily, but many alcohol and drug dependent people who commit crimes may be compulsorily detained. We do not necessarily think this is a good policy, although it is probably better than custodial care in a penal institution. However, being compulsorily detained does not preclude their voluntary submission for help. Nor does it mean that we should not continue any therapy recommended. It simply means that it may not be as effective.

The mental health nurse may come into contact with dependent clients more frequently in the community these days. This creates a greater difficulty for her, as such clients will continue to be influenced by their peer groups, friends and associates, who may have their own reasons for encouraging their dependency. However, it could be argued that this is a more realistic situation for therapy, as in residential care settings the client is one step removed from the situation to which they will inevitably have to return. The principles and skills required to help these clients are not significantly different from those required in residential settings, but simply more constrained, with the client facing temptation throughout the therapeutic process.

Nurses dealing exclusively with the dependent client may well become disenchanted and cynical. This is of course very human and natural, but we recommend that nurses be aware of the possibility and its consequences, recognizing that once such an attitude has developed, the nurse's usefulness to the client is seriously limited. Positive strategies to prevent this need to be devised, and we suggest that nurses in this environment should develop strong skills of debrief and group support.

PRINCIPLES AND SKILLS REQUIRED

No matter how little motivation the client shows to change, the nurse must show the core conditions of empathy, warmth and genuineness. She must continue to listen accurately to both his verbal and his non-verbal behaviour. To establish an empathic bond with the client is the only secure way of knowing when he requires the encouragement and support he needs to change his life.

The nurse needs to be skilled at challenging the client's discrepancies from a positive position, challenging the strength of his resources when he is feeling down and unable to fight back, e.g.:

Client: 'I don't think it's really worth it, I've lost everything, my wife, children, job, house, what's the point of going on?'

Nurse: 'You're feeling a little down, reflecting on all your losses, but in a way doesn't it prove something that you survived all that and are still game for another try? All those things you say you've lost are still within your grasp if you succeed this time, aren't they? Or were you being dishonest earlier when you said that this is what you have been aiming for?'

The nurse needs to raise the client's esteem whenever possible by reinforcing his strengths, especially in view of his uphill struggle – noting his resolve, how well he is looking, his ability to go into town without going for a drink. Eventually, he may be able to go into a bar and order a soft drink. All these strengths require positive reinforcement in the form of genuine regard. Even if the client regresses and has a drink, concentrate on how well he did for so long, rather than punishing him for his failure.

The most important skill is being able to communicate the trust and faith the nurse has for him, and that that trust cannot be shaken even by a setback or disappointment. One word of caution: the nurse must not fall into the trap of becoming the client's drink substitute when adopting this approach. It would be easy for the nurse to begin to feel sorry for the client; and by being overly 'sympathetic' rather than empathic, she may reinforce his 'dependence' on her. This dialogue shows how the nurse must continually put the responsibility back on to the client to prevent dependence:

Client: 'I really don't know what I'd do without you, nurse; when you're here I feel so secure, I don't ever feel the need for a drink. I don't even think you would mind if I did have a drink would you?'

Nurse: 'I sense you're beginning to doubt yourself and are putting the responsibility on to me. I have enough trust in you to know you will succeed in giving up drinking if you want to, and yes, I would mind if you had a drink, because I'd be disappointed that you had lost faith in your resolve. I trust you can give up drinking but I need to remind you that you're giving up for you not me.'

This approach needs to be tactful but firm, otherwise the nurse may become a replacement crutch for the client's emotional instability. The client needs to walk on his own.

Role-play techniques may occasionally be helpful, where clients can enact the emotional situations that precipitate a bout of drinking, and through this enactment find alternative strategies for dealing with their emotions. The nurse's role in this would be of great value, due to her closeness to the client. Any role-play situation may be emotionally tense, and knowing a nurse well may help this technique to be less threatening.

It may be seen that the nurse must practise all her behavioural and counselling skills to be an efficient helper with the dependent client. It is an exhaustive and frustrating task, but none the less the rewards for success with clients like Frank are incalculable, and the satisfaction of helping the 'unhelpable' is immense.

SUMMARY

Many drugs, including alcohol and tobacco, are capable of causing both physical and psychological dependence. This dependence is not predictable in, nor inevitable for, any individual: dependence can develop in almost anyone. It follows from this argument that the effective treatment of the drug addict or alcoholic should begin with an understanding of the client as an individual. This understanding can easily be jeopardized by prejudiced views and attitudes held by nurses. It is not enough to want to help. Helping requires the nurse to believe that the client can be helped and to have faith and trust in the client, whether this is the first or the 50th attempt to control his dependence.

We have suggested that it is the nurse's task to stimulate attainable goals for clients, and to encourage the restoration of longer-term aims and even distant dreams. This approach is necessary to rekindle the client's belief in himself.

Probably one of the most important implications for the nurse is the need to avoid cynical attitudes developing within herself. We are aware that this is not easy, but any cynical approach will undoubtedly sabotage the client's self-esteem and undermine any possible successful outcomes. Skilled challenges aimed at the client's discrepancies of thinking and behaviour are strong medicine, and should be respected as such. There is a significant difference between inviting the client to see himself more clearly by skilful challenge and destructively telling him what you think in cold hard terms. Challenging skilfully can only be successfully achieved from a position of empathy and, similarly, this is achieved from listening to both verbal and non-verbal communication. The nurse needs to raise the client's self-esteem wherever possible by reinforcing his strengths, not continually pointing out his weaknesses. If the nurse is able to do this effectively and communicate how much faith and trust she has in him, it will help him to be independent. This latter point is most important, for it may help to avoid the potential trap of the nurse becoming a substitute for the drug the client has become dependent upon.

Finally, it is worth mentioning that we have concentrated on an abstinence programme which, we believe, remains the more common practice in dealing with dependent clients. Some clinicians are of the opinion that clients dependent on alcohol may be rehabilitated to some form of continued social drinking, in perhaps the same way as a heavy smoker may cut down, and registered drug addicts are maintained on lower-dose opiate substitutes. Although we have no personal experience with this approach, we see no reason why it may not be possible with some individuals. We would, however, recommend that the same skilled approach be undertaken.

FURTHER READING

Davidson, R., Rollnick, S. and MacEwan, I. (eds) (1991) *Counselling Problem Drinkers,* Routledge, London.

Dawtry, F. (1968) *Social Problems of Drug Abuse*, Butterworths, London.

Edwards, G. (1982) *The Treatment of Drinking Problems: a Guide for the Helping Profession*, Blackwell Scientific Publications, Oxford.

Edwards, G. and Grant, M. (eds) (1977) *Alcoholism: New Knowledge and New Responses*, Croom Helm, London.

Edwards, G., Jaffe, J. and Arif, A. (eds) (1983) *Drug Use and Misuse: Cultural Perspectives*, Croom Helm, London.

Heather, N. and Robertson, I. (1981) *Controlled Drinking*, Methuen, London.

Jaffe, J., Peterson, R. and Hodgson, R. (1980) *Addictions: Issues and Answers*, Harper and Row, London.

Kennedy, J. and Faugier, J. (1989) *Drug and Alcohol Dependency Nursing*, Butterworths, London.

Kessel, N. and Walton, H. (1979) *Alcoholism*, Penguin Books, Harmondsworth.

Kinney, J. and Leaton, G. (1983) *Loosening the Grip: a Handbook of Alcohol Information*, 2nd edn, Mosby, St Louis.

Rix, K. and Rix, E. L. (1983) *Alcohol Problems: a Guide for Nurses and Other Health Professionals*, Wright, Bristol.

Smith, R. (1982) *Alcohol Problems*, BMA, London.

Williamson, P. and Norris, H. (eds) (1984) *Personal Skills Training for Problem Drinkers: A Counsellors' Guide*, Aquarius, Birmingham.

Willis, J. (1974) *Drug Dependence*, 2nd edn, Faber and Faber, London.

Working with people expressing aggression in residential settings

13

Katherine has been in residential care for twelve years. She has become obese from prolonged use of major tranquillizers and institutional food. It is unusual to see her without a cigarette in her mouth or walking jauntily around eating a sandwich or sweets. It is possible that Katherine would not be noticed in a long-stay ward or mental health unit, except for the fact that whenever there is an incident she can usually be found in the midst of it. She has almost achieved notoriety within the care system. Staff are warned how unpredictable she is: if the fire alarm sounds, someone will remark, 'Oh, it's probably only Katherine'; when a pane of glass breaks, people expect Katherine to be the cause; if a client or member of staff has been attacked, inevitably Katherine has been 'at it' again.

Katherine is 32 years old, has been married and divorced, has a child, and both elderly parents are still alive, but she has not seen any of these people for some years now. Trained nurses, doctors and other professionals are wary of her, so it is not surprising that her family became disenchanted many years ago. Yet when time is taken to get to know her, she becomes more than just a manifestation of an undesirable behaviour pattern: she is a warm, caring and sensitive individual. She does not consciously intend to hurt anyone, but simply finds great difficulty in controlling her emotions. She can sometimes be seen in great distress, crying bitterly into a tissue, and if she is listened to she will tell how frustrated and depressed she is about her life. She will say how helpless she feels, with despair in the knowledge that she will probably spend the rest of her life in residential care.

Katherine is not perhaps typical of the aggressive client, but neither is she untypical. She represents and exposes a powerful phenomenon that can be observed in many institutions among residents considered to be aggressive: people tend to behave according to other people's expectations of them. We have to emphasize, however, that this is not so in every case. People become aggressive for almost as many different reasons as there are aggressive people, and consequently it is important to investigate the causes, as they hold the key to dealing effectively with the aggression. It is always more difficult to find the cause when the client is distant from the nurse, if the nurse is afraid, hesitant or withdraws from the relationship. The client's problems and needs can never be fully understood and dealt with if a poor rapport exists.

Aggression can take many forms. It is sometimes seen as a physical and violent attack upon a person or object, but more commonly it is a verbal explosion of emotion directed at someone or something. Even in more 'normal' adult interactions raising of voices indicates an aggressive intent and heightened emotion. Even more subtle is when self-mutilation, depression and sulky behaviour manifest as symptoms of aggression turned inward.

PROBLEMS AND NEEDS OF THE AGGRESSIVE CLIENT

The client expressing aggressive behaviour patterns desperately needs help. It is probable that violence occurs because there is no other route to express the seething emotions that exist within that individual: it is despair due to an inability to find alternative, more desirable, strategies to vent feelings that results in violent behaviour.

The client may feel misunderstood, isolated, lonely, frustrated, and in the absence of a constructive means of communicating this, he acts out his feelings in aggression.

IMPLICATIONS FOR THE NURSE

The nurse has many responsibilities in dealing with aggressive and violent behaviour, and it is useful if she can organize these mentally before an incident occurs, rather than after. If she can do so it may well assist her effectiveness in any aggressive interaction.

Responsibility for the client

The nurse needs to help the client to resolve his problems, and protect him from himself or others. This will include an honest appraisal of knowing what limits she will set on behaviour before she considers restraint. Does she have the courage, resources and willingness to risk taking direct action which may jeopardize her relationship with the client? If conflicts exist on the issue of restraint, she may need to challenge her beliefs, attitudes and thinking in this area until she is very clear about her limits. Restraint is, unfortunately, sometimes necessary, and this is a reality we have to face, but when it is used it is important that its use is critically evaluated:

- Why was it necessary?
- What motivated its use? Staff anxiety for the client? Other clients? Themselves?
- What other strategies were available? Were they inappropriate? Why were they inappropriate?
- What exactly happened? Cause? Effect?

- How did we all feel? Staff, clients with person restrained?
- How do we all feel now?
- How could it have been prevented?
- How can we prevent its recurrence?
- What action should be taken now?

This is only a sample of the type of question that should be asked following incidents and restraint; it is up to the team to devise their own according to their unique situation.

PRINCIPLES AND SKILLS REQUIRED

It is important that the cause of the aggression is sought in every incident. This may best be done by the use of reflecting the client's feelings as seen through non-verbal behaviour, and by facilitating discussion through an open question, e.g.: 'I can see you are very frustrated and angry about something, Katherine, I wonder if you feel able to talk to me about it?' 'I would like to understand how you feel.' 'Tell me what's really bothering you.'

It is also important that a relationship of trust remains throughout every incident – facilitated through honesty. Here the nurse needs to be totally honest about what she has in mind. If, for instance, she intends to get help to restrain the client and give an intramuscular injection, she must not mislead him into believing she just wants to talk, e.g.: 'Katherine, I can see you're very upset and I think you need some medication. You refuse to talk calmly to me about what's troubling you, and frankly you are frightening me and I fear for people's safety.' 'I've sent for some help to give you an injection, but I hope you will agree to have it without force.' 'I hope you will believe me when I say I'm only trying to help you.'

This interaction may be unrealistic if the client is likely to react to it violently, but it needs to be said even if it is during actual restraint. The nurse needs to be frank and explain her actions to ensure some rapport remains.

Even during physical restraint the nurse may facilitate a caring relationship. Conversation with the client should not cease, even during restraint. If the nurse is able to continue talking in a calm soothing voice, explaining what is happening and why, much of the rapport may be saved, e.g.: 'Katherine, I'm sorry it has come to this. When this happens it means we've failed. If you feel you can't talk to us and allow us to help without incidents like this, then something must be wrong.' 'I hope when you are feeling calmer we can talk and you may be able to explain how you felt and explore more productive ways of dealing with your feelings than aggression.' 'I'm going to give you this injection now; I know it's difficult but if you can try to relax a little it won't hurt so much. It will help you to feel more relaxed and we'll stay with you till you are able to feel calmer.'

In situations of verbal aggression a skilful approach may divert any actual violence. The principles and skills here are as follows.

Absorption

The nurse should be able to absorb any hostility or abuse directed at her without reacting. Obscene language may cause offence but it will not cause physical harm; however, retaliating or showing offence may well precipitate an actual physical attack. We suggest that the nurse raise her awareness of exactly what may make her unable to absorb verbal abuse and deal with it in safe role-play type situations.

Distraction

Nurses may be able to distract clients who are verbally aggressive by switching the conversation completely, by putting on some music, or by using of humour if the client is known to be susceptible to this.

Approach

The nurse's approach may be all important. She should be non-threatening, and to facilitate this the following suggestions may be useful:

- A low posture – preferably sit near to the client;
- Hands in pockets – or similar;
- Helpless posture may help;
- An open frontal approach is recommended wherever possible;
- A congruous smile may help alleviate the client's fear that the nurse's approach heralds physical force;
- Maintain eye contact to establish a willingness to listen, without constant staring which may be interpreted as confrontation.

Reassurance

Positive verbal reassurance may be very helpful, e.g.:

- 'I'm trying to understand.'
- 'I'd like to listen to what you have to say.'
- 'Please don't feel threatened, I'm not going to hurt you.'
- 'I really do care – I want to help you.'

Disclosure

Somehow, probably as a legacy from the custodial days of mental health care, a belief has developed that the nurse should be fearless. We are not at all sure about or impressed with this. In many ways it detracts from the empathic, genuine and caring attitudes which need to be demonstrated. Far better, perhaps, to say to a client, 'I'm trying to understand how you feel, but at the moment I'm frightened that you may hit me', rather than the cool 'hard' approach that can be interpreted as challenging, taunting and an invitation to physical confrontation.

We suggest that the nurse disclose what she feels to the client, whether it be fear, dismay or disappointment, provided it is honest and not devisive, and at the same time communicates sufficient confidence to convey the fact that the nurse is able to take control if the client wishes it. We believe that this will close the gap between the two, form a bridge and strengthen an existing, but perhaps fragile, rapport.

General principles which may help prevent a violent incident

Observation of the client's behaviour may forewarn the nurse of a potentially violent incident. There may be many telltale signs, such as scowling, pacing, shouting, clenched fists and so on. Knowing the client well is the nurse's most effective weapon.

The team of nurses must be working as a team, and there should be good communication so that there is consistency of care. There is nothing more frustrating for any individual than to have conflicting instructions or advice. If this situation exists, frustration will eventually build up and a violent reaction can be anticipated.

Safety valves: in any well run ward or mental health unit there must be some established method of being able to express frustration, fears or general 'moans'. Clients' meetings or group discussions may be useful to help defuse situations before they become violent issues.

If it begins to look as if a violent incident may be imminent, the person closest, with the best rapport with the client, should normally be directed to deal with the situation. Any known antagonistic agents, i.e. particular people, should be removed.

ATTENTION-SEEKING BEHAVIOUR WHICH TAKES AN AGGRESSIVE FORM

Suffice it to say here that the nurse needs to know the cause of behaviour in order to facilitate its change. When aggression results from a client seeking attention, many factors will determine the response:

- Is the aggression likely to harm the client or another person?
- Is an extinction programme established (see p. 63)?
- What course of action is available other than reinforcing the undesired behaviour by attention?
- Can attention realistically be withheld long enough for some positive behaviour to emerge, so that this can be linked with attention?

In all cases of aggressive behaviour the nurse will be called upon to use her knowledge, discretion and judgement, and the above suggestions are intended only as a guide. In reality the nurse must find her own appropriate strategies for the unique individual in her care.

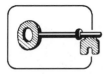

KEY CONCEPTS

1. It has been shown that aggression may take many forms. Physical violence, verbal abuse, hostility, self-mutilation, depression or sulkiness may all be manifestations of aggressiveness.

2. Primarily the client's problems centre around an inability to communicate effectively. If he is unable to use appropriate strategies to deal with emotions such as insecurity, loneliness, despair, frustration and uncertainty, frank aggression may be the result.

3. It has been suggested that the client requires understanding and someone to listen to him; he may subsequently be able to understand himself more clearly. It is only when he is able to do this for himself that he will be able to formulate new strategies to cope with his feelings.

4. The nurse's responsibilities are to herself, her colleagues and the client. It is possible that these responsibilities can only be discharged successfully by the use of restraint on occasions. When these situations arise, the nurse should be able to restrain effectively with the minimum force, and subsequently investigate by critical evaluation the necessity for such action.

5. The skilled nurse will be able to maintain the client's trust by remaining honest, and avoid violence by absorbing abuse, distracting the client and using appropriate positive reassurance. We would conclude by adding that this altruistic approach is only possible in an established climate when the nurse truly cares for the client, has tried to form an empathic bond and is open enough to share with the client her feelings and hopes for more positive ways of dealing with the causes of the aggression.

FURTHER READING

COHSE (1977) *The Management of Violent or Potentially Violent Patients: Report of a Special Working Party Offering Information, Advice and Guidance to COHSE Members*, COHSE, Banstead, Surrey.

Lorenz, K. (1970) *On Aggression*, Methuen, London.

Ownes, R.G. and Ashcroft, J.B. (1985) *Violence: a Guide for the Caring Professions*, Croom Helm, London.

Story, A. (1979) *Human Aggression*, Penguin Books, Harmondsworth.

Working with children $\boxed{14}$

To appreciate the complexity of a child's world and its influences, an understanding of the normal milestones of development and the child's family system is required. It is not our intention to explore in any depth the psychological, physical or social background of any particular child problem, but rather to give some guidance as to how general principles of care must be applied in a special way to children because of the nature of the child's state of development. Whether a child is seen at home, attends a mental health unit or is admitted, each is frequently perceived as a symptom of failed care approaches in the family system. It is often a last resort to admit a child, and in our opinion this should remain so, as prolonged absence from a normal family unit can produce more maladjustment than it is designed to relieve. However, there are times when it becomes clear that the child and the family, no matter what intervention takes place, are in such turmoil with each other that some space between them is necessary. The particular challenges involved in work with children on a day or residential basis have led us to concentrate on these particular means of intervention. For example:

> David's behaviour had become increasingly demanding. He would change from a state of withdrawal to a state of hyperactivity, with frequent temper tantrums. He suffered from encopresis and had a fear of men. The decision to bring him into the unit was due to the fact that his presence at home was causing a strain on his mother, who directed her frustration at her boyfriend, who in turn regularly hit David in the face, on one occasion causing severe bruising and bleeding. David's father, who has since left the household, also had a history of violence, mainly directed toward David's mother. Admission was brought about shortly after David had caused severe bruising to his 2-year-old stepsister. David was 6 years old. In this case, it seems that both David's and his family's safety was in jeopardy, and the space provided by admitting him gave a chance for the multidisciplinary team to assess the situation without the fear of further risk to David or his sister. During the first 48 hours David was totally withdrawn, refusing to speak and cowering or moving away from any approach made towards him by any male member of staff. It took a long time before he could appreciate and enjoy the security of a loving and trusting relationship.

The following is a list of the more common difficulties a child may present to the community mental health nurse or on admission to a child or adolescence unit:

- Abuse
- Anorexia
- Behavioural disorder
- Elective mutism
- Enuresis
- Psychosomatic states
- Language and learning difficulties
- School phobia/refusal
- Autism
- Encopresis
- Hysterical behaviour
- Obesity
- Depression/suicidal
- States of deprivation/failure to thrive.

PROBLEMS AND NEEDS OF A CHILD

Although each individual is unique there are predictable milestones to development, each with its accompanying needs. At different ages the individual can be placed on a continuum of dependence on or independence from the family in order to meet these needs. The family, whether it be traditional nuclear, single-parent, remarriage, adoptive or multigenerational, is the primary source to fulfil the young child's need for the security of protection, love, nurturing and identity. This dependence changes over time as the growing child begins to develop his own resources and independence. As progress through the individual lifecycle raises the changing demands of adolescence and adulthood, the family unit needs to be stable enough to provide support yet flexible enough to adapt to different circumstances. Some children fail to have their basic needs met, and the nurse must be alert to the signs of neglect or abuse and clear about their role in child protection systems. Other children encounter difficulties in managing the tasks of the individual lifecycle, or suffer the consequences of being in a family that has difficulty in adjusting to the transitions of the family lifecycle. The nurse must appreciate that when a child's difficulties warrant intervention by a nurse or multidisciplinary team, he or she is likely to experience this as yet another traumatic event in a long history of confusion, conflict or rejection. Particularly when time away from the family situation is indicated, the child can view the admission as another way of telling him that he is trouble, a burden, worthless and should be rejected. It is therefore necessary for the nurse to make herself accessible to the needs of the child, in order that she may provide the warmth and acceptance that has been so lacking until then in his life. Figure 14.1 illustrates some common problem areas with children in care away from their own families, and the needs that counteract these. The following is a list of questions or statements that a child of 7 or 8 might ask himself when he finds himself in care:

Why am I here, I don't understand? – Confusion

What is going to happen next? – Anxiety

What is going to happen to me? – Fear

Why can't I stay with my mum/dad? – Rejection

What should I say or do? – Conflict

It doesn't matter, anyway, no-one can hear/understand me. – Frustration

SKILLS REQUIRED

The skills required are developed from an awareness of the needs of children in distress. They involve understanding what the child is trying to say and being able to communicate in his own language. The child, when communicating, does not always take into account the needs of the listener. For example, a 7-year-old may talk about an event but not the background or build-up to that event, thus making full grasp of the story difficult. The listener therefore needs to be able to ask appropriate questions in order to clarify the full meaning. Another important aspect when listening to a child is to take note of the non-verbal communication, as this is particularly strong, accurate and expressive. For example, observing a child playing with dolls may convey more about concerns, conflicts and anxieties than questioning would. When communicating with children the nurse 'must have an awareness of the developmental stage in relation to the child's ability to understand and think at certain degrees of complexity'. Young children are often very concrete in their thinking and often believe they have caused certain events, hence the common feeling of guilt often expressed by children who have experienced parental divorce or

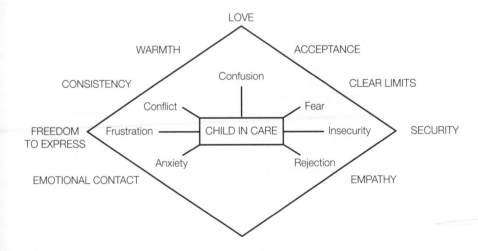

Figure 14.1   The problems and needs of a child in care

separation. It is for this reason that it is vital for the adult to check understanding again (Norbeck, 1980).

The requisite skills are:

- Crisis skills
- Teaching skills
- Boundary setting
- Reasoning skills
- Exploratory skills
- Creative communication
- Conveying acceptance.

These can be remembered by using the mnemonic *Children's Traumas Become Repressed Causing Endless Agony.*

Crisis skills

There are times when the child loses control and vents his feelings through some destructive act. As with dealing with any aggressive incident, harm to others or himself must be prevented. The skill in this situation is gaining control in the quickest and safest way possible. If a child's safety is at risk this may involve physical restraint; if so, it should be used with the minimum of force and ample opportunity should be given for the initial physical contact made by the nurse to restrain the child to be converted into a warm embrace, thereby enabling him to relax in a secure environment. It may be necessary to remove the child to a place where there is less stimulation and less attention. This should be done for a minimal time only. In all incidents, a thorough exploration of the causes and consequences is essential, in order to establish alternative ways of behaving. One specific skill in the area of crisis intervention is that of distraction. This is used to gain immediate cooperation or obedience by the child. It involves telling the child what to do rather than what not to do, and intervening sufficiently loudly to gain his initial attention, in order to give the command. This 'resetting mechanism' clears the channel for the child to focus attention momentarily away from the destructive set. For example:

> After hearing a commotion in the TV lounge, the nurse on entering saw Peter about to throw a cup at another boy. Her response, 'Peter put that cup down now' was sufficiently loud to startle Peter into hesitating, allowing the nurse to stand in front of him and take the cup away.

It is important during an incident like this to allow the child to express his frustrations in another way, ideally verbally expressing his anger or acting it out in some form of activity room where he can vent pent-up feelings safely.

Teaching skills

These involve enhancing the child's environment in order to maximize his awareness of the things around him. It is necessary for the nurse to be enthusiastic about activities and choices, giving the child every opportunity to use his powers of judgement in order to make decisions. Giving the child a choice will increase his sense of autonomy and may reduce the need to defy. For example, by asking what the child wants to wear it may be possible to avoid the issue of whether or not to get dressed. Conversely, unnecessary choices should be avoided, as they may lead to additional conflict. For example, rather than say, 'Do you want to go for dinner now?' say, 'It is time for dinner now'. Maintaining the child's interest and pointing out the value of activities may give him a sense of purpose and increased self-esteem. All too often children are given toys and a room and told to play. This is satisfactory only to the extent to which the materials given and the supervision offered are sufficient to generate and enhance the child's imagination.

Boundary setting

This is the consistent application of clearly defined and totally understood behavioural boundaries, sometimes referred to as 'limit setting'. If boundaries are left for the child to discover, this may lead to his feeling guilty over the behaviour and unsure about further loss of control, fearing potential retaliation and/or punishment and rejection. However, clearly set boundaries offer a sense of security to the child, increasing his confidence for self-expression and exploring other directions. Some boundaries are based on avoiding injury to others or himself. Others could be reality issues such as time limits and property limits. Ginott (1964) proposes four steps to successful limit setting:

- Recognize the child's feelings or wishes and help him to express them as they are: ('You feel angry, and you'd like to hit me').
- State clearly the limit on the specific act: ('Hitting is one thing I won't allow you to do', or 'I won't let you hit me').
- Point out other channels through which the feelings can be expressed: ('You can hit or kick the pillow').
- Allow the child to express resentment or anger for having his behaviour restricted or redirected.

These four steps can be applied to any area where boundaries must be applied and should always be negotiated and clearly communicated on an individual basis to ensure that their meaning is fully understood.

Reasoning skills

This relates to the nurse's ability to explain, enabling full understanding on the part of the child. In order to do this, the nurse must consider the child's developmental level and anxiety levels. There is a need to be sensitive to what the child is anxious about and to appreciate what the likely outcome of an explanation will be. Consider the effects of these two explanations on a 7-year-old child about the same event:

'Tom, I want you to come and sit with your mum and dad and have a chat with Bill the doctor, Shirley the lady doctor, me and Dave the other nurse, is that OK?'

'Tom, I want you to sit in on a session of family therapy so we can all express what's going on and see if we can make things better.'

The latter's use of ambiguity and 'foreign' language is much more likely to cause fear and resistance than the former, where the intention is clear.

Exploratory skills

These skills are aimed at helping the child to explore his own feelings and thoughts and to express them. This is a two-way process and particularly important with children, as they need to know what others are thinking and feeling. The nurse can elicit the child's thoughts and feelings in many ways, often the more imaginative the better. Rather than direct questioning, generate interest in the topic first through wishes or fantasy, or by allowing the child to correct the adult's incorrect information. The saying 'Actions speak louder than words' is particularly relevant here. Physical contact and hugging to convey acceptance is very powerful. If the child feels anxious about communicating feelings verbally, then alternative outlets could be using play or puppets; even just being with them can serve as a bridge for the message.

Creative communication

Understanding the value of play, art, exercise, drama and other forms of creativity and their use in the therapeutic regimes of children in residential care settings is essential. These activities can have several functions at each developmental level:

- Development and mastery of specific motor skills;
- Expression of imaginative or symbolic content;
- Repetition and working through of inner conflicts.

The nurse's role in relation to these activities can be either as a participant or as an observer. The nurse must ensure that she does not interfere with any 'working through' process by the child: just being there is usually sufficient to offer support during anxious moments or times of skill acquisition. These times offer a chance for the child to be himself, expressing thoughts, fears, conflicts or desires freely. The nurse could also express her own world through this medium, and by sharing with the child may enhance the bonding sufficiently to engender trust. From this the child's confidence may grow and his readiness to disclose and share may increase.

Conveying acceptance

Counteracting the child's feelings of rejection can be started by conveying acceptance to the child through the nurse–child relationship. The nurse must be open and honest with the child about the relationship and also consistent, especially in the form of communication. This can be shown through the use of the skill areas mentioned above, but can be summarized as follows (Norbeck, 1980):

1. Providing a safe environment;

2. Providing developmentally appropriate equipment and activities;
3. Positioning oneself at the same level as the child;
4. Engaging in appropriate activity as the child directs;
5. Being with the child and attentive to him;
6. Talking in language appropriate to the child;
7. Respecting the child's need for social distance;
8. Respecting the child's pace of activity;
9. Demonstrating warmth and concern for the child.

If the nurse can accept the child as a valued member of society, someone who needs love, warmth and security, then she can begin to rebuild what is often perceived through the child's eyes as a shattered and fearful adult world.

FAMILY INVOLVEMENT

It is seldom necessary to care for a child in isolation from the family: a child's problem will mostly involve the family in some way. Even in cases of abuse (physical and sexual) it will be necessary and wise to involve the family, where appropriate and possible, in the therapeutic programme (see chapter on Sexual abuse). Most of the therapeutic intervention should incorporate the needs of the parents and siblings. This may occur in several forms.

Mothering groups and fathering groups

This is where the respective parents gather to talk about their roles and relationships, offering each other different perspectives on the mother–child or father–child relationship. The nurse may play the role of prompter and information-giver to help the group work together.

Family groups

Here the whole immediate family is invited together, with a specific therapist and/or a nurse. The family dynamics, relationships, issues and conflicts are aired openly in order to maximize the opportunities for communication between the parties and reduction in barriers. Other activities the nurse is likely to be involved in when working with children, both in mental health units and at home, are those supportive and therapeutic activities aimed at helping the whole family as well as the child, e.g. individual counselling of parent or parents; marital work; helping the parents work or play with the child; teaching and modelling for the parents; and generally offering a consistent support system where the parents can feel confident and safe to communicate anything that may be of benefit to the child and family.

IMPLICATIONS FOR THE NURSE

Working with children can be very emotionally and physically demanding. The nurse must be aware of the possible consequences of what often is a very close relationship with a child. The following is an outline of the most common mechanisms which, if the nurse is unaware of them, may interfere with the giving of care.

Overdependency

This is where the child takes to the accepting nature of the environment to such an extent that the thought of anything outside it fills him with dread, thereby impeding eventual independence.

Emotional involvement

When the nurse becomes particularly attached to a child to the extent that she finds it difficult to view the situation objectively, her judgement may be compromised and cause additional conflict within the ward team. The continuous demands a group of children will make on a nurse will depend very much on how realistic the nurse is. If she provides uncensored attention, she will not survive. It is therefore imperative when caring for children to be aware of the emotional demands made and the limits to which you can give. Feelings of inadequacy, frustration, ambivalence and anger are all common emotions experienced by the nurse towards staff, self and the children.

It is necessary to accept these as normal processes and have the channels to explore them in a supportive staff environment in order to protect yourself, thus increasing the likelihood of consistent delivery of care to the child.

CONCLUSION

The child in care may look upon the carers as a substitute family. The nurse must find a balance between being mother or father, brother or sister, advocate and nurse. It may be that she can amalgamate all these roles into one, but this is acceptable only to the extent to which she can satisfy the demands a child may make on one particular role, within the constraints of her own professional judgement. The common factor to all these is the need for affection and love. To be able to give this, often in the situation of personal attack and what may seem like endless frustration, is a very valuable personal asset. Finally, we have tried to identify specific skills the nurse may need to use when caring for children within a mental health setting. There is a wealth of material that revolves around the skills described; we hope our description is sufficient to stimulate you into further study.

FURTHER READING

Bhoyrub, J.P. and Morton, H.G. (1983) *Psychiatric Problems in Childhood. A Guide for Nurses*, Pitman, London.

Calam, R. and Franchi, C. (1987) *Child Abuse and its Consequences*, Cambridge University Press, Cambridge.

Carpenter, J. and Treacher, A. (1993) *Using Family Therapy in the 90s*, Blackwell, Oxford.

Dallos, R. (1991) *Family Belief Systems, Therapy and Change*, Open University Press, Milton Keynes.

Davenport, G. C. (1991) *An Introduction to Child Development*, Collins Educational, London.

Hsu, L. K. G and Hersen, M. (1989) *Recent Developments in Adolescent Psychiatry*, Wiley, New York.

Jacobs, M. (1986) *The Presenting Past*, Open University Press, Milton Keynes.

Klein, J. (1987) *Our Need for Others and its Roots in Infancy*, Tavistock, London.

Skynner, R. (1990) *Explorations With Families – Group Analysis and Family Therapy*, Routledge, London.

Skynner, R. and Cleese, J. (1984) *Families and How to Survive Them*, Methuen, London.

Street, E. and Dryden, W. (eds) (1988) *Family Therapy in Britain*, Open University Press, Milton Keynes.

Treacher, A. and Carpenter, J. (1981) *Using Family Therapy: a Guide for Practitioners in Different Professional Settings*, Blackwell, Oxford.

Wilkins, R. (1989) *Behaviour Problems in Children*, Heinemann Nursing, Oxford.

Wilkinson, T. R. (1983) *Child and Adolescent Psychiatric Nursing*, Blackwell Scientific Publications, Oxford.

15 Working with elderly confused people

Mrs Garland's admission was the culmination of several months' gradual deterioration in her behaviour. Her family had coped quite well up to now, but recently Mrs Garland had been wandering about at night, turning the gas on without lighting it or cooking things and leaving them to burn. What seemed to be the last straw for her daughter, who had been caring for her, was when her mother squatted in a corner of the kitchen and defecated. This resulted in the daughter approaching the doctor with pleas for help. Mrs Garland had been on the waiting list to come into the elderly assessment unit, but this increase in deterioration had warranted immediate admission, as her daughter could no longer cope and Mrs Garland was a risk to herself and others.

On admission, Mrs Garland was accompanied by her daughter and son-in-law. They were taken to the reception lounge and offered a cup of tea. It was usual for the nurse in charge and another to introduce themselves and record essential information and to give the relatives and the client information they would need. Mrs Garland was sitting next to her daughter. She seemed nervous and was continually fidgeting with her dress, pulling it up to her face.

'Do you take sugar Mrs Garland?' She looked towards the nurse with a vacant gaze. 'Go away.' She got up and walked towards the window. 'What is this place?'

'I've told you, Mum, it's a place where you can rest and get better.'

'There's nothing wrong with me, take me home.'

The nurse intervened, 'Come and sit down, Mrs Garland and have a cup of tea and then we'll explain everything.'

'Where's my Billy?'

She started to cry. Billy was her husband, who had died four years ago. By this time her daughter was becoming distressed. In an effort to distract Mrs Garland, the nurse took her hand.

'Come on, Mrs Garland, I'll show you our garden, it's lovely out there.'

Her mood changed quickly and she seemed to go with the nurse quite willingly. The remaining nurse then spent a considerable time with the daughter helping her explore a whole range of feelings, varying from frustration and anger to guilt and sadness, until she could accept the situation sufficiently in order to leave her mother in the unit with some sense of personal relief and reassurance.

This progressive loss of contact with reality, highlighted by intellectual, emotional and memory disturbances, is a manifestation of 'dementia'.
The following describes the symptoms and gives examples of behaviour illustrating them.

Memory disturbance

At first, Mrs Garland became absent-minded and forgot things like appointments, items of shopping and where she had left things in the house. This, however, progressed to seeing someone one day and forgetting that she had seen them the next, or setting out to do the shopping and arriving back late at night, via the police, distressed, saying, 'I got lost'. Her memory for recent events had become extremely bad, but during this period she would recall past events of her childhood and early adult years very well. Recently she had started confusing dates, events and anniversaries: she could not recall whether her husband had died one year or four years ago, and occasionally she had stated that he was not dead. This severe memory disturbance results in a major manifestation of confusion.

Disorientation in time, place and person

The disorientation in time illustrated by Mrs Garland's wanderings at night is quite common, and an extension of this is the complete reversal of the sleep pattern, i.e. asleep most of the day and awake during the night. Disorientation in place is often highlighted by the constant questioning of 'What is this place?' or 'Where am I?', despite persistent answers and reassurance. This particular aspect is extremely frustrating; the insecurity, anxiety and fear often results in anger and frustration.

Probably the most disconcerting form of disorientation is that of 'person'. This becomes distressing, especially for relatives who visit the client, who turns and states, at best, 'I am not who you say I am and I certainly don't know you' or, at worst, gives no response or acknowledgement of their presence at all.

Emotional disturbances

Mrs Garland's sudden change from crying to contentment at being shown around the garden demonstrates the 'emotional lability' that is often present. This is the inappropriate switching of extremes of emotion from sadness and crying to euphoria and laughter. Others, however, may exhibit a shallowness of emotion and lack of responsiveness. Associated with the confusion, especially early on in its development where moments of insight are apparent, are anxiety and depression, which can dominate the client's mood.

Intellectual impairment

The first signs of this occurring are usually seen when the client finds it difficult to make decisions, or chooses inappropriately. The ability to make judgements diminishes rapidly and the ability to think in abstract forms becomes difficult.

It can be seen from the description of these behaviours that someone experiencing this devastating process can be transformed into someone hardly recognizable by those closest to him. These changes often exacerbate an already fragile body, resulting in an individual who is probably the most difficult person to nurse in terms of the physical and psychological demands made upon the limited resources available. This brings a challenge to all those who undertake this particular caring role.

PROBLEMS AND NEEDS OF THE ELDERLY CONFUSED CLIENT

The problems and needs of the elderly confused are often considerable, varying from the basic needs of nutrition and warmth, through those of love and belongingness, to esteem. It is therefore imperative that when assessing such clients priorities are taken into consideration and the best use of resources made. There is a variety of assessment forms available, all of which are designed to establish the physical, psychological and social needs of the client.

Physical

A thorough medical assessment on admission is required in order to establish the extent of the client's physical wellbeing and also to eliminate a variety of other causative agents which can cause confusion, and which would mean a different course of treatment and care. Two other causes of confusion in the elderly are toxic states and depression, which would warrant alternative regimens of care. Nursing observation in this area should be related to physical needs and ensuring that safety factors are considered. An elderly confused person who is very unsteady on his feet is agitated and restless. Because of this the potential danger of falling is very real, so it becomes a priority to assess the degree and cause of immobility in order to rectify the problems if possible, and also to minimize the extent of restlessness. Particular attention must be paid to all the essential needs of the elderly confused because each one is at risk from self-neglect, due to the incapacitating nature of the 'dementing' state. Assessment and planning of the individual's needs for nutrition, elimination, hygiene and sleep is vital in every case.

Psychological

Imagine yourself in a building where you wander round finding that every room you come to is different and you can never return to the room you set off from. In each room there are people whom you have never met before, yet they seem to know you and tend to coax you from one area to another. When you try to speak to them the message comes out garbled and when they speak to you it seems like a foreign language. Some of these people pull at your clothes, enter into your bathroom and sometimes even your toilet area. Food and drink are thrust at you at any time during the day and if you don't eat it then someone will spoonfeed you. How would you react in this situation?

It is not surprising that many elderly confused clients are agitated and distressed, as for them it must be something like this: a world of strange places and faces, not knowing why they are there and yet being helpless to do anything about it. This situation invariably leads to the psychological problem of:

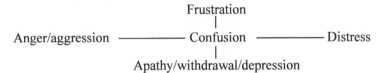

Their needs in relation to these problems are those of reassurance, repetitive explanation and clarity of action, all conducted in an atmosphere of acceptance, without condemnation and ridicule.

Social

The nurse should never assume that, because the client is grossly disorientated, what could be perceived as more complex needs do not exist. The need for pride, dignity and independence is high in all of us, but possibly more so in the elderly. The fear of losing these must be very distressing, and it is therefore up to the nurse to be sensitive to this and provide every opportunity for the individual to maintain independence, through which pride and dignity can be maintained. By a careful choice of activities the nurse can generate some course of usefulness in the client, thus avoiding possible isolation. It is a common mistake to underestimate people's insight and capabilities, especially when they are living with those whose orientation is limited to the vague acknowledgement of their surroundings. It must be stressed that each individual must be cared for on his own merits.

IMPLICATIONS FOR THE NURSE

When caring for the elderly, the nurse is confronted with the reality of 'human decay'. The progressive deterioration of these clients is inevitable, and no matter what the nurse's interventions may be she cannot change this. This may cause feelings of helplessness and despondency in the nurse, and may even progress to questioning the futility of maintaining this quality of life. There are serious ethical questions that the nurse must personally explore until a value can be found that is conducive to the maintenance of life and enhancing the quality that remains, by dedicated and skilful care. The dangers of working in this area without exploring and coming to terms with the reasons and personal demands may be reflected in the nurse's approach to her clients. She may, as a defence, withdraw emotionally and deal with her clients in a mechanical and impersonal way, without the 'giving' that is essential in any therapeutic relationship. It only takes one or two individuals with this sort of attitude to have a negative effect on a whole residential community. It is particularly important that morale is maintained as high as possible, so that an air of hopeful optimism can be reflected on to the clients.

No matter how well staffed residential care or mental health units are, the physical and psychological demands made upon the nurse are considerable. The pressure of dealing with the essential needs of clients and working in a team aiming to finish in time for another event to start, i.e. being constrained by the unit routine, increases the likelihood of nurses taking short cuts and sacrificing their quality of care for the number of tasks completed. Ensuring adequate staffing levels and using an individualized nursing care approach will help minimize the risk of this occurring. However, in reality we live in a society where care of the elderly will always be given limited resources, partly because of the ever-growing demand but also because of the lack of importance and value we give to our ageing population. Despite what often seems a gloomy picture, nurses can and do gain tremendous satisfaction from caring for the elderly confused, as illustrated in this quote from a student nurse writing about her experience with the elderly:

> The last three months have instilled in me a new sense of tolerance, responsibility of care, and knowledge which I hope will continue to grow in me. I almost feel guilty because I have got so much out of this experience, and if I have given a part of what I have taken, then I think I have justified my stay there. (Anne, 1982)

PRINCIPLES AND SKILLS REQUIRED

The major areas of skills necessary to care for the elderly confused effectively are non-verbal, verbal, psychomotor, group and management skills.

Non-verbal skills

The nurse must utilize every personal asset she has to enhance communication with the client. This involves the effective use of non-verbal skills: talking in a tone of voice that is conducive to his hearing, which does not necessarily mean intensity; enhancing contact by the appropriate use of touch; listening face to face, with eye contact; being close, with an open posture; and leaning towards the client all show non-verbally that the nurse cares and wants to be involved.

Verbal skills

Verbal skills encourage the client to communicate through his confusion. The nurse must allow the client to express his fear and desires no matter how confused they are, and at the same time she must be sensitive to his feelings and needs. The verbal skills are those related to specific questioning, clarifying and giving repetitive explanations. These must be exercised without patronizing, for it is easy to fall into the mistake of playing the role of parent as opposed to helper.

Psychomotor skills

If one were to analyse the physical tasks involved in caring for someone who was virtually helpless, they would vary from the large movements of lifting to the intricacies of applying a sterile dressing. Indeed, the role of the mental health nurse can seem diverse, but the common factor when carrying out these psychomotor skills is the attitude of the nurse and the manner in which they are conducted. Whenever a physical task is performed, be it feeding the client or assisting him to the toilet, there is always a need for the use of appropriate verbal and non-verbal skills in order to facilitate socialization.

Group skills

Group skills involve being aware of the needs and abilities of each individual within the group and coming up with a formula that will be sufficient to facilitate a common interest. With the elderly confused the common denominator is often the past, mainly because that part of memory is often more intact than the recent, and it leaves them with a sense of reality. Reminiscence therapy is conducted as a part of 'reality orientation'. Other group activities related to reality orientation serve this purpose of socialization well, and at the same time stimulate and help maintain the client's usage of resources at its maximum.

Management skills

Most relevant management skills are related to being in control of the environment. Besides the essential management of resources, i.e. manpower and facilities, there are specific skills involved in making the most of limited resources to the benefit of orientating the elderly confused. By utilizing the skills of the care team it is possible to create an environment which is bright, colourful, functional and clean. The sensible positioning of signs and the use of any aid to reinforce reality will help orientate confused residents, e.g. calendars, clocks, menus, activities sheets, directional arrows and nameplates are all materials that can be used in a continual reality orientation programme.

SUMMARY

As our residential care homes and long-stay elderly units become filled with our ageing population, the demands made upon the personal resources of the nurse increase. As the elderly progressively deteriorate, the skills to cope with this become stretched. It requires tremendous dedication and application to care for those that require so much yet who appear to many to give so little. Yet they do give: they give with their eyes, their touch, their smiles and their confused acknowledgements of gratitude. And, who knows, there may be more going on in those minds than we think. Therefore, let us assume the best possible state rather than the least; after all, we will be old ourselves one day.

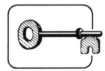

KEY CONCEPTS

1. The progressive loss of contact with reality, highlighted by intellectual, emotional and memory disturbances, is a manifestation of dementia.
2. This severe memory disturbance results in a major manifestation of confusion, i.e. disorientation in time, place and person.
3. It is imperative that when assessing these clients priorities are taken into consideration and the best use of resources is made.
4. There is a need to pay particular attention to all the essential needs of the elderly confused, because each one is at risk from self-neglect due to the incapacitating nature of the 'dementing' state.
5. It is not surprising that many elderly confused clients are agitated and distressed, for they are living in a world of strange places and faces, not knowing why they are there yet being helpless to do anything about it.
6. When caring for the elderly, serious ethical questions must be explored until a value can be found that is personally acceptable and conducive to the maintenance of life and enhancing the quality that remains by dedicated and skilful care.
7. The skills required to nurse the elderly effectively are:
   - verbal and non-verbal skills that enhance communication;
   - psychomotor skills that involve physical contact and are used to satisfy the physiological human needs;
   - group skills to enhance socialization and potentiate remaining memory and reality;
   - management skills to create an environment that minimizes the chances of confusion and enhances reality orientation.

FURTHER READING

Barton, M.A. (1983) Reaching the patient (nursing elderly patients with dementia). *Geriatric Nursing*, **4**(4), 234–6.

Browne, K. (1984) Confusion in the elderly. Nursing: the add-on. *Journal of Clinical Nursing*, **2**(24), 698, 700–2, 704–5.

Chenitz, C. (1983) The nurse's aide and the confused person. *Geriatric Nursing*, **4**(4), 238–41.

Easterbrook, J. (ed) (1987) *Elderly Care: Towards Holistic Nursing*, Edward Arnold, London.

Holden, U. and Woods, R.T. (1982) *Reality Orientation: Psychological Approaches to the 'Confused' Elderly*, Churchill Livingstone, Edinburgh.

Hollingham, P. A. (1990) *Care for the Elderly*, Penguin, Harmndsworth.

Mitchell, R. G. (1983) Confusion (causes and treatment). *Nursing Times*, 13 April, 62–64.

Scrutton, S. (1989) *Counselling Older People: a Creative Approach to Ageing*, Edward Arnold, London.

Wolanin, M.O. and Phillips, L.R. (1981) *Confusion: Prevention and Care*, Mosby, London.

16 Working with people who are dying

This chapter seeks to share with you our strong convictions that nursing the dying client can be a rewarding and insightful experience. Understanding the stages of dying is only the beginning of a whole area of study we believe the mental health nurse is most appropriately qualified to undertake. It is included in this text because we feel it is an area offering potential personal growth through self-awareness, and contains within it some essential principles and skills which ought to be within the mental health nurse's repertoire.

It has been observed by Kubler-Ross (1978) that people pass through stages of dying. These stages are extremely important for nurses to understand if good care and skilled interactions are to be implemented with dying clients. The five stages most commonly observed are denial, anger, bargaining, depression and acceptance.

Although these stages follow a generally accepted sequential order, it should be pointed out that individual clients may not necessarily follow them in sequence. It is quite possible for a client to experience denial after depression, for example, or anger after depression. Some clients may appear to have reached the final stage of acceptance, and still regress to depression or anger from time to time. It is an extremely useful guide to the process of mental adaptation to the concept of death, but the point we are stressing is that it is not an immovable, inflexible progression.

We are suggesting that it is the skilled nurse's job to enable the client to work through these states whenever they occur, towards acceptance, at his own pace, with as little trauma as possible and as constructively as possible. Each stage of the process is a normal healthy reaction, and should never be considered otherwise. However, to be fixed in any one stage is not only unhelpful but may also be counterproductive to the natural healing processes that lead to a peaceful natural death.

The observant nurse used to dealing with the terminally ill client is able to recognize each stage and be prepared for the behaviour associated with it. The person who may be involved with informing clients that they have a terminal illness may be regarded as courageous, but because the mechanism of denial is usually the initial response to such news, seldom is this person confronted with more than stunned silence or incongruent laughter. The disbelief of the reality of oncoming death is far more likely in most clients than sorrow or depression.

Anger, on the other hand, is commonly directed at the nurse, professional carer or close relative. The feelings of the client are actively focused on the unfairness of his dying when others far less deserving are to remain alive. The sudden insight into the things undone and unsaid, the appreciation of all the wonderful people, places, aromas, sensations, tastes and activities that he is to be deprived of is unbearable. Why him? What, after all, has he done to deserve this? It is not hard to imagine our own indignation and anger to appreciate this stage of the dying process. It is probably in this stage that most unresolved anxiety occurs. This does not necessarily reflect only the fear of physical pain, but also the emotional pain. How difficult it must be to have the constant reminder every day that before long you will never see your children, your wife or your home again. This is a continual torment, raising anxieties that cannot be quelled and anger that cannot in justice be directed at anyone or anything. This mixture of anger and anxiety is extremely difficult to deal with, for the intensity of the injustice potentiates the anger and the intensity of the anger prevents any action taking place. This in turn creates anxiety, which maintains the inactivity. However, as anxiety is usually a self-limiting phenomenon most people break out of this vicious circle and progress to bargaining.

Bargaining is the person's first attempt to control the events that appear to have overtaken him. Some method of action is needed to buy time to undertake all the things undone, unseen and unsaid. The only course open to the client is to make bargains with himself, his God and his beliefs that he will be better, not make the same mistakes, or make amends in some way if only he can be granted more time. Although this may sound somewhat unrealistic, almost like fighting reality with fantasy, it is in our opinion a very constructive stage. The realization that time to act is the thing that really matters, to contemplate in fact what the time is really for, and how best each second can be maximized is what leaves the client able to go on. Nurses are often involved in bargaining, and in many cases they may be distressed by questions – sometimes almost desperate pleas – of: 'If I give up smoking now, nurse, will I live long enough to...? Is there anything I can do to just hang on long enough to...?'

It is our belief that these questions should not be shrugged off but dealt with seriously and honestly, no matter how painful this may be for both parties. Without honesty from professionals, how are the terminally ill ever going to be able to make plans of a realistic nature and make purposeful choices?

Depression may be the beginning of a fatalistic, although angry, acceptance that whatever happens, or whatever the individual tries, death is inevitable. If the bargaining stage has been short-lived, then the depressive stage may be longer. This could be due to the reflective thought and analysis that are usually dealt with previously, but now have to occur under the realization of depressive finality. However, if a lengthy bargaining process has taken place the depressive aspects may be very short. It is our assumption that it is inevitable that reflective thought in either stage will more often than not result in the same conclusion: if death is inevitable for everyone, but I have the knowledge of how soon mine is to be, I have an advantage in being able to use what's left of my time constructively. I intend to waste none of it on regrets, but spend all of it purposefully, usefully and to the full.

This, as Kubler-Ross suggests, is 'the final stage of growth'. This final stage of acceptance can be viewed as the most meaningful insight life has given the individual. Many clients share with nurses the realization that it is only with the approach of death that they have learned to appreciate life. To learn how to live, to live one day at a time, to appreciate everything, every experience, as if it may be their last, is indeed worthwhile. How many of us would be able to say, if we were struck down today, that we have no unfinished business to complete? For instance:

- Would my children know I loved them?
- Would I have said sorry for the things I've done and left undone?
- Will the loved ones I leave behind understand how unhappy I would be if they grieved for me?

Perhaps when we consider the advantages the terminally ill client may have in dealing with these issues – albeit having this thrust upon him – we would refrain from pitying him lest we forget to learn from him.

The elderly client may have very similar stages to progress through, although it is generally accepted that there is less anger and the first stage of acceptance is reached more readily. It may be presupposed that your entire life could be considered as the whole process through the stages: in youth and adolescence death is ignored, denied; the concept of death in middle age is met with anger and bargaining; in the elderly progressing towards death is a depressing finality, but with much more emotional contentment, stability and fulfilment of unfinished business, acceptance is more commonly seen. This analogy may perhaps clarify why the death of children and young adults has such a profound effect on nurses. Yet especially in children, the anxiety, despair and anger we feel is not necessarily shared by the client. The concept of fear associated with death is in some ways a learned behaviour, for until this century death was not such a taboo subject. Even today, many cultures and societies do not treat death as such a terrible and apprehensive finality. To transfer our anxieties on to children may be seen as an unnecessary burden on them, and to discuss death openly and frankly may be a policy worth careful consideration.

Nurses dealing with terminally ill children are invited to reflect on these words written by Kubler-Ross (1978):

> It is hoped that all the children of our next generation will be permitted to face the realities of life. It is hoped that we will not 'protect' them as a reflection of our own fears and our own anxieties! It is hoped that we adults are beginning to have the courage to realize that it is our fear that we project on to the next generation. Once we have courage enough, we can acknowledge honestly that there are problems, and we can solve them if we have someone who cares and who facilitates the expression of our fears and guilt and unfinished business. If we can do this, we can empty our pool of repressed negativity and start living fully and more harmoniously.

Children who have been exposed to these kinds of experiences - in a safe, secure and loving environment – will then raise another generation of children who will, most likely, not even comprehend that we had to write books on death and dying and had to start special institutions for the dying clients; they will not understand why there was this overwhelming fear of death, which for so long covered up the fear of living.

PROBLEMS AND NEEDS OF THE DYING CLIENT

The client who is terminally ill requires skilled nursing of a very high standard. Although the physical care of each client may be completely and effectively dealt with, it is not uncommon to see the psychological care that is, in our opinion, so important, largely overlooked. Years of controversy surround the principal issue of whether the client should be told when he is diagnosed as having an incurable disease. We would pre-empt this debate by asking how we will know whether he even wants to know, if we do not take time to find out? Most nursing approaches that fail do so because the nurse fails to appreciate the needs, values and wishes of the client. Never is this factor more pronounced than when nursing the terminally ill. Nurses and doctors who consider it their role to cure appear to feel personally guilty, lacking in some way, perhaps a failure, when confronted by a client they are unable to 'cure'. Often the error they commit is to defend their position by avoidance and pretence, rather than facing issues and dealing with them effectively. They may not be able to cure, but they are most certainly able to help if they are possessed with sufficient personal resources and the requisite caring attitudes.

It is our hypothesis that the dying client requires the following:

- Honesty from his carers;
- Permission to grieve for his impending loss;
- Support to work through the stages of dying;
- Information that is as accurate as possible to enable realistic plans and goals to be formulated;
- To be part of the decisions made about him; at least, to be allowed to voice his opinions on issues that concern him personally, e.g. where he is to be nursed; whether his life should be prolonged (use of antibiotics); how alert he should be in contrast to how much sedative/pain relievers he may need/want;
- A knowledge of how his death/dying is affecting the emotions of other humans around him – not only his relatives and friends but also the professionals caring for him;
- To be able, should he choose, to discuss in an open climate how he feels about his death. To have around him at his death the people he wants in attendance.

In simple terms, to die with dignity.

IMPLICATIONS FOR THE NURSE

Should all clients be told fully about their illness when it is of a terminal nature? Some clients already know but simply want concrete affirmation. Some demand to know and others do not wish to know at all. In fact, the latter will employ denial whether you tell them or not, so it may not even matter. In the final analysis all clients will know, whether 'officially' informed or not; it is usually only a question of timing.

So, when should clients be told? The answer is, when they want to be told. If the nurse is a skilled listener, has formed an empathic bond with the client and cares, the client will indicate when he is ready to be told. If, on the other hand, the nurse does not form a meaningful rapport, she will be constantly avoiding contact as she carries a dreadful fear of being asked 'Am I going to die, nurse?' The nurse who really listens to her client and understands him will know, when this question is asked, whether it is an honest request requiring a realistic answer or whether it is a plea for reassurance and hope. Either requires a skilful answer, but it is our contention that the deeper the relationship the easier that skill becomes. Attesting to this concept, Kubler-Ross (1978) cites an unidentified social worker, quoted by Wahl, as saying:

> I know he wanted to talk to me, but I always turned it into something light, a little joke or some evasive reassurance which had to fail. The client knew and I knew, but as he saw my desperate attempts to escape, he took pity on me and kept to himself what he wanted to share with another human being. And so he died and did not bother me.

This, we suggest, is a typical example of how fragile our own emotions surrounding death may be. The client in this case is so strong and the professional so weak that it would seem right to pity us from his position. Maybe this strange reversal of role epitomizes the powerful influences that occur in the knowledge of one's own finiteness.

To be successful at caring for the dying, the nurse should have fully explored her own feelings about death. How does she feel about her own mortality; does she pity the client through a raging fear of her own death; or can she be peaceful and confident in the knowledge that dying is only a final stage of life? Looking closely at how we feel about death may not be pleasant, but is a realistic option that a self-aware professional may need to take. It may answer many questions about how we behave with the dying client:

- Do we identify the death of a child with the prospect of losing our own children? Is this why we react so violently on these occasions?
- Do we falsely reassure the dying client, not to comfort him, but to comfort ourselves?
- Do we shun the subject of death so readily because it upsets people, or because the subject is so close to our only personal certainty?
- Do we feel that to be open and honest about death is in some way tempting fate; that talking about it will hasten our own?

If even some of this strikes chords of recognition, then perhaps it is not difficult to understand why dying clients are 'screened off', or nursed in side wards, have minimum contact from very 'busy' nurses, and that the chat we've been meaning to have with Mr Jones never materializes.

It may be helpful to you at this point to know that we are not implying criticism of the nursing care currently employed with terminally ill clients. We are stating that in our past professional careers we have used avoidance and pretence, and are now so unhappy with our performance in the light of new insight that we hope to enable others to see a better, more effective way of caring.

Often difficult situations make an honest and open relationship almost impossible. It is important that these situations are dealt with effectively to maximize effective care. One example is when relatives express a wish that the client should not be told of the terminal nature of his illness. This situation is extremely difficult, and may need some time to be resolved. Although it is unwise to generalize, we wish to emphasize that anything which interferes with the nurse–client relationship may reduce its effectiveness and value. The relatives need to be made aware of the significance of their wishes. They need to be told that to be dishonest in an attempt to shield the client may significantly reduce the quality of care that he will receive, not, perhaps, physically but in the psychological support he could be offered. It can be pointed out that denying the client information will rob him of his independence, the ability to plan and to finish off his life's business. They should be asked how they will cope with direct questions from the client, and how their attempts to shield him will affect their relationship. Finally, they may be asked what the nurse should say if asked about discharge, test results and similar difficult questions. Although this may seem rather hard on relatives, it should be remembered that they are in fact taking responsibility for an individual, so they should know what this entails. In the light of lucid explanations and insight, the implications of their often ill-considered wishes may make them change their minds. When a relative is adamant, the nurse may offer an undertaking not to inform the client directly, but we believe it would be most unwise to guarantee non-disclosure, when in her professional judgement it may be in the client's best interests.

It is our belief that this approach will generally prove effective in situations similarly difficult, such as with other nurses, senior professionals, medical officers and administrators. In principle, when a nurse is asked to be dishonest with a client a sacred trust may be broken, interfering with an empathic relationship, which in turn will detract from good care. We believe that when anyone interferes with good nursing practice they must be challenged.

PRINCIPLES AND SKILLS REQUIRED

Denial

When information is given to clients which confirms the terminal nature of their illness, but their reactions seem to contradict this, it is reasonable to assume that some degree of denial is taking place. The nurse's interactions should not change during this stage, and she should continue to be honest and open and to work towards the client. Sometimes difficulties exist when unrealistic goals are discussed; this may make the nurse uncomfortable and potentiate avoidance, so other strategies need to be employed. Take the following examples:

Client: 'When I go back to work I shall have a lot to catch up on. When the course of radiotherapy is finished, I'm going to try jogging again. If I can just put on some more weight, I'll regain my strength and go home.'

In theory the nurse should not reinforce the denial stage by playing along, but it is extremely difficult to dash a person's hopes and dreams to the ground, no matter how unrealistic they are. The example above may engender an extremely high charge of emotion within the nurse. It would be easy to be overwhelmed by a wave of sympathy or pity for the individual, and resolve it by simply replying, 'Yes, that's a good idea'. It would, however, be wrong of us to advocate this, as it would be wrong to condone the abrupt or brusque response: 'Don't be silly, you'll never be able to do that'. Instead, we would suggest that an honest yet empathic reply is more sensible and therapeutic:

Nurse: 'I can see you feel hopeful of being able to do that, and I would love to share your hope, but under the circumstances I wonder how realistic it is?'

This response has the advantage of not denying the client's feelings of hope, but neither does it reinforce his denial. It is not overtly sympathetic, which would distract the client from himself to perhaps feeling sorry for the nurse. It leaves a little scope for the client to shrug it off and continue denial if that is his need. Finally, and probably most powerfully, it shows the client that the nurse is not interested in pretence, but is prepared to be helpful and professional no matter how difficult and uncomfortable that makes her feel. This is a healthy beginning on which to base a future close, open and trusting relationship.

Anger

The terminally ill client has every right to be angry at the injustice in his life, After all, why should this happen to him? Why him? is the question that may continually torment him, for there appears to be no satisfactory answer to this inflicted frustration. There are so many things left to do; he should be angry at someone or something responsible for his misfortune. In logic there is no focus for this anger, so the client either projects it outwardly on to people around him, or inwardly to himself. The outward projection of anger is a profoundly more healthy reaction, as internalized anger tends to manifest itself as deep and intractable depression, which may result in premature and unnatural death in the form of suicide. The skilled nurse will therefore have to deal effectively with this anger, as she needs to be able to absorb it and accept it usefully. The client who learns the patience, tolerance and acceptance of his nurse also learns to trust her, disclose to her and share his final stage of growth with her. The nurse who has the qualities required to go through this stage with her client receives as her reward not only the trust of her client, but also an insight into how close a nurse and client can become. Contrary to popular belief, this does not make losing the client more difficult, but less traumatic, for there is no guilt to feel, only sadness at the natural passing of someone who was close.

So, how should the nurse facilitate the client venting his angry feelings? First she needs to identify them, and if she knows her client well she will identify anger in his tone of voice, facial expression, posture and the attitudes he is able to express. The nurse must somehow communicate her permission to the client, to be able to say, not necessarily verbally, that it's OK: 'I understand you're angry'; 'I understand your anger, and in some ways share it; if it's directed at me, that's OK too'; 'You have a right to be angry and it's better out in the open than simmering inside.'

Open statements which share the nurse's ideas should be openly discussed: 'I know you're feeling angry at everyone, I'm trying to understand and accept your bitterness, but unfortunately I'm human too, and I need you to tell me every so often that it isn't me personally and maybe release your anger in other ways.'

Knowing that you understand and are accepting his emotions may be very helpful to the client at this point. You may be able to show him ways of directing his energy into constructive areas, such as writing about the things that make him feel angry, or talking to others about how caring for the terminally ill could be better. Useful strategies simply to help the client dissipate his anger would include physical pursuits such as plasticine modelling, the use of a punchbag/pillow, ball games, art work (especially finger painting). If a client says, 'I just feel like shouting or screaming', the nurse may feel inhibited about encouraging this – after all, clients screaming in a ward would not help the confidence or peacefulness of other clients. Finding an appropriate place to facilitate this should not be completely dismissed, though, as this strategy may be most helpful for some clients. Most of these ideas will require tailoring to the individual client and institutional needs. Some clients may not be as mobile as others, some activities may only be appropriate for outdoors, and the latter requires either a soundproof room or a very isolated area.

Openly verbalizing and accepting the need to pass through this stage may in itself accelerate the process.

Bargaining

Clients will often involve nurses in bargaining, e.g.: 'If I stop smoking, will I have a few extra months, nurse?' The skilled nurse will attempt to make this rather vague statement more specific. A straight answer would probably be 'no', or at best a 'maybe'. A more empathic answer demonstrating the skill of concreteness may be the most helpful reply here: 'Am I right in thinking you're anxious because you may have less time left than you need, and stopping smoking is the one thing you think you have some control over?' Pause. 'I'm not really sure about the smoking, but perhaps it would be helpful to look at how best your time could be spent.'

These types of response may enable the client to make productive steps forward in this stage, and help him to see how best his 'bargain' with himself can be made. The vain hope of more time 'if I...' can be made productive by converting it to 'If I do... first then I may have time left for....'

Striking bargains with themselves, their God, or whatever else they believe in, is a necessary step towards acceptance. If the nurse is able to achieve something concrete from this stage, to develop plans and priorities, then we suppose she will do so through using the skills more fully dealt with in progressive responding (see p. 40).

Depression

Unlike clinical depression, which has roots in pathological mental functions, this stage of dying is the culmination of an emotional journey leading to an inevitable conclusion. Depression may be a short or a long stage, depending upon the personality of the individual and his environment. The skills the nurse requires in this stage are fully discussed in Chapter 6 on depression, but additionally she needs to be able to communicate the knowledge that this depression is not pathological but natural and normal. It is the client's grieving process for the loss he is about to experience. It is the quiet reflective stage, where there is no hope or denial, just the depths of despair in the knowledge that before long, life and all its values will be taken away. The nurse needs to spend time with the individual showing she cares, reassuring him by reflecting his strengths, his qualities and his resources, showing by her presence that he still has a lot to offer, that his wisdom, humour, smile, touch and conversation have a value to her and anyone else in contact with him. This can be emphasized by simply being with the client, holding his hand, smiling, making eye contact and with empathic and reinforcing verbal messages, e.g.: 'I know you feel down at the moment, but I do miss your smile'. 'You look really low today, it almost makes me feel sorry for you, but do you remember you said I should never do that?'

Or by gentle challenges: 'I remember you complaining a week or so ago that you had so little time, now you keep saying there's nothing left to do and you don't feel like doing anything. I'm a little puzzled.' This should not be an attempt to bludgeon him out of his depression or get him to 'pull himself together', but to remind him gently and continually that you are with him, that you trust and accept him, and that you have confidence in him. He will work through this stage.

Acceptance

When the client reaches acceptance the nurse's task is nearly complete. This is a time for listening to the client in order to share in his growth. He has reached the point where each new day is a bonus to be lived to the full, in the knowledge that death is inevitable and need hold no terrors. The unfinished business is completed and all that is left is to appreciate fully each precious second of life. Perhaps we may learn from the client that to value each moment as if it is our last is the secret of exploiting the full potential of our life.

The stages are not arbitrary barriers which need to be fully broken down and the spaces between them fully explored. There is bound to be a blurring between stages. The nurse should always expect the unexpected: anger to occur in denial; some denial in bargaining and so on. The principal skill in helping the dying client must always be an empathic acceptance and an awareness of needs.

Finally, an important factor in caring for the dying client is the acknowledgement of hope. Hope in the denial stage has been considered, along with the need to balance hope and the inevitable reality of death without crushing the energy that hope brings. Once the client has accepted his own inevitable death, hope can be seen from other perspectives. Egan (1994) tells us to listen to our clients for an echo of hope. This may sound fine in the physically healthy, with no immediate threat to life, but it is an equally important consideration in the care of the dying. The skilled nurse will have developed the appropriate antennae for eliciting the client's hopes, which may be to have a pain-free day, see their daughter married or to enjoy the flowers of spring. If these hopes are realistic, then the nurse may foster the energy that they bring and celebrate it with the client and their family. Many clients will feel helped by a belief in God and life beyond physical death, perhaps seeking and benefiting from pastoral care. Those without firm religious beliefs can also be helped by enabling them to share their views and the forces and values which have driven them throughout their lives, their construal of life, or their belief system, e.g. pacifism, socialism, humanism and so on. The nurse is in a strong and privileged position to explore these personal and spiritual dimensions in a non-judgemental and caring way.

In current times few people suffering from a terminal illness die at home, but for those who choose to be cared for in this way, in familiar surroundings and in the midst of a loving family, peaceful death can be achieved. Macmillan, Marie Curie and District Nurses are highly skilled in the holistic care of the dying and their families, particularly with the ever-increasing developments in pain control making a significant reduction on the need for hospital or hospice care. It is an excellent reflection on good practice that these nurses often continue to support families following the death, and help them further on their bereavement journeys.

SUMMARY

The principles and skills of nursing the dying client are to:

- Own your own feelings about death;
- Understand the stages of death;
- By not avoiding contact, achieve an honest, open relationship based on a mutual empathic understanding;
- Be able to make concrete the client's vague plans, and thereby control anxieties within him;
- Avoid robbing the client of his independence, overcompensating for your own feelings and giving false reassurances;
- Support the client through the stages of dying by communicating the client's resources, strengths and your own confidence in him;
- Through your experience and knowledge, to facilitate the venting of his emotions by whatever strategies are available and appropriate;
- Continue to listen, accept and learn to understand the client and grow from this learning.

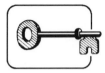

KEY CONCEPTS

1. It is extremely important to understand the stages of dying if good care and skilled interactions are to be implemented with clients who are dying.
2. The observant nurse used to dealing with terminally ill clients is able to recognize each stage and is prepared for the behaviour associated with each.
3. Realization that death is inevitable and imminent may facilitate appreciation of life.
4. The concept of fear associated with death is in some ways a learned behaviour.
5. To transfer our own anxieties on to children could be viewed as an unnecessary burden to them.
6. Most nursing approaches that fail do so because the nurse does not appreciate the needs, values and wishes of the client.
7. To be successful at caring for the dying, the nurse should have fully explored her own feelings about death.
8. Anything that interferes with the nurse–client relationship may reduce its effectiveness and value.
9. A person interfering with good nursing practice should be challenged, whoever they may be.
10. Be prepared to help the client sustain hope when it is realistic. Be facilitative in enabling the client to express his belief system, undertaking this in an accepting and non-judgemental way.

FURTHER READING

Caughill, R. E. (1976) *A Dying Patient: a Supportive Approach*, Little, Brown, Boston.

Corr, C. A. and Donna, M. (1983) *Hospice Care: Principles and Practice*, Faber and Faber, New York.

Dickeson, D. and Johnson, M. (1993) *Death, Dying and Bereavement*, Open University, Sage Publications, London.

Herth, K. (1993) Hope in the family care giver of terminally ill people. *Journal of Advanced Nursing*, 18, 538–48.

Kubler-Ross, E. (1970) *On Death and Dying*, Prentice-Hall, Englewood Cliffs, New Jersey.

Kubler-Ross, E. (1975) *Death. The Final Stage of Growth*, Prentice-Hall, Englewood Cliffs, New Jersey.

Kubler-Ross, E. (1978) *To Live Until We Say Goodbye*, Prentice-Hall, Englewood Cliffs, New Jersey.

Nursing Times (1978) *Care of the Dying*, 2nd edn, Macmillan, London.

Stedeford, A. (1984) *Facing Death, Patients, Families and Professionals*, William Heinemann Medical Books, London.

Thompson, I. (ed) (1979) *Dilemmas of Dying: a Study in the Ethics of Terminal Care*, Edinburgh University Press, Edinburgh.

17 Working with people experiencing bereavement

Pain is inevitable in such a case and cannot be avoided. It stems from the awareness of both parties that neither can give the other what he wants. The helper cannot bring back the person who is dead and the bereaved person cannot gratify the helper by feeling helped. No wonder both seem dissatisfied with the encounter. (Murray-Parkes, 1976)

Raymond's face contorted into a painful but controlled grimace, as he forced inside him the emotions he was violently wishing to suppress. He reached out for the chair arm and sat down, as if his legs could no longer bear his weight. His head bent forward and his hands seemed to come up only just in time to catch it. Colour began to return to his knuckles, which until now had been almost continually clenched. The charge nurse repeated his statement as if he were unsure that he had been heard: 'I'm very sorry, there was nothing we could do, your father was already dead when the ambulance arrived in casualty.' There was something similar to panic and confusion inside Raymond's head – he felt so many emotions he had not realized it was possible to feel at the same time. He felt like shouting angrily, but there seemed no point; he felt like crying, but what would that achieve? Perhaps it was a mistake, perhaps they'd got it all wrong, but he knew this was only a vain hope. He continued to feel angry, afraid, confused, yet dulled, somehow numb. He began to realize that he was behaving strangely, rocking backwards and forwards in the armchair, and now acutely aware that the charge nurse was still standing over him. 'What can I do?' he thought, 'I'm expected to do something, say something, but I can't, I don't want to, I don't know what to do.' 'I'm sorry, it's such a shock. I'll be OK in a moment, just give me a little time, I'll be OK. Thank you', was all he could manage. It seemed so feeble but it took tremendous effort just to get those few words out. 'I'll leave you for a while then', said the charge nurse, quietly closing the interview room door. The charge nurse had undertaken this task many times before, but it never quite became routine and he was, as always, relieved to leave the room.

Raymond's response to being informed of his father's death could be viewed as reasonably typical, but every individual will react differently. Within the first few minutes of hearing news of a death of a close relative, any of the potential emotions of grief – shock, disorganization, denial, depression, guilt, anxiety, aggression and acceptance (see p. 204) – may be evoked. Any nurse who has been exposed to bereaved relatives will know the sense of helplessness and the anxiety that is always around in such situations. Being prepared for the variations in behaviour of grief-stricken people may help the inexperienced nurse cope more effectively. Probably the most unexpected response is that of anger and resentment directed at the nursing and medical staff. This response, although not common, usually follows the initial shock, and is generally an attempt to resolve feelings of guilt that may be associated with the death. The fact that the bereaved was not present at the time of death, has in some way not fulfilled promises, has not said or done things they feel they should have, may result in this guilt being projected on to the unfortunate person present. 'Why didn't you make it clear he might die?' 'Why didn't you phone me sooner?' 'Why did you let him die?' can be expressed most violently and can be very distressing to the unprepared nurse.

Frank denials and disorganization can be difficult to deal with in ward situations: the relative who simply refuses to believe the news and insists on visiting the deceased; or the bereaved person who becomes so distraught, confused and distressed that the nurse is right to fear for their personal safety. To allow a person to leave the premises in such a mental state may be foolhardy, and all attempts to dissuade the individual from leaving should be made until they have recovered from the shock.

It is also appropriate to bear in mind that some other circumstances may parallel bereavement behaviour. A person may suffer similar emotional trauma and behavioural extremes when going through divorce proceedings, unemployment, when informed of some chronic illness process, loss of a limb or other bodily part, or when burdened with sudden responsibility in adolescence. It should be remembered that it is just as feasible to grieve the loss of a spouse, a job, health or childhood as it is the death of a close person. The factor common to all these losses is our attachment to them, which can be seen as both physiological and psychological. Bowlby (1980) suggests that the nature and degree of the attachment is significant when considering the depth or magnitude of the grief.

It may, then, be reasonable to assume that many causes of reactive depression are associated with a loss of some important or valuable asset in the individual's life. Many middle-aged and elderly individuals grieve for their lost fertility and youth long before they grieve the death of someone close to them. The bereaved individual may be seen in many disguises and manifesting very different behaviours; the skilled nurse is able to detect the grieving process, understand it and deal with it appropriately.

It is useful to consider the term 'grief' and to place it in context with two other commonly used terms, mourning and bereavement. Grief is a highly intense feeling of suffering, with well defined cross-cultural, psychological and physical characteristics. Grief is consistent across peoples, and as such is arguably a universal experience. Grieving can, however, be significantly shaped by the process of mourning. This is far more culturally determined, often with prescribed ritualistic patterns of behaviour which are socially accepted as normal. Since we now live in a far more culturally enriched society, it is important that as nurses we are aware and respectful of differing ways of mourning. Bereavement describes the person's total loss experience and encompasses both grief and mourning.

THE NEEDS OF THE BEREAVED

As Raymond portrayed, the essential need of a bereft individual is time – time to adjust and come to terms with a significant loss. Many people are tortured by anxiety feelings following the death of a spouse, largely due to fear of the unknown. Tasks and responsibilities that they now face, which have previously been dealt with by the deceased, are now barriers to their peace of mind. There now exists a vacuum, an empty place, which somehow has to be filled. There may well be much resistance to this initially, which may create additional difficulties. For example, the widow with a young family to care for may need help from the eldest child to take some of the burden of everyday life away from her. Simple tasks like babysitting, washing up and minor domestic chores that her husband may have helped with may now be displaced on to the elder children. This may make her feel inadequate or guilty for asking 'too much' of her children. It is often these very practical issues, and the subsequent emotional intensity that they stimulate, that prevent the individual coming to terms with a loss. The mental equilibrium of the individual needs to stabilize sufficiently to enable a rational appraisal of the situation and acceptance that life is going to be different. There will be difficulties to overcome, and to succeed in overcoming them vacuums have to be filled. There will be new people to meet, different approaches to consider and substitutes to be made. To reach this rational stage effectively, the individual must have dissipated her anger for the unfairness of her loss, shed the guilt that is implicit in most bereavement situations, and begun to accept her anxiety as a real thing and focus it upon tangible problems. Sadness and depression take a great deal of time to ease, but they will be more speedily dissipated when tangible issues are worked on. When practical issues begin to be solved, the collateral influences on mood are removed and depression may lift much more quickly. For example, when a person is very anxious about the future without her deceased husband, whether she can cope, and additionally becomes upset and confused when she remembers past encounters, a vicious circle exists which somehow must be broken. First steps may be to ensure the person is having a reasonable amount of sleep, eating a reasonable diet and generally looking after herself. This may sound trite or obvious, but a meal, a hot bath, a change of clothes and a good night's sleep are good starting points for solving problems. Sorting out priorities, resources and possibilities may require some assistance from friends, relatives or neighbours, but generally these are fundamental beginnings for bereaved individuals to refashion their lives.

It is important to remember that the grieving process takes time, and that it is a natural process which cannot be rushed. It may take many months, and possibly up to two years, for a bereaved person to return to 'normal' life. If people are given the right constructive help to deal with their emotions and practical problems, we believe this time will be usefully spent and fewer people will suffer pathological grief syndromes later on.

IMPLICATIONS FOR THE NURSE

The nurse should be able to appreciate the emotions and likely behaviour that the bereaved relatives of her clients may be experiencing. She should not shy away from difficult emotions with the bereaved, but facilitate their expression and deal with them effectively. To be able to do this, the nurse may have to consider how she would cope with a personal bereavement and the difficulties she might encounter. Even for the nurse who has suffered a bereavement, it is useful to look again at the needs she had and how best these were fulfilled. We must, however, urge one caution with this approach – what may have been right for the nurse should always be tempered with empathy for the unique individual being helped. The nurse should not develop one inflexible or stereo-typed approach, but be aware that individuals have different needs and require different responses. Many times we have been asked how a relative should be told of a person's death. There is, of course, no simple answer: the skilled nurse will know how best to handle the situation. The charge nurse in the origi-nal illustration favoured the 'tell them and leave them approach'. This may be a good method for some individuals, but to observe relatives' reactions and see how much support, discussion, debriefing or privacy they require and act accordingly would be a more flexible model. Similarly, there is no 'safe' way to actually say that the person has died.

Some people will be upset by euphemisms such as 'passed away', and most by a blunt 'Mr Brown is dead'. This perhaps is why 'I'm not sure how to break this news to you' is favoured by many. It allows for the relative to respond with whatever euphemisms they wish. The old joke 'Take one step forward all you soldiers who think you've got a father', said the sergeant; 'Where do you think you're going to, Brown?' shows how one imaginative mind focused on telling bad news. We do not recommend this, but it does illustrate that the most difficult and serious tasks become trivialized by humour in order to make them more acceptable to us. It also illustrates that breaking bad news should be envi-ronmentally planned if possible. A quiet room with an easy chair, where there will be no distractions from ringing phones or people coming in and out, is far more suitable than the parade ground or, for that matter, the middle of a dayroom or dormitory. The environment should at least offer a vehicle for privacy and appropriate support if necessary. Preferably, nurses involved in breaking bad news to relatives should arrange to have a sufficient amount of time to spend with them should the need arise.

It should also be noted that community staff tend to work more autonomously than their hospital counterparts, and that consequently direct access to support is not always possible. Working with the bereaved is not only highly satisfying, it is highly demanding. It exposes the nurse to a whole cock-tail of emotions that she may have to contain. As a consequence of this it is imperative that anyone working with this client group receive regular and skilled supervision (see Chapter 4). Within this process care should be taken to ensure that no personal material of the nurse is being 'revisited' by triggers in the client's disclosures. Thus if her work with the person creates distress for the nurse, there should be adequate opportunities for a thorough debriefing to alleviate this and ensure the continued effectiveness of the therapeutic process.

PRINCIPLES AND SKILLS REQUIRED

Information giving

The relatives will usually require certain information following a death: whether there is to be a postmortem, how to obtain a death certificate, collection of property and such like. It is unlikely that any relative in a distressed state will remember much of what is being said, so it is of great importance that the nurse considers what needs to be said verbally and what information should be in written form.

If at all possible, information should be given to friends, neighbours or other individuals not so closely involved. It should be the nurse's intention to help the bereaved, not to add to a burden by additional tasks at this time.

Occasionally relatives may ask very searching questions at this point: 'Did he die in pain?' 'Did he ask for me?' 'Who was with him?' Some of these questions require answers, others are purely rhetorical. In any event, the nurse confronted with them may feel very uncomfortable, for she will undoubtedly not have the answers to all of them – some may be unpalatable and she may be tempted to tell white lies. Almost stock phrases have crept into nursing vocabulary to cover these events, such as: 'He was made as comfortable as possible.' 'He didn't regain consciousness.' 'He didn't appear to be in pain and died quite peacefully.' These may not always be entirely honest, but are designed to ease the distress of relatives at a time when the harsh realities may be intolerable. We believe that nurses should always try to be honest and preserve the integrity of a relationship whenever possible, but using these particular euphemisms wisely and judiciously may in these circumstances be acceptable.

The relative who refuses to believe in the death of the person and becomes agitated and distressed may need very skilled handling. A firm but gentle approach is needed to restore a calm and genuine understanding of the situation. Generally such individuals exhibit an almost panic reaction and require appropriate nursing interventions. Firmly comforting the person with a guiding arm and directing them to a seat is usually effective, as is continuing to talk in a calm, soothing voice, saying 'Things will be OK', 'There's no cause for alarm', 'You simply need a little time', 'We are here to help you' and similar supportive statements. With this type of response it may be necessary to spend some considerable time counselling the person both before and after visiting the body, should this be the elected course of action. We believe that relatives who do visit the body, and are helped to release some emotions at this time, are generally benefited in the ensuing grieving process.

Interaction skills

The bereaved relatives will require essentially the basic skills of counselling (see Chapter 2):

- Attend – show the individual you care by listening attentively to what he has to say.
- Listen carefully to facts about the deceased so you can share important insights into his loss.
- Reflect – his emotions so he appreciates the complex emotional factors currently affecting him.
- Clarify – his confusion, contradictory beliefs, attitudes and emotions, so that both you and he can see discrepancies in self-blame, and anger at the death.
- Summarize – in the hope that a clearer picture of the entirety of the emotional components will enable a focus of action to be formulated.
- Challenge – or facilitate self-challenge when it is obvious that he is being too hard on himself and pursuing self-defeating strategies.

Customs and fashions change over time, and one in particular surrounding death is the custom of viewing the body. At one time nearly all funerals took place from the home, with the body lying in the front parlour. More recently, it has become the custom to leave the body in a 'chapel of rest' at the undertaker's premises. This distancing sometimes results in relatives and friends not visiting the body at all. We believe this is a crucial factor in the development of pathological grief syndromes and the precipitation of unnatural taboos concerning the cultural aspects of death. We sincerely believe that every effort should be made to give relatives and friends the opportunity to visit the body to say their final farewells in private. When the person dies in hospital or some similar institution, relatives should be offered a chance to see the body as soon as possible. It seems reasonable to prepare the body in the customary fashion – wash, shave, change linen, brush hair and remove any drips, tubes or other medical artefacts – before allowing visits. It certainly should not be a facility available exclusively in clinical morgues or chapels of rest, but if possible viewing should take place in the setting where death occurred. Nurses escorting relatives to visit a deceased client may skilfully 'model' emotional disclosure that may be beneficial to the bereaved. To illustrate this, the following life situation of one of the authors is described.

> Entering the side room, I saw my father lying on a bed with a sheet pulled up to his neck. His face was blanched and a little contorted as though his death had not been painless. He had obviously been dead for many hours. My brother stood by my side. His relationship with my father had not been as good as my own, and I knew he was feeling guilty and distressed over the death. I began by finding my father's hand and, holding it, I said, 'I'm sorry, father, I wasn't with you when you died, I should have spent more time with you and I feel very guilty now I look at your body lying there cold and lifeless, but I know you knew how much I loved you, and how much you were loved by everyone. I know you'll forgive me, so I'll say my final goodbye now.' My

brother listened to this, and as if enabled by my unembarrassed disclosure of emotion, broke down in tears, touched his father's hand and spoke to him with an open and tender emotion that had not occurred between them for many years.

A nurse cannot hope, on such a brief meeting with relatives, to have the same empathic understanding as a man may have for his brother, so it would perhaps not be appropriate or possible to facilitate so much emotion with relatives, who are after all largely strangers. It is, however, valuable to facilitate a monologue from the relative to the deceased client if possible. In a similar vein the nurse may speak to the client in the presence of the relatives before leaving, e.g.: 'I've brought your sons to see you to say goodbye – I'd like to say goodbye as well. I've nursed you for some weeks now and you've not complained. We all feel guilty that we could not have helped you more, but I think we did our best. We'll miss your smiling face. I'll leave you with your loved ones now.'

This might appear rather bizarre, embarrassing or even ridiculous, but it is designed to facilitate the release of emotions within the bereaved which may prove to be a healthy start to the grieving process. The nurse undertaking this modelling may well feel uncomfortable; she may even receive some odd looks from colleagues and relatives, but the potential good is a priceless gift to the bereaved person, who can benefit immensely. Following a visit to the deceased, the relatives should be seen again before they leave, to ensure they are coping adequately. The nursing skill here is listening to the emotional content of the bereaved and responding accordingly. Some relatives may be so distressed and unable to cope that they require referral to other agencies. Nurses should endeavour to have resources available for these eventualities: social worker, community nurse, family doctor, telephone numbers of friends or neighbours who may be helpful. National organizations such as CRUSE may be helpful in offering specialized counselling for the bereaved. Once the client has died, the nurse's overall responsibility shifts to the care of the relatives. This care may only be minimal or transient, but none the less it should be proficient – professional and efficient.

SUMMARY

1. The nurse needs an awareness of the stages of grieving in order to prepare herself for the potential emotional components of the interpersonal exchanges encountered in bereavement.
2. The nurse must be able to absorb anger directed towards herself or the institution, should this arise.
3. The nurse must have an ability to be patient, to allow emotions to be released and to listen and show empathy.
4. She should use her skills of non-verbal behaviour, especially touch, tone of voice and posture, to help the bereaved, especially if they are shocked, agitated and distressed.
5. Information given should be clear, and preferably written. It should be given to the person most likely to understand and employ it.

6. The nurse should not avoid the bereaved but give all the skills she has to them. This may include modelling 'debriefing emotions' with both the deceased and their relatives.
7. The nurse should have 'contingency resources' for referring distressed bereft individuals for continuing care.

KEY CONCEPTS

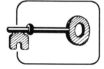

1. Once the client has died, the nurse's overall responsibility shifts to the care of the relatives.
2. It is important that the nurse does not shy away from difficult encounters with the bereaved. Every individual will react to traumatic news of a death in a different way.
3. The nurse should not develop one inflexible or stereotyped approach, but be aware that individuals have different needs and require different responses, and being prepared for this variation in the behaviour of grief-stricken people will help the inexperienced nurse cope more effectively.
4. The potential emotions of grief are shock, disorganization, denial, depression, guilt, anxiety, aggression and acceptance.
5. It should be remembered that the grieving process takes time and is natural.
6. It may be helpful to remember that some other circumstances may parallel bereavement behaviour, such as going through a divorce, unemployment or chronic illness.
7. It is often the very practical issues and the subsequent emotional intensity that they stimulate that prevent the individual coming to terms with a loss. For example, 'What am I going to do about bills, the funeral, my job, the children', etc.
8. Relatives who visit the body may require help to release some emotions at this time.
9. In connection with the latter, it follows that some relatives may be so distressed and unable to cope that they require referral to other agencies.

A BEHAVIOURAL PROPOSITION FOR DEALING WITH INTRACTABLE AND PATHOLOGICAL GRIEF: GRIEF THERAPY

Grief is a common component of human behaviour: it would be unusual, if not impossible, to go through life without at least one experience of grief. Additionally, it can be argued that there are degrees of grief. For example, the loss of a pet in the formative years of life may seem the end of the world to a child, while in later life the adult may well be upset but be more philosophical about the event. Losing your mother at the age of 96 may well be more acceptable than the sudden death of a spouse in a road traffic accident. The degree of grief relates directly to the suddenness, closeness and intensity of loss for each individual in any situation.

The mental health nurse will be familiar with death through both her professional contact – the client and his relatives – and unfortunately through the inevitability of being human, and her personal experiences and thoughts. Whichever is uppermost in her mind is unimportant, however. What is imperative is that she has an awareness of and an openness to her feelings about death. Before any therapy is attempted for the grieving person, the nurse/therapist must have a depth of understanding and an awareness of her own mortality and her own reactions in grieving situations, or at least an ability to control them.

Grief therapy, although one of the most potent of all behavioural strategies, is in our opinion one of the most traumatic and potentially hazardous. It would serve no good purpose whatsoever to have the nurse in a shattered emotional state as well as the client.

The basic concept that grief therapy is founded upon is that, as mentioned earlier, each individual progresses through a grieving process, which can be expressed in commonly recognized stages. It is thought that those people who remain in a grief-stricken state and subsequently exhibit symptoms of mental illness are those who have not progressed through these stages adequately. The following are the most commonly accepted as being the stages of grieving in more detail:

- *Shock:* The initial response to being told of a death. This may include physiological responses such as nausea, vomiting and fainting, or psychological traumas such as withdrawal, apathy, confusion or disinhibition.
- *Disorganisation:* An inability to think clearly, to arrange the simplest plan. Such disorganization often takes the form of ritualistic 'searching' behaviour.
- *Denial:* This is the complete disassociation of the knowledge of the death, an inability to believe, despite the facts. This is often like total amnesia for the event.
- *Depression:* Usually the result of denial breaking down and the finality of the knowledge sinking in, often accompanied by feelings of unworthiness, helplessness and poverty of ideas.
- *Guilt:* A component that no death can escape. Not only feelings of blame for the event, but also that the bereaved has survived.
- *Anxiety:* Often connected with coping without the deceased, not being able to control events, including fears for self.
- *Aggression:* From irritability to anger, directed not only towards yourself or significant others (i.e. doctors and nurses) but also to the deceased for having deserted you.
- *Acceptance:* Believing that all has been done that can be, saying a final goodbye, committing the deceased to memory and continuing with life.
- *Reintegration:* Restarting and eventually, perhaps, replacing, finding substitutes for the deceased and relegating the past and concentrating on the future.

The therapy proceeds on the premise that each of these stages needs to be worked through, but first it is important to be sure that therapy is appropriate. The therapy is traumatic, and as such, may have risks attached; it is therefore suggested that it be used only in severe cases of intractable grief. The natural grieving process can take anything up to two years, so at least this period should have elapsed before therapy is contemplated.

The process of therapy should be explained to the client in detail, making no pretence that it will not be painful, and stressing that it will require total co-operation with the nurse. There must exist a relationship of trust and one of high motivation on the part of the client to be free of grief.

Dr Ron Ramsey, who has researched and treated many clients in intractable grief syndromes, maintains that a specific contract should be drawn up, the main areas being as follows:

- The client must commit himself to complete the therapy.
- During the therapy he will not commit suicide.
- He will not physically assault the therapist.

Once this is achieved, the process somewhat artificially takes the client through the six most troublesome stages of grieving to move him quickly to the final process of reintegration, consequently resolving the grief.

The first stage the client is asked to consider is denial. This is done by confronting the facts. The nurse may use artefacts to aid this stage, such as the death certificate, newspaper notices, letters of condolence etc., asking questions such as 'How long has your child been dead?' 'Do you believe your child is dead?' and subsequently making statements for the client to repeat: 'My child is dead.' 'I will never see her again.' 'She has gone forever.' 'Her body is in the ground.'

Asking the client to read out loud the death certificate, the notice in the paper and letters may also be necessary. This brings about a cathartic reaction in the client and reinforces the facts to him. Although this appears very cruel and traumatic, its effect is to release the emotion, which is clearly important in the treatment. Furthermore, it may be necessary to help the client now physically to discard personal items used by the deceased – to throw away items such as soft (even favourite) toys or clothes, perhaps even a wedding ring in the case of a deceased spouse. This helps to consolidate the knowledge that they are not coming back, that he or she is not just away but dead. As may be imagined, this stage can be very distressing, and for both client and nurse it requires tenacity and perseverance.

It should also be noted that if the client blindly obeys without the release of emotion – sobbing, agitation and some resistance – the nurse should be suspicious that he has not indeed passed through denial, and continued effort must be maintained until such time as the nurse is sure the client has accepted the death. Once this denial has broken down, the client will be left in a state of depression and the nurse must try to support him through this.

A common misconception regarding supporting a depressive person is that the nurse should be sympathetic. In fact, related to behavioural principles, sympathy is a positive reinforcer: most people find sympathy rewarding, and therefore the great danger is to fix the depressed behaviour by this reinforcement. Certainly in grief therapy something much more productive than sympathy is required.

The nurse should in fact highlight the main areas of the emotional state for the client – to heighten awareness – then move on to a more productive phase. Empathic responses may help here, such as: 'You feel sad now because you now realize you have lost your child for good.' 'You feel helpless, perhaps even unworthy because you can't bring him back.' This empathic feedback will help maintain the trust and rapport between the nurse and the client, which could have been damaged during the first stage. The client should be encouraged to verbalize his feelings, but with positive supporting statements added to them, e.g.: 'I do feel helpless', then 'Yet this is quite normal, and I will get over this. I am capable of coming to terms with these feelings.' 'I do feel sad', then 'But I will get better.'

When the nurse is confident that the client is happy with these statements, progress should be made into the third stage: guilt.

It should be explained to the client that all humans are fallible, that to be perfect is impossible. There is no bereaved person who does not feel remorse in some way; even a saint will feel guilty after the death of a close one. He will still feel he could have done more, said things differently, expressed his emotions openly. This perhaps is the one thing that will help the client unlock the guilt he still has – 'It's not too late'.

It is our experience that the locked-in emotions of guilt are probably one of the most important factors in grief syndromes. The key to this lock is to facilitate the verbal expression of the things left unsaid. The nurse should seek some focus of contact with the dead person, a photograph, the graveside, whatever the client has that will help him to be in touch finally with the deceased. Prompts can be used, in fact modelled by the nurse at this point to facilitate this release, e.g.: 'I'm sorry for the things I could not do when you were alive.' 'I loved you very much – perhaps I didn't tell you just how much I loved you.' 'I'm sorry I wasn't able to say goodbye – but I'll say it now.' 'I miss you very much, but I have to get on with my life now - so goodbye.'

These verbalized emotions addressed to a photograph are very powerful indeed, and allow the final breakthrough for the client. It is always amazing just how much relief the client accomplishes from a session such as this.

If possible during this session, the final stages should be attempted. Using the same technique, any residual anger or aggression can be dissipated using statements such as: 'You hurt me so much when you left me.' 'I hated you when you died, leaving me with so much unsaid, so much undone, left me to cope.'

These verbalized expressions are usually enough to take the client up to the final stages of acceptance, leaving the nurse only to complete the treatment by reinforcing how much better he is feeling now he has resolved his grief, ending on positive statements for the client to practise, such as: 'Although I'll always remember you, you have to be part of my past now, I have my life to restart.' 'My husband/child/mother needs me now, I have to begin again.' There is no finer satisfaction than reaching this stage, and comparing the withdrawn and pathetic soul at the beginning of the therapy to the hopeful, refreshed client at the end. During the therapy the client and the nurse have lived through tremendous traumatic emotions, and at times they will both have had their doubts, but in practice the therapy is so powerful and successful that it will have proved to be most worthwhile.

It is impossible to state how long this therapy will take. For some clients it may take days only, for others much longer. This therapy should not deter neighbours, chaplains and voluntary organizations, e.g. CRUSE (national organization for bereaved families), helping individuals through bereavement counselling in less formal settings prior to admission to a mental health unit; we do not deny their importance, or detract from their success. However, so often in our experience clients with intractable grief syndromes are undiagnosed, and consequently unhelped. Clients suffering pathological grief are often admitted to mental health units or referred to community mental health nurses with varying degrees of depression. It is only when an empathic bond is built with the client that an accurate picture is revealed and the potential benefits of this therapy are realized. For this reason, it is our opinion that the therapist most able to carry out this technique is the community or residentially based mental health nurse. In any event, the person needs to be thoroughly conversant in behavioural principles and sound counselling techniques.

CONCLUSION

This chapter was intended to stimulate your interest in helping the bereaved relative or the client suffering grief in other, perhaps more covert, manifestations, e.g. divorce, amputation etc. It is hoped that the text, and the sharing of our personal insights and experience, have influenced you to undertake an intelligent and sensitive approach to bereaved people. Having introduced the concepts of grief, we ended the chapter with a behavioural programme specifically constructed to help clients suffering from pathological forms of grief. We cannot stress strongly enough that the introduction to grief therapy is not an open invitation to practise it. It must be clearly understood that grief therapy should be used only in states of protracted and pathological grief by an individual who is trained in behavioural techniques. It is our view that it would be most unwise to begin this therapy without consultation with the responsible medical practitioner, an established empathic relationship and the informed consent of the client. If these criteria are met, it is our belief that the therapy can produce remarkable benefits for the client, and should not be denied to those in need.

The dying client and the bereaved will always represent a consistent part of the mental health nurse's practice, and it is hoped that this chapter has in some small way helped you to help this client group further.

FURTHER READING

Bowlby, J. (1980) *Attachment and Loss, vol 3: Sadness and Depression*, Penguin, Harmondsworth.

Cook, B. and Phillips, S. (1988) *Loss and Bereavement*, Austen Cornish Publishers Ltd, London.

Dickeson, D. and Johnson, M. (1993) *Death, Dying and Bereavement*, Open University, Sage, London.

Dunlop, R. S. (ed) (1978) *Helping the Bereaved*, Charles Press, London.

Leick, N. and Nielson, M. D. (1991) *Healing Pain, Attachment, Loss and Grief Therapy*, Routledge, London.

Murray-Parkes, C. (1976) *Bereavement: Studies of Grief in Adult Life*, Penguin Books, Harmondsworth.

Staudacher, C. (1987) *Beyond Grief – a Guide to Recovering From the Death of a Loved One*, New Harbinger Publications Inc., Oakland CA.

Schiff, H. S. (1979) *The Bereaved Patient*, Souvenir Press, London.

Tatelbaum, J. (1989) *The Courage to Grieve, Creative Living, Recovery and Growth Through Grief*, Cedar Books, London.

Worden, J. W. (1993) *Grief Counselling and Grief Therapy*, Tavistock, London.

Worden, J.W. (1991) *Grief Counselling and Grief Therapy: a Handbook for the Mental Health Practitioner*, Routledge, London.

Working with institutionalized clients 18

Some years ago David was admitted to hospital with a diagnosis of anxiety/depression, following an attempt to commit suicide. David remained in hospital for over 15 years, yet this was not due to his anxiety or depression but because the institution was the only place he felt safe and secure. More recently David has been 'decanted' into the community into a residential care home. However, any attempt to converse with him about the subject of living more independently is met with a blank stare, an anxiety attack or an aggressive response. Although he now lives in the community he remains 'institutionalized'.

David has become institutionalized to the extent that his original diagnosis is mild in comparison to the debilitating state in which he now finds himself. Other than on the issue of his independent living, David is obedient, compliant and complacent to an extraordinary degree. His mask-like features would persuade the observer that he was suffering from Parkinson's disease. This would be equally supported by the blank expressionless eyes and the shuffling gait. The giveaway clues of his actual disability can be easily observed when his chair in the day room is taken by an unsuspecting stranger, or a new care assistant changes his routine for some reason. It is then that his blank eyes become expressive and David becomes animated, for his security and safety are threatened.

For many years David's choices and decisions have been largely made by other people. Having accepted that David's judgement was impaired due to his initial mental illness, it is still a sad reflection of the care he received that his decision making was excluded, even to the simple decision of what time he should go to bed. From almost the first day in hospital, David's routine was set. What time he would arise, what he ate, where he slept, what occupied him, even how he should be entertained, were influenced almost totally by what someone else felt was best for him. This has not significantly changed since he has been 'residing in the community'. It can be noted by observation that even within a short period of time in an active acute mental health unit or day hospital, patients will adopt predictable patterns of behaviour. If these behaviours are reinforced by the figures of authority, i.e. the staff, they tend to be repeated. The newly admitted client, even if fully aware of his wishes, needs and his own assertiveness, may still be subject to anxiety and insecurity in a strange environment. The tremendous psychological pressures of the 'group' (other clients), 'authority' (the staff) and the established routine for him to comply and blend in will be extremely difficult to resist. Institutional behaviour is essentially behaving as the controllers of the institution expect and demand a member to behave.

In his (1959) book *Institutional Neuroses*, Russell Barton considers many causes and effects of the lack of choice within a client's environment. We support Barton's ideas and add that it is the authorities' expectations of patients' behaviour that tends to stereotype, confine and constrict individuality. The following is a short list of just a few expectations staff may have. Any thoughtful nurse may easily double this list.

- Clients should comply with staff regulations (? regardless of whether they are explained, reasonable or difficult).
- Clients should not complain (they are here for treatment, for their safety, to be looked after, and we're trying to help, aren't we?).
- Clients should adapt to the standards of the institution (whether this is improvement or decline).
- Clients should be grateful (we are helping them, aren't we?).
- Clients should be... (substitute here almost any emotional description, and add) when... (a time considered suitable in our values, e.g. clients should be 'happy' when told 'good' news; clients should be 'tired' when it's bedtime).
- Clients should share our values about life, death, health and illness (at least).

The list can become endless. Such intractable staff attitudes, whether 'good' or 'bad', are their attitudes, and we suggest that the only therapeutic attitude to have concerning expectations of clients is: 'I expect clients to have different attitudes from mine and I respect their entitlement to have and keep them'. To expect people to be the same, to fit in, to be 'normal' and to have similar standards and to accept this is, in our opinion, as likely a cause of institutionalization as any suggested by Barton.

How long does it take to become institutionalized? This is a question often asked. There is no set or standard answer, as it will depend largely on the forces for and against such a situation. Some clients will be more resistant to complying with the institution, and some institutions will be less influential in making clients comply. To be fair, some progressive institutions are very aware of this problem and take active steps to avoid institutionalization developing.

It is not in any case an 'all-or-nothing' concept, it is a process. It begins on the first contact with an institution, and ends only when contact is broken with that institution. The effects on the individual exposed to this process, as previously intimated, can vary tremendously. It is not entirely confined to clients: some staff may show signs of institutionalization relatively quickly, and in some cases most severely. To look at the specific factors that affect the development of pathological states of institutionalization would require a longer discussion. We recommend that students interested in this area read both Barton's work and the work of Irving Goffman (see Further Reading).

PROBLEMS AND NEEDS OF THE INSTITUTIONALIZED CLIENT

It is ironic that probably one of David's biggest problems is that he has very few fundamental needs. His needs are almost entirely catered for by the institution. His primary needs of food, shelter, warmth and comfort are indefinitely available without any anxiety that they will ever be withdrawn. Even some of the higher-order or complex needs, such as belongingness and companionship, may be supplied in the residential environment. It is only the very highest human needs of self-respect, self-esteem, prestige and what Maslow (1971) calls self-actualization, that the institution fails to supply.

It is, in fact, exactly these that the client who has become institutionalized lacks; he has been bereft of self-esteem and self respect, and he has been robbed of his humanity in his higher expectations. His dreams have become mundane or non-existent, and he has lost the motivation to strive for the ultimate goals of personal satisfaction that Maslow aptly described as self-actualization. David's problem is not that his basic needs are not met – it is that they are. It is because he no longer suffers any anxiety, because he experiences no challenge, that he feels no sense of satisfaction. Having no prospects for the future, no plans and no expectations deprives an individual of his hopes and desires. Without incentive to fulfil basic human needs, the individual human spirit is deprived of motivation and dies, just as a flower dies without water. As if to substantiate the truth of this statement, the institutionalized client is often described as 'dehumanized'. We take this to mean having lost the human spirit, leaving only the body shell.

The client needs to be restored somehow, to have this human spirit rekindled, to have his dignity, his hopes and his dreams returned to him. What we must remember, however, is that if the process of robbing David of his humanity took 15 years, we must not expect to restore it in seven days. The process of 'rehabilitation' for David will not be a simple task. It may be painful for both parties to engage on a project that neither may fully enjoy, and many payoffs are indefinite and distant.

IMPLICATIONS FOR THE NURSE

The first crucial factor the nurse needs to be aware of is that her approaches to each client must be flexible. Having respect for a client means much more than simply calling him 'Mr'. Respect means that you are aware of his rights as an individual, that you consider him to be a unique human being and that you will not cut across his values; to understand that what he holds to be valuable, no matter how silly it appears to you, must be respected. This may mean that on some occasions the individual's wishes will clash with the customary routine and the nurse's expectations of client behaviour. Rather than immediately dismissing this refusal or non-compliance as awkward or unreasonable, take a few minutes to contemplate exactly how unreasonable it is and, more importantly, how unworkable it really is. Sometimes clients' suggestions are not at all silly and it is recognized that listening to their views can bring about significant and desirable change. Adopting a flexible approach will probably do no more than offset some of the institutional processes in the more acute clients, and it will have much less effect on the longer-stay clients. Understanding this from the outset may help nurses become less frustrated, for if they are expecting startling results from simply altering their approach they will undoubtedly be disappointed.

Another factor nurses need to be aware of is the risks that a 'rehabilitation' approach requires. There are many risks nurses must take if they are intent on restoring a client's dignity, and the first is perhaps the damage to their own prestige. Nurses become nurses primarily, we believe, to help clients. Unfortunately, all too frequently the nurse's concept of 'helping' means making the individual dependent upon her. Stepping back from the client and encouraging him to take more responsibility for himself, refusing to give advice and insisting on his making his own choices may initially result in damage to the nurse's self-image of her helping skills. It is only after several months of gradually observing the client become more independent that the rewards received from such 'non-behaviour' can be appreciated. A further risk the nurse takes with this approach is the threat of reducing standards. It is often used as a convincing argument that when the nurse stops working on the client, the client stops too. In other words, if the nurse does not insist that the client has a bath, he will probably not have one at all. Fundamentally we disagree with this philosophy. We consider that although in practice this is largely what happens, it is used quite unfairly as an example. It fails to take account of the fact that the institution incapacitated the individual in the first place, that before the institutionalization process took place the individual was quite capable of taking responsibility for his own bath. It would be ridiculous to remove an engine from a car and replace it with pedals and then exclaim, 'See, I told you it wouldn't work on its own if we stopped pedalling'. It seems to us that the exponents of the argument for nurses doing everything for clients in order to stop standards falling are saying exactly this. Standards of dress, hygiene, table manners and the general tidiness of the environment may indeed decline, and obviously some degree of monitoring and subsequent persuasion may be necessary, but surely this is a very small price to pay for beginning the process of restoring the client's motivation, self-respect and decision-making ability.

Dispensing with the role of parent and entering into a more equal partnership with a client can increase the risk of anxiety feelings within the nurse. This is perhaps because operating from a superior position had in the past engendered a feeling of security. When instructing or directing from a position of superiority it is not necessary to understand or explain the reasons for such prescriptions. Once you enter into an equal partnership with a client, it is possible to be challenged. It may even be possible that you are wrong, and that, on introspection, no valid reasons can be found for some of the things you have been doing. Who knows, some of the traditions which have been respected perhaps need to be challenged?

Is it possible to imagine the ramifications of the following brief dialogue?

Nurse: 'Mr Brown, could you come along for a bath please, it's Thursday night again.'

Client: 'I'm sorry, nurse, although I would really like to please you, I'm not sure I care for a bath tonight, and definitely not just at the moment as I'm having a conversation with Mr Smith.'

Nurse reports to the officer in charge: 'Mr Brown refuses to have a bath.'

Officer in charge: 'Oh does he, I'll soon see about that.'

Some nurses may recognize some of this dialogue, if not all of it. We appreciate that Mr Brown would be a very unusual client to be so unreasonable, resistive and uncooperative, but none the less we would be most happy to see many more Mr Browns.

PRINCIPLES AND SKILLS REQUIRED

We believe nurses need to be skilled in the following areas:

- Knowing and accepting the individual's values. This will entail the nurse listening to the client, spending time with him, and trying to understand how he feels about himself and his life.
- Encouraging the client to make choices. This requires some behavioural skills (see Chapter 3), especially using positive reinforcers and the shaping process to reward successive approximations towards independent choice.
- This process may begin by adding at least one choice to each daily activity, and gradually increasing them, e.g. increasing the choice of bedtime from 10 p.m. to 11 p.m. and varying the times during the week; one choice of food at mealtimes increasing to several choices; proceeding eventually to choice of clothes, activities and recreation.
- Ensuring that the client remains secure when faced with choices he is not used to. This will involve a special relationship which is trusting and open, but without being restricting, advising or oversupportive. Establishing such a relationship can be extremely difficult, and can only be achieved by being sensitive to the client's anxiety levels and understanding what he can cope with. It particularly involves the use of non-verbal reassurance, especially gestures of encouragement and touching when appropriate, without encouraging dependence.
- Being able to accept the negative feelings of hostility and aggression should the client feel insecure. Not reacting to displays of temper caused through frustration, but by verbal skills helping the client ventilate his feelings, and sharing your own.
- Being able to model and teach mature and intelligent decision making. This requires the nurse to behave appropriately in various situations and explain to the client why it was appropriate (see 'Social skills training', Chapter 3). Facilitating intelligent decision making can be demonstrated by sharing your own recent domestic decisions with the client. This should illustrate how appropriate choices are made by choosing from a larger rather than a smaller list of options, and linking the choices with possible outcomes or consequences.

- Being aware of the interactions responsible for reducing independence. To be able to reduce these and deal with the adverse emotional reactions within yourself. Objective self- awareness is probably the surest way of preventing yourself making the client more dependent. One way of achieving this self-awareness may be by recording the day's events in a diary, and evaluating how frequent and how necessary each of your daily interactions is in relation to client independence.
- Being sensitive to the client's needs for higher values of self-respect, individuality and purpose. This is achieved by constantly updating your ideas about each client. Try to forget how they behaved last year or last month, and concentrate on their currently undeveloped potential.
- Facilitating, both verbally and non-verbally, increasing responsiveness between the client and the real world outside the institution. This means encouraging clients to write letters, read newspapers, catch buses and generally proceed away from rather than towards reliance on the institution. Smiles of surprise are usually far more reinforcing than apathetic shrugs of the shoulders.
- Being able to let go of your responsibilities for the client once he is able to retake possession of his own destiny.

CONCLUSION

We hope this chapter has helped you to see that helping clients does not always mean doing everything for them, and that institutions tend to rob people of their individuality, independence and uniqueness, and that it is the nurse's job to try to restore these. Developing empathy with the institutionalized client is difficult because he is so far away from the nurse's own orientation. The nurse who is very independent and capable often has difficulty accepting that her client may be able to develop these characteristics too, if given the opportunity and the appropriate skilled help.

Successfully nursing the institutionalized client can be extremely rewarding, but requires patience, positive attitudes and trust in the human being's potential. We hope this brief chapter has stimulated some insight, challenged a few attitudes and offered some useful guidelines to nurses engaged in this difficult and frustrating area of care.

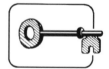

KEY CONCEPTS

1. It can be noted by observation that, even within a short period of time in an active acute admission ward, clients will adopt predictable patterns of behaviour. Institutional behaviour is essentially behaving as the controllers of the institution expect and demand a member to behave.
2. The authority's expectation of clients' behaviour tends to stereotype, confine and constrict individuality.
3. Some clients will be more resistant to complying with the institution and some institutions will be less influential in making clients comply.

4. Institutionalization is not entirely confined to clients: some staff may show signs of institutionalization relatively quickly and, in some cases, most severely.
5. Having no prospects for the future, no plans and no expectations deprives an individual of his hopes and desires.
6. Institutionalization robbed David of his humanity over 15 years; we must not expect to restore it in seven days.
7. Respect means that you are aware of the client's rights as an individual.
8. Unfortunately, all too frequently 'helping' means making the client dependent upon the nurse.
9. Some of the traditions which have been respected perhaps need to be challenged.

FURTHER READING

Barton, R. (1959) *Institutional Neuroses*, John Wright, Bristol.

Goffman, l. (1968) *Asylums*, Penguin Books, Harmondsworth.

Goffman, I. (1974) *Stigma*, Penguin Books, Harmondsworth.

Morgan, R. and Cheadle, J. (1981) *Psychiatric Rehabilitation*, National Schizophrenic Fellowship, Surbiton, Surrey.

Paine, T. (1982) *Rights of Man*, Penguin Books, Harmondsworth.

Shepherd, G. (1984) *Institutional Care and Rehabilitation*, Longman, London.

Townsend, J.M. (1976) Self concepts and the institutionalisation of mental patients: overview and critique. *Journal of Health and Social Behaviour*, **17**, 263–71.

Extending Knowledge and Skills

PART

3

Community skills 19

Thomas has been in and out of mental health departments for many years. He has had many therapies and therapists. He expresses quite convincingly that each community mental health nurse (CMHN) who visits him will be his last. His life has had many painful experiences, he is unable to deal with life's stresses, he finds great difficulty in forming relationships with women, and generally feels life is hardly worth living. Although Thomas had a good job as a teacher and meets interesting and stimulating people, he remains isolated and wholly unable to trust himself to be open, with the subsequent risk of being let down again.

Elsie is reaching her sixties and has had several children, now all grown up. Her husband left her years ago, and she now lives alone in a council flat. She is permanently anxious and frequently depressed. When the CMHN visits she is nearly always tearful following a crisis with her family, or agitated as she is about to enter one. The root of her problems seems to be her inability to control her conflicting feelings. Her children abuse her kindness by demanding support from her at one period then ignoring her and having no contact with her for several months. One of her children is constantly in trouble with the law, another frequently dumps all her children with her and runs off. Elsie is left feeling constantly afraid of excessive demands and being unable to cope, or despondent because she feels rejected and deserted. She appears unable to communicate these feelings due to contrasting anger and guilt.

Joan is in her mid-thirties, married with a teenage daughter. Previously Joan had had a homosexual affair which, when discovered, caused extreme reactions within her marriage. Her husband, understandably perhaps, became rather suspicious, resentful and bitter. Joan, paradoxically, became extremely jealous and smothered her husband. As if she expected some ironic revenge to be meted out, she felt insecure and anxious, expecting him to leave her. After many admissions to mental health units with anxiety and exhibiting intense jealous reactions, it appears that these symptoms have run their course, and Joan seems to have dealt with both her jealousy and her anxiety, and now feels resentful towards her husband for what she suspects has been his enjoyment of her difficulties. She has become bitter in the awareness that he has used her infidelity as a weapon against her, and deliberately increased her insecurity and jealousy to make her more dependent upon him. It is apparent that the family and marital tensions have reached a critical point.

ROLE OF THE COMMUNITY MENTAL HEALTH NURSE

It may be apparent in viewing the brief case histories above that in each case the CMHN has a difficult, yet different, role to play. Thomas requires a friend's support, a therapist's advice and a counsellor's understanding; Elsie needs someone to show her that she can cope, and that she is needed, to reinforce the realities of life so she can realistically help her family, and also realize and understand their ungratefulness. Joan, her husband and her daughter require a skilled family therapist, an arbitrator, a defuser and a social worker. In later stages of distress, the CMHN may find herself having to intervene in highly emotive issues that would not normally be the province of the nurse. As if this role were not demanding enough, she must also be able to deal professionally with the administration and monitoring of medicines, have the skills, knowledge and resources of a social worker, and the practical application of a skilled manager.

IMPLICATIONS FOR THE NURSE

It can easily be seen that the role of the CMHN is multifaceted. Taking this a little further, it is not hard to imagine that the nurse requires a considerable repertoire of skills and resources to fulfil that role. The nurse employed in such a role must therefore be able to offer an eclectic approach – a unique approach for each unique situation – and be resilient enough personally to withstand the pressure of such a totally demanding occupation. The main pressures upon the CMHN, or any professional working alone, need to be fully understood by both the nurse and her employing authority to ensure that they do not impair her effectiveness.

Isolation

The CMHN is an autonomous professional, often working on her own with no personal feedback from colleagues. Although CMHNs may work in teams and have team meetings, the actual interpersonal exchanges between nurse and patients will be isolated from other observers. In a residential situation, although interactions may be personal and unobserved, a collective opinion is none the less formed within the confidentiality of the staff room. These opinions take the form of how difficult, unreceptive or even downright awkward some patients appear to the majority of the staff. This subjective information is at least of some help or comfort to more inexperienced and insecure members of staff, who may otherwise believe that they are 'doing it all wrong'. This collective subjective feedback is not available to the community nurse, so other strategies have to be used.

Trust

The CMHN must have confidence in her own abilities, and sufficient experience in successful therapy to be able to trust in her own personal resources. She should not be so arrogant as to believe she will always be right, or always know best, but neither should she be so self-doubting that she is hesitant and procrastinating. The community nurse's job is based on a clarity of action, a sensitivity to needs and a discriminating ability to judge situations correctly. This difficult balance can only be achieved if the individual has a highly developed sense of trust in her own senses, and not only knows that she is able to deliver the appropriate approach, but can sense when she is unable to.

Self-analysis, evaluation and self-awareness

Having no accurate objective feedback on her own effectiveness, other than her patients' progress, the community nurse needs to reflect on her work performance and self-needs from time to time. It is most important that she analyses what she is trying to achieve with each patient, what she is actually achieving, and to what extent the outcomes are dependent on herself. To reflect actively on her own needs to achieve progress, knowing she is succeeding and that she is coping with the job, is by no means an insignificant ability that she requires to develop. The autonomous nature of the job dictates that the nurse is self-directed and self-aware but, more importantly, that the direction is accurate and the self-awareness realistic. Being industrious and energetic towards an inappropriate goal is obviously counterproductive, but many caring individuals fall into this trap because they are blinded by the fact that they are 'busy' and always 'rushing about' organizing. Similarly, the nurse's self-awareness may be depressing and demotivate her; she may feel that 'Whatever I try fails'. The problem here is that without information from other professionals, it is difficult to bring reality into the situation. The failure has become 'personalized' rather than being realistically assessed. It may require someone to point out that whatever and whoever tries in these circumstances, they are bound to fail. It is imperative to stress this particular aspect of self-awareness at this point: self-awareness may potentiate a depressed mood because it lowers the defences and gives more insight. People concentrating on self-awareness may find greater difficulty in using mental mechanisms such as projection and rationalization (see Freud, 1958). It is for this reason that self-awareness should be tempered with reality constructs, e.g.: human beings are human; it is impossible to be perfect; faults recognized can be changed, but not all at once; and faults recognized should not be punished, simply rectified steadily. As we also point out in the supervision model, it is just as important to recognize one's strengths and qualities as it is to focus on one's weaknesses. Our fundamental belief is therefore that if self-awareness creates depression, then the appropriate dose of reality has not been adequately mixed with it.

Debrief

The term debrief is used specifically to indicate 'the frequent expression in a safe environment of emotion which, once verbalized, can be examined and dealt with more objectively'. For a more formal scheduled debriefing, supervision should be sought on a regular basis (see Chapter 4).

A skill which it is essential for the community nurse to learn is how to debrief. It is always difficult to discuss with another person the intimate fears of our own limitations; to be able to admit to feelings of insecurity, inadequacy, embarrassment or simply not knowing something we believe it is expected that we should know. It is, however, one of the few simple ways of maintaining an individual's mental health. To harbour these negative feelings, to foster them and allow them to infiltrate her confidence will eventually undermine the nurse's efficiency and personal wellbeing. Unfortunately, many nurses feel debriefing is simply 'dumping' problems on to someone else. We, on the contrary, believe that this disclosure, which after all requires considerable courage, honesty and trust, does not place a burden on the listener but allows her to share the problems. It facilitates a reciprocal arrangement so that common feelings of high intensity and considerable anxiety can be identified and dealt with by mutual support.

It is our belief that the autonomous professional should endeavour to practise debriefing skills on a regular basis with a colleague, supervisor or friend, if she is interested in her own wellbeing and personal efficiency. We believe this should be at least a monthly programmed meeting, and may be made more powerful if it is group- facilitated in working terms. Debrief meetings have the added benefit of allowing a cohesive group team to emerge, directed towards honest appraisal, self-awareness and personal effectiveness, which in turn is client-orientated. It is in the supervising nurse's interest to schedule these meetings within the work programme and to facilitate them in a non-authoritarian, confidential and trusting environment. The group may be facilitated by an outside agent (professional group facilitator, psychologist, counsellor) initially if this is thought to be beneficial, or depending upon the method of group interaction desired (drama therapy, group discussion, T-group, group counselling). Whichever method is used, and whether an outside agent or a group member facilitates the group, they should seek to be ongoing, non- threatening and relaxed to be most successful. Any group meeting for debriefing would be advised to meet frequently initially, and then vary the frequency according to need. It is becoming more accepted that debriefing groups are a necessary part of effective working life in a stressful occupation. Organizations, from multinational companies to small pressurized sales-type businesses, are increasingly recognizing the need for debriefing sessions. Social workers, teachers and counsellors are becoming committed to setting up professional support groups. It seems to us that in this particular area community nurses may learn from their example.

Debriefing skills require the nurse to disclose facts concerning her behaviour in certain situations and how she felt about them. It is a two-way process, in that the disclosure must be listened to accurately without judgement or condemnation. The process of relaying this information to another in an atmosphere of support may be sufficient to enable the nurse to work through her anxieties. However, there are times when she may require more than listening and support. The frustration of working and making decisions on her own can sometimes cause a saturation of ideas, which may in turn reduce motivation. In such a case, a group of people coming together for debrief is particularly useful in that experience and ideas can be shared. The listeners in a debrief group must be careful not to give advice, while at the same time not letting this deter them from sharing ideas, in order for the discloser to look at her situation from a different perspective. The skills of self-disclosure and information giving 'borrowed' from the counselling model could be useful in helping a group share experiences without being directive.

Before terminating a debrief relationship, whether it is just two people or a group, it is important to allow the discloser to state how she feels now, having had an opportunity to share her experience. This may in fact bring out more issues that need to be dealt with, so if time is a constraint current feelings need to shared at least 15 minutes before the end of a session, so that the person concerned is not left emotionally confused. Although not always appropriate, the end should aim towards a positive outcome, which may vary from every-one feeling 'great' to 'Let's see what develops and bring it back to our next meeting', emphasizing the importance of a continual support system.

SKILLS OF COMMUNITY MENTAL HEALTH NURSING

The counselling skills described earlier are a sound base for practising mental health nursing in the community. The formation of rapport from an empathic base cannot in our opinion be faulted as a starting point, but there are some significant differences between residential and home nursing.

Control of the environment

The patient in his home is no longer so dependent upon the nurse. Often he is more self-directed and independent, and the contrast with his behaviour in resi-dential care can often be striking. The nurse is not able to control the environ-ment as she may wish. When a patient invites the nurse to sit down, it is in a chair, in a room and at the time of day that the patient decides upon. Practical problems emerging from this may be distractions such as the television remain-ing on, or friends, spouse or neighbours interrupting. The patient may decide to sit away from the nurse and make meaningful communication more difficult; in short, barriers to good communication may be created which the nurse cannot control. If the nurse's relationship with the patient is strong enough, these barriers may be discussed and dealt with relatively easily; if not, then the nurse needs to work very hard indeed to establish a deeper relationship.

The nurse working in the patient's home must be sensitive to and respect the individual patient's cultural norms. For example, some patients may be quite offended by nurses asking to use the toilet. They may be embarrassed, for if the bathroom is upstairs it may be considered strictly private. Although this may seem strange to some nurses, breeching this type of cultural conditioning may result in the patient being out the next time the nurse calls. Being able to interpret and understand non-verbal signals in socially sensitive situations such as a patient's home is an invaluable skill. This skilful sensitivity will prevent many damaging behavioural interactions occurring.

Another contrast necessary to appreciate when involved in patients' homes is the closeness or intimacy of involvement that it often precipitates. One's home is sacrosanct, with only 'special' people generally invited inside, unless they are on errands of business. The CMHN is in the position of having one foot in each of these particular camps. The skill in this situation is using the special nature of being invited into the home to its maximum advantage while simultaneously maintaining a professional purpose. In other words, the CMHN will be the friendly professional, not a professional friend. Counselling skills concentrate very keenly on the patient finding his own solution to problems, with the nurse taking a catalytic role, and in the patient's home situation (such as those seen in the case studies) problems may be so acute that the nurse may feel that advice, persuasion and solutions are quite legitimately her prerogative and are necessary. Although we appreciate the pressure upon the nurse to resort to this approach, we strongly urge caution, for quickly offered instant 'solutions' are often grasped by the patient but seldom result in positive outcomes, and are therefore not realistic. An example of this type of situation would be the following:

Joan: 'I think what it really amounts to is I don't love my husband any more. In fact, I don't really like him. Do you think I should leave him? Would you write to the council for me, and help me get a solicitor?'

Joan requires much more here than an instant answer. Is she asking the nurse for reassurance for a course of action she has decided upon, or is not sure about, or is she hoping the nurse will say, 'No, you shouldn't'? The skilled nurse will know her patient sufficiently well to be able to share her doubts about the question: 'I'm not really sure why you're asking me, have you decided already, are you unsure, or do you want me to say no?' Or she may offer a simple challenge: 'I'm not really sure that it matters what I do or think; I'm wondering if you've really thought it through yet yourself?'

The nurse may decide that offering new perspectives on the issues may be useful: 'I think you know that whatever you finally decide, I will support you as much as I can, but there are perhaps other factors to consider. There is your daughter, financial issues and your job. Perhaps you haven't thought this through yet?'

Or she may want to contrast leaving with staying: 'Well, Joan, what are the things that make you want to leave, and the things that make you want to stay? Let's see if you can list them, then we can go on to things that will help either course of action be better.'

This is leading to a 'force-field analysis' approach (see page 48) and may be followed up with open suggestions of resources which may be helpful: marriage guidance, social services, single-parent family associations.

It should be stressed that these options are not given as advice, but simply as information and resource knowledge for Joan to choose freely.

It may be felt by the nurse that Joan's problems involve the whole family so fundamentally that she needs to see them together. Observing how they interact, how communications become unclear and how emotions are repressed within the family group may open up other options for solving their difficulties. The skills required here are basically family therapy skills, which are closely related to those used in counselling. Other approaches that may be considered include behavioural-based therapy, or a transactional analysis approach (see Further Reading).

Elsie's case requires the CMHN to be familiar with the principles and skills of behaviour therapy. Certainly the nurse needs to establish a rapport, but it is important that her non-verbal communication and her desire to be helpful do not reinforce Elsie's helplessness. Helping Elsie deal with her anxiety may involve teaching her how to relax (see Chapter 3) and perhaps helping her reward herself positively for her decision-making behaviour. Being able to say 'no' to excessive demands made upon her and subsequently not feeling guilty for refusing requests may be a significant advance for her. Taking a behavioural approach while simultaneously helping Elsie to see herself more clearly by using counselling skills may be the most appropriate nursing interventions.

Helping Thomas may require the most intensive and continuous therapy. Thomas seems to be testing each therapist until eventually his prediction of them failing with him comes true. Somehow the skilful nurse has to be able to get through to him that it is his responsibility to become well, and that this should be important to all parties. Not playing games with him, and expressing to him the anxieties and practical problems with his case, may be ways of challenging him helpfully. To raise Thomas's self-awareness of his previous dependence on his therapists, and his subsequent feelings of disappointment and rejection, may make the nurse–patient relationship more honest and open. The nurse needs to be able to evaluate realistically how he can be helped, what he expects of her and what goals he hopes to achieve. The main skill demonstrated with Thomas will be the skill of immediacy (see p. 45) operated from the core conditions of warmth, genuineness and empathy (see p. 20). The relationship formed between Thomas and the nurse is to be the most therapeutic tool in his care. To experience a relationship where he is free to explore his feelings and be exposed to honest feedback of his presentation of himself may be powerful medicine. In a climate of trust he may be able to take risks in exposing his feelings, in the knowledge that he will receive accurate feedback in a non-threatening and non-punishing way. He may find this difficult at first, or in fact give up. As long as it is reinforced as his decision to give up, that it is his responsibility for his own future that he has decided, then even this may be a positive step forward. Should he maintain the relationship it will require the nurse to use her judgement of his stability, for at some time in the future she will need to encourage Thomas to transfer his learning to the real situation outside therapy. At this stage in Thomas's development he may require tremendous support and reinforcement, but care must be taken not to encourage him to be dependent, or to be so sympathetic as to reinforce any failures he may encounter.

In Thomas's case the nurse does not set out to be the paragon, to be all-understanding or the perfect role model; indeed, this may spoil the effect. The nurse represents honest feedback for a learning purpose, and one thing Thomas needs to learn is that human behaviour is human, fallible and, on occasions, disappointing. Taking risks in relationships can have negative results, but generally the payoffs outweigh the disappointments. If the nurse can teach Thomas this, and allow him to look at his own behaviour and previous experience openly and honestly, then some advances in his wellbeing may be anticipated.

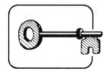

KEY CONCEPTS

1. The nurse must be able to deal professionally with the administration and monitoring of medicines, have the skills, knowledge and resources of a social worker and the practical application of a skilled manager.
2. The nurse requires a considerable repertoire of skills and an eclectic approach – a unique approach for each situation. This is especially important, as the CMHN may find herself having to intervene in highly emotive issues that would not normally be the province of the nurse.
3. The autonomous nature of the job dictates that the nurse is self-directed and self-aware, and it is for this reason that the CMHN must have confidence in her own abilities and sufficient experience in successful therapy.
4. A skill which it is essential for the community nurse to learn is how to debrief. This skill is particularly stressed because the actual interpersonal exchanges between nurse and patients will be isolated from other observers and this may result in there being little support or objective feedback in difficult cases.
5. The community nurse's job is based on clarity of action, a sensitivity to needs and a discriminating ability to judge situations correctly.

SUMMARY

The Community Mental Health Nurse may have many difficult roles to play, but her primary role will be to maintain an empathic rapport in order for the patient's needs to be satisfactorily fulfilled. The nurse must be aware that the patient may be more self-directed and be in the process of restoring some independence, and it is vital that this is not taken away by well-meaning advice, which reinforces dependency.

If the nurse operates from a position of understanding, she will be sensitive to the cultural uniqueness of the patient, be able to read his non-verbal cues accurately, and respect him as a person. It is important to remember that the balance between being a friend and a professional is a tenuous one, and it has been suggested that the nurse should seek to be a friendly professional, not a professional friend. Once the appropriate climate of helping has been established, by which we mean the correct balance between the nurse's support, the patient's independence and the demands of society as represented in the community by friends, neighbours and significant others, the nurse can be more effective. It is the nurse's role at this point to use her skills to enable the patient to make appropriate choices and wise decisions. We suggest that simple challenges, offering new perspectives, and using techniques such as force-field analysis and immediacy skills (see Chapter 2) are probably the most useful in these situations. To help the patient successfully, the nurse should have a sound knowledge of the resources available in the community, accurate information that may be helpful, and understand the principles of the more common therapies such as transactional analysis, cognitive behavioural therapy, behaviour therapy, family therapy and counselling.

Finally, in order for her to continue as an effective helper, the community nurse needs to seek strategies that will maintain her sensitivity yet not rob her of confidence, and seek objective appraisal of her ability and skills within a supportive climate. For this reason we strongly recommend support groups, debriefing sessions and regular effective supervision.

CONCLUSION

Community mental health nursing is the largest area of mental health service delivery and it is our hope that this short chapter may be useful to readers interested in this area. Our aim was not to create an exhaustive piece of work to be used as a reference text, but simply to outline the interactive skills and implications for nurses operating outside the confines of residential care settings. It is true, of course, that not all CMHNs will operate autonomously as we suggest. Some will be heavily involved in mental health education, running groups, and as part of the primary health care team. An important part of any professional's work is in relating to and complementing other allied workers in the field, whether they belong to voluntary agencies or to statutory bodies. These were not omitted because we consider them to be less important, but simply because this volume cannot hope to cover them in any depth. In consequence, what is presented here is intended as an introduction to a body of knowledge and skills and a foundation for development.

FURTHER READING

Brooker, C. (ed) (1990) *Community Psychiatric Nursing, Vol 1*, Chapman & Hall, London.

Brooker, C. and White, E. (eds) (1992) *Community Psychiatric Nursing, Vol 2*, Chapman & Hall, London.

Butterworth, C. A. and Skidmore, D. (1981) *Caring for the Mentally Ill in the Community*, Croom-Helm, London.

Carr, P., Butterworth, C. and Hodges, B. (1980) *Community Psychiatric Nursing: Caring for the Mentally Ill and Handicapped in the Community*, Churchill Livingstone, London.

Jansen, E. (ed) (1980) *The Therapeutic Community Outside the Hospital*, Croom-Helm, London.

Pollock, L. C. (1989) *Community Psychiatric Nursing: Myth and Reality*, Scutari Press, Harrow.

Reed, J. and Lomas, G. (eds) (1984) *Psychiatric Services in the Community (Developments and Innovations)*, Croom-Helm, London.

Sladden, S. (1979) *Psychiatric Nursing in the Community: a Study of a Working Situation*, Churchill Livingstone, London.

Human sexuality 20

Janice M. Russell

In order to be sensitive to the needs of the individual, nurses need to address various issues of sexuality, some general and some quite specific. Sexuality is more than the physiological acts of sex, and to be comfortable and skilful in dealing with this aspect of clients' needs and care, it is important for the nurse to explore issues relevant to her own sexuality. Moreover, it is being increasingly recognized that adverse sexual experiences such as abuse and rape may be fundamental to the client's condition, and may become the focus of intervention. It is also the case that HIV prevention and infection will increasingly become an issue, both in hospitals and within the community.

To facilitate self-exploration, then, and to introduce the bare bones of the salient issues of this topic, this chapter will give a brief outline of the following:

- Concepts of sexuality, sexual health, and sexual prejudice;
- Physiological aspects of sexuality;
- Psychological aspects of sexuality;
- Sociocultural aspects of sexuality;
- Gender identity and sexual expression;
- HIV/AIDS;
- Potential problems: mental illness, mental disability, lifecycle, physical disability;
- Sexual harassment.

SEXUALITY, FEARS AND PREJUDICES

Sexuality is generally thought of as involving the whole person. The term was first coined in the late 19th century (Heath, 1982) and differs from the word 'sex', which is generally used to denote a physiological act. Sexuality is conceptualized as being a part of our identity, and human sexuality includes the biological, sociocultural, psychological and ethical components of sexual behaviour. In other words, sexuality is an intrinsic part of our being. Sexuality influences our thoughts, actions and interactions, and is involved in all aspects of physical and mental health.

A major part of human sexuality and sexual identity is sexual expression. The freedom for sexual expression is acknowledged and reflected in the World Health Organization's statements concerning the elements of sexual health. These are:

1. A capacity to enjoy and control sexual and reproductive behaviour in accordance with a social and personal ethic.
2. Freedom from fear, shame, guilt, false beliefs and other psychological factors inhibiting sexual response and impairing sexual relationships.
3. Freedom from organic disorders, disease and deficiencies that interfere with sexual and reproductive factors (WHO, 1975).

In recognizing the elements of sexual health the nurse will need to facilitate the individual in optimizing their chances of achieving them. In order to do this effectively, she needs to be able to listen skilfully and communicate in an accepting and non-judgemental manner. How well she is able to communicate with the client will depend upon the degree of her self-awareness and acceptance.

Most people in society will carry both ignorance and prejudice concerning sexuality, which shows in different ways. Consider your personal reactions to the following statements:

Gay men should be allowed to foster children.

Straight people are only straight because they've been brainwashed.

Clients needing institutional care have the right to sex, either with each other, with visiting partners or through masturbation.

Sex between people with mental health problems should be prohibited.

All four statements reflect attitudes which hold some degree of prejudice and pose some ethical questions about sexuality. It may be interesting to return to them at the end of the chapter.

Whatever our personal attitudes about sexuality, we have no right to inflict them on those we nurse, or to punish them for sexual beliefs or practices that differ from our own. Equally, there is no reason why nurses should have to put up with sexual prejudice from their clients, and there is a fine art to respectful challenging where this is the case. More will be said about this later.

Where nurses do find difficulty in accepting aspects of sex and sexuality it is not helpful to be self-judgemental, rather to raise awareness and knowledge and to seek appropriate support so that the interests of the client may be best met. The following is offered in this spirit.

PHYSIOLOGICAL ASPECTS OF SEXUALITY

An understanding of the human sexual response cycle is useful to the nurse dealing with sexual function or dysfunction, whether the cause be physical or psychological. Masters and Johnson (1966) provided a useful blueprint of this cycle of response observed in humans. A summarized account of their pioneering work may be found in Belliveau and Richter (1971).

Briefly, Masters and Johnson suggest that human beings go through four phases within the sexual response cycle. These are the **excitement phase**, where both genders experience increased muscle tension and genital vasocongestion; the **plateau phase**, where engorgement and slight changes in the size of the vaginal opening and coronal ridge occur; the **orgasmic phase**, where, preceded by increased muscular tenseness, both genders experience orgasm through rhythmic contraction, usually combined with ejaculation in males; and the **refractory phase**, where the clitoris and labia return to normal in women, and penile erection is lost in men. The length of the refractory phase before further stimulation can occur varies according to age and circumstance.

This information rests on clinical observation of human subjects in the laboratory. The unfortunate title of Belliveau and Richter's (1971) book would suggest that psychosexual dysfunction (i.e. failure to meet these criteria in one's sexual life) means that one is inadequate. Sadly, many people who do experience sexual difficulty or lack of fulfilment carry the extra psychological burden of feeling exactly that. Much hype exists around sexuality, and individuals often feel pressurized to perform to some outside standard, rather than discover what is mutually satisfying for themselves and their partners.

It is also important to stress the context of sexual functioning, and in this respect Masters and Johnson's paradigm is of limited use and the danger in their physiological–reductionist viewpoint is that those who do not function 'to the textbook' do indeed feel inadequate. Further, sexual counselling which focuses only on the physiological will have limited use, given that the individual's psychological state will influence their degree of responsiveness.

In recognition of these limitations, Kaplan (1974) offers a tripartite paradigm of sexual functioning where the notion of desire is seen as important to the whole process, and Schnarch (1991) proposes a 'quantum model' of sexuality where he suggests the notion of a total arousal system as being important. In other words, twiddling the right knobs or pushing the right buttons only has value where the people involved are free from fear and inhibition, either of past internalized experience or of the present situation. Schnarch also makes the point that the 'right' physiological responses can occur with little or no subjective pleasure being experienced. In other words, we must take account of the whole person in issues of sexual action and interaction.

Nevertheless, it is useful to note some of the common dysfunctions which human beings encounter, and to acknowledge that most people, whether they have mental health problems or are 'normal', will experience at least one of these at some point in their life. It is also useful to look at some of the myths around sexual activity which misinform our views and experience.

COMMON PROBLEMS OF SEXUAL DYSFUNCTION

Female

- Primary orgasmic dysfunction (never having achieved orgasm);
- Secondary orgasmic dysfunction (having achieved orgasm in the past but with current inability to do so);

- Vaginismus (vaginal muscular spasm making the vagina impenetrable);
- Dyspareunia (pain during vaginal intercourse);

Male

- Impotence, or the inability to achieve effective erection;
- Premature ejaculation (N.B. this means the male is unable to exercise any control over orgasm, which may be after ten seconds of stimulation or ten minutes);
- Ejaculatory incompetence – failure to ejaculate.

Counselling approaches and behavioural programmes have been seen to achieve considerable success in helping people resolve these problems. It must be emphasized, however, that some people may never technically conquer the dysfunction but may come to accept and develop their current sexual behaviour to a level of fulfilment. Many people conceptualize their problems in relation to myths and pressure, and it is important that the nurse does not problematize that which is acceptable to the client. Some common myths which affect sexual behaviour and expectations are:

- Both partners must have an orgasm.
- The man's orgasm in heterosexual sex signifies the obligatory end to the proceedings.
- A woman is most likely to climax through intercourse than with any other kind of stimulation.
- There are many different kinds of orgasm for women - clitoral, vaginal, G-spot and, 1992's contribution to the debate, the U-spot.
- Men with erections must be satisfied or something terrible will happen to them.
- Heterosexual intercourse with mutual orgasm, perhaps followed by a cigarette, is the norm we must all aspire to.
- Masturbation is harmful and a second-best activity.
- Only men masturbate.
- We must have sex at least three times a week.
- The bigger the penis, the better the sex.
- Everybody else is having a whale of a time.......

PSYCHOLOGICAL ASPECTS OF SEXUALITY

Various theories have been offered as to how we develop our sexuality, and implicit in these theories has been some kind of developmental norm. A précis is offered below, with a brief critique as a cautionary rider. Theories of human sexuality can only ever derive from informed speculation, and they are not to be read as rigid blueprints for norms and deviations.

Perhaps the most influential theory on sexuality derives from the work of Sigmund Freud. Freud adopted an instinct-based approach, with the sex drive being seen as one of the primal human instincts, which are physiologically based. He coined the word **libido** to describe the sensory manifestation of the sexual instinct.

Freud (1930) produced a developmental model of human sexuality which posits that sexual energy is expressed through different bodily zones, oral, anal, phallic and genital. Moreover, these zones were, in his view, appropriate to different stages of development, from birth to maturity.

Oral stage

Freud saw this as a major source of infantile gratification, as evidenced by thumb sucking. It would assume a varied importance at different stages of life, through the use of food, drink and smoking. The oral zone also remains a pleasure site during acts of sex.

Anal stage

This includes any activity which is stimulating or gratifying to the anus, whether through defecation, increased muscle control, or using the anus as an erogenous zone.

Phallic stage

This describes the child's awareness and exploration of its own genitals.

Latent stage

Freud speculated that from about the age of four, the child's sexual impulses become sublimated to intellectual and social growth.

Genital stage

Freud hypothesized that from puberty onwards, the erogenous zones become focused on the genitals, and the sexual impulse becomes other-directed rather than self-directed.

Freud then went on to suggest that many problems in adult life are related to an excessive or inadequate level of gratification at different stages of psychosexual development. A Freudian psychoanalyst, for example, may explain an adult's smoking habit as an unfulfilled need for oral gratification, or may describe a person who likes to be very controlled as an anal retentive.

Freud's theories have offered helpful insights, but it must be remembered that they are themselves culturally influenced and must not be read too rigidly. Freud's response to young women disclosing sex with their fathers, for example, was to ascribe unconscious motivation to the women and to dismiss the claims as fantasy. His theory of normal sexual development has also been used to discredit homosexuality as abnormal, and as a psychological condition best cured. Freud also saw male heterosexuality as the norm, so that his theories of female sexuality were limited, with the female genitals being seen as more the absence of a penis than existing in their own right. Such assumptions had a pervasive effect until more challenging theories developed over the last twenty years.

In contrast to the psychoanalytic theory, behaviourists, spearheaded by the work of Skinner (see Chapter 3), claim that sexual activity and thought processes are patterned through a measurable psychological response to stimuli. Much of adult sexuality has been developed through learning and conditioning throughout childhood, within the cultural norms of the individual. This approach has been beneficial within sex therapy, and with treatment for sex offenders, where the conditioning response to stimulus may be altered.

Maslow (1970) suggests that human sexuality is one of the basic human psychological needs for the survival of the species. He also relates human sexuality to other higher-order needs, so that sexual fulfilment and freedom of sexual expression may be seen as part of the self-actualization process. This underlies the concept of sexual health referred to earlier.

This synopsis is offered as a taster of the traditional theories of sexuality which have informed much psychiatric theory and practice to date. The nurse is encouraged to explore different theories and to develop an eclectic understanding and practice. She is then better able to use whatever is appropriate for different clients in different situations, and to utilize the relevant psychological theory.

Sexuality, as stated earlier, is an aspect of self. In understanding more about your own sexuality you increase your understanding of self-concept and self-image. This enhances nursing practice, where the nurse is able to be more self-aware and relaxed in the use of her skills with clients where there are sexual issues.

SOCIOCULTURAL ASPECTS OF SEXUALITY

Just as our ideas and experiences of our sexual selves are psychologically influenced, so they are also socially influenced.

Through various media and practices, for example family, school, religious institutions, legal system, peer groups and mass media such as TV, magazines etc., we are given strong messages about what shape our sexuality should take, and even what shape our bodies should be to be sexy. This gives a social construction of sexuality to which we are expected to adhere, so that people who do not are seen as deviant.

Since the Kinsey reports (1948, 1953), there has been increased information available about sexual preferences and practices within the western world, which have helped to dispel some of the myths about sexuality and have widened the scope of 'normal' sex. The last thirty years have also seen various degrees of challenge to sex role stereotypes, primarily through women's liberation movements and the gay liberation movement. There is considerable political backlash to this trend, however, and society still chooses to 'mould' boys and girls into certain ways of behaviour. It is, however, more acceptable today in certain ways to adopt alternative lifestyles to the norm. Considerable institutional and legal pressure remains, however, for those who fall outside it, to which the nurse needs to be sensitive.

The narrowness of the western norm, and confirmation that it is socially rather than 'naturally' constructed, may be found by looking at the practices of other cultures, for example:

- The Kerabi bachelors of New Guinea practise homosexual anal intercourse as a part of puberty rites.
- The Toda of India permit women to have several lovers and husbands.
- Hopi Indians keep boys and girls aged 10–20 apart.
- Polynesians see love as the 'life force'. There are no words in their language for sexually obscene, indecent or impure, nor are there words for illegitimate, adultery, bigamy or divorce.
- Mojave Indians have institutionalized homosexuality to the point of imitating each other's roles, with transvestism being commonly accepted.
- Trobrianders permit specifically genital play between children (see Hogan, 1980; Oakley, 1985.)

Recognition of these potential differences perhaps enables the nurse to accept the choices and values held by any one individual.

GENDER IDENTITY AND SEXUAL EXPRESSION

Having identified the narrowness of the 'norm', it is perhaps useful to briefly identify the range of sexual preferences the mental health nurse may be working with, or indeed experiencing.

Heterosexuality

Heterosexuality means sexual attraction for the opposite sex, and generally speaking is subject to the least bigotry from society. Heterosexuality may be problematic in the form that it takes, however, for example subjection to sexist practice and attitudes, pressure to be monogamous, and the pressures of some of the myths identified earlier.

Homosexuality

This is sexual attraction for one's own sex. Homosexuality is now considered to be a fairly clinical term and is sometimes considered offensive: 'gay' and 'lesbian' are often used as more easily acceptable and proud terms for many members of this group. Just as with heterosexuals, gay relationships take all sorts of forms – long-term, short-term, monogamous and polygamous, and sexuality is only one part of a gay identity. Not all gay or lesbian people will have had the courage and support to come out, i.e. to be overt about their sexual preference, and the nurse must be sensitive to the stigma that clients have already experienced.

Bisexuality

This means those who are sexually attracted to members of either sex. One argument suggests that we are all capable of sexual arousal and satisfaction by either sex, and that it is cultural conditioning which makes for unilateral choice. Whatever the case, it seems likely that many people will have had a sexual experience, even just in terms of arousal, with members of both sexes.

Transvestism

This is the practice of deriving pleasure or increased sexual arousal from cross-dressing. We might note that it is a lot easier for women to adopt traditionally male garb and style than vice versa.

Trans-sexualism

A trans-sexual is a person who identifies psychologically and culturally with one sex while being physically a member of the other. This can be a frightening and isolating experience, and the client may feel unsupported. Counselling intervention can help the client in making difficult choices, and medical and surgical intervention is possible so that they can eventually achieve the desired identity.

POTENTIAL PROBLEM AREAS

Since sexuality involves so many different aspects it is not surprising that there are many potential problem areas, particularly in a society where it has become so commercialized and hyped. This section notes some of the areas with which the mental health nurse might be faced.

Developmental

Some potential problem areas are life-stage related; for example, in childhood psychosexual development may be contaminated through parental messages. Adolescence may feel overwhelmingly sexual, and young people may have difficulties over masturbation, pornography, pressure to perform and guilt about sex. Children and adolescents are vulnerable to sexual abuse, and more will be said about this later.

In adulthood, there may be relationship difficulties, infidelities, lack of sexual fulfilment, family pressures, ignorance about sexual functioning and technique. In later adulthood women may experience a change with the menopause, which may be of a depressing nature connected with feelings of loss, or of a liberating nature as they enter a new phase of life. Men too experience change as their frequency or intensity of sexual arousal diminishes. In later life, the human response system in both genders changes, manifesting in less vaginal lubrication for women and less frequent erections in men. There is no reason why elderly people may not still experience sexual fulfilment, if they remain reasonably healthy. Society often does not recognize this, and such ignorance may itself be a pressure or source of fear as people get older.

Adults with learning difficulties

For adults categorized as having learning difficulties, one of the philosophies of care is that they have access to as full and normal an environment as possible. The success of such a philosophy will vary depending on all sorts of variables, and we must acknowledge a wide range of conditions which are conflated under the term 'learning difficulties', ranging from the underpotentiated individual to those with severe brain damage.

Nevertheless, the needs of these groups of people for love and physical affection are the same as those for the rest of the population, and there will be the same degree of differences in sexual interest and orientations. Society has generally tried to control the sexual activity and expression of those with identifiable mental limitations. Extreme examples of such control include enforced sterilization, contraceptive injections, instant removal of babies and enforced termination.

On a more insidious level, however, it is the everyday response of carers to those with learning difficulties which can inhibit or encourage freedom of appropriate sexual expression. There may be difficulties involving inappropriate masturbation, sexual acting out or issues of contraception, but for many clients there is a potential for them to be taught to appreciate sensuality, to make responsible choices and to handle feelings in an appropriate manner. It may even be argued that enforced denial of the client's right to be sexual and to have sexual expression is ultimately damaging and even, at the extreme, potentially dangerous. Again, the task for the nurse is to be self-aware and accepting, and discussion of her feelings and attitudes towards those with learning difficulties may be useful.

Physical conditions

There are a variety of physical conditions which interfere with the transmission of sexual stimuli. Loss of physical function does not mean loss of sexuality, and there are numerous issues to be considered which will challenge the skills and awareness of the nurse. Those with physical disability may need psychological help in the form of support or counselling, for self or for self and partner. They may also need physical help, either through physiotherapy or literally through being aided to make sexual contact. Some of the issues around this area, all of which challenge the nurse, are:

- Coping with congenital conditions, e.g. spina bifida, cerebral palsy;
- Coping with changed body image, e.g through colostomy, limb loss;
- Coping with loss of motor ability, e.g. paralysis, cerebrovascular accidents;
- Coping with sensory loss, e.g. blindness, deafness, multiple sclerosis;
- Coping with impaired functioning, e.g. heart conditions.

In such situations nurses need to be able to listen accurately and to help free the client from embarrassment. The task is to approach the difficulty from an integrated perspective, where the needs of the whole person are taken into account, and sometimes where creative thinking comes to the fore.

Sexuality and mental illness

Sexuality and mental illness may be seen as related to some extent, in the sense that each may contribute to the other, i.e. some conditions of mental illness have consequences for aspects of the client's sexuality, while some mental illness may be seen as having its root cause in sexual issues, e.g. long-term impotence or sexual abuse (see Chapter 21).

Often, however, particularly in residential settings, the client's sexuality is ignored or dismissed, due to embarrassment, ignorance or even fear. There are, however, several major areas that the nurse must be familiar with if she is to cope effectively with the sexuality of people with mental health problems. These are:

- The effect of the mental problem on an individual's sexuality;
- The effect of the institutional environment on an individual's sexuality;
- The effect of any treatment for mental health problems on an individual's sexuality;
- The effect of the nurse on an individual's sexuality.

The effects of mental illness

It is difficult to generalize about the effect of mental illness on sexual functioning. However, there are some generally recognized patterns which are specific to certain symptoms. Schizophrenia is a manifestation of a set of symptoms that affects the total personality. Its effect on one person, then, will be different from that on another. From the early onset of symptoms, sexual functioning may be affected in various ways, ranging from a lack of or decrease in sexual desire, to hypersexuality or bizarre and unreasonable sexual behaviour, when symptoms such as delusional or hallucinatory experiences influence the thought patterns of the individual. Either instance may have drastic effects, not only for the client but for any partner in a sexual relationship. In this instance the nurse must be able to reassure the people involved about the nature of the client's illness and its relationship to sexual activity.

Clients who experience severe mood changes, from depression to mania, will also experience a reciprocal change in sexual drive, literally from depressed libido to manic activity, sometimes of an inappropriate nature. In these instances, the nurse may be in a position not only of offering information and reassurance regarding the nature of the changes, but of making interventions to protect the client from activity based on poor judgement and, on occasion, to protect those around them. Knowledge, awareness, skilled intervention and support are essential to the nurse who finds herself in this situation. She may also have to help her client come to terms with their own activity following a manic episode, with skilled listening and acceptance.

It is generally thought that any severe emotional state affects sexuality (Kaplan, 1974), although the relationship between the stress and the level of activity is not clearly understood. Schnarch (1991) makes the point that a certain anxiety level will inhibit some individuals while being necessary for the sexual functioning of others, and perhaps this could be so for more extreme stress conditions. Whatever the cause and effect of the emotional state, the degree of concern from the client about these effects will vary. One woman being treated for depression was relieved to be able to overtly state that she had no interest in sex, having endured an unsatisfactory sex life for years (and here perhaps the relationship was reciprocal). Others may be devastated by a reduced or heightened libido. The important aspect for the skilled nurse is to be aware of the difficulties and to work inside the client's value system as far as possible and appropriate, while retaining ethical practice. At the least the client may be reassured about their condition, and might even gain insight if some aspect of their sexual activity or experience is a contributory factor to the mental illness.

The effect of institutional care

There are various types of institutions for the care of people with mental health problems: care homes, hostels, group homes and even some bedsitter accommodation still carry with them the constraints of institutions. All too often, these institutions can take responsibility for individual care too far, to the extent of depersonalizing and regularizing clients' behaviour so that they are left with little choice to make, and little opportunity to make a decision. This pattern can also relate to staff attitudes towards sexual behaviour within residential settings.

In hospitals, community hostels and residential care homes, clients' sexuality can often be ignored. Single-sex environments may discourage mixing with the other gender. Masturbation may be discouraged, and there are often no facilities for personal sexual expression except in the toilet areas. Dormitories are often impersonal and sexual activity between clients is prohibited, and often treated with anger and disgust. Such attitudes are incompatible with high-quality care. Certain questions must be asked to explore institutional attitudes to the sexual needs of the client:

Should sexual activity be allowed 'in-house'?

Should facilities be provided for this to occur?

How practical are 'conjugal visiting' rooms, i.e. rooms set aside for clients to be alone with their partners without fear of disturbance?

Which clients are to be allowed to express their natural drives?

How are we to facilitate this?

Do we provide appropriate sex education for long-stay clients?

Do we offer sufficient opportunity for contraceptive counselling?

How willing are we to facilitate the use of contraception?

Akhtar, Crocker and Dickey (1977) implied that some sexual activity might be tolerated but identified certain limitations. They stated certain criteria for assessing the appropriateness of sexual activity, considering issues of informed consent, impaired judgement and mental ability. Ultimately, however, each individual should be assessed and limitations set where potential harm may be experienced.

The effect of mental health treatment

A major component of mental health treatment may be the provision of medication to counteract the symptoms of certain disorders. Many of the drugs involved have side-effects related to sexual functioning, some of which are summarized below.

Phenothiazines, e.g. chlorpromazine, thioridazine

Many of these agents produce impotence or ejaculatory difficulties, including absence of ejaculation and painful ejaculation. Amenorrhoea, galactorrhoea and loss of libido are other commonly expressed side- effects.

Tricyclic antidepressants, e.g. amitriptyline and trimipramine

As depression resolves sexual activity usually resumes, but continued use of these antidepressants has been known to cause impotence and ejaculatory difficulties. Delay in orgasm has been experienced by some women.

Hypnotics–sedatives

These are generally known to have a depressing effect on the central nervous system, consequently reducing the effectiveness of sexual activity.

Chloridiazepoxide (Librium)

Although less frequently prescribed nowadays, this has been associated with a delay or failure to ejaculate.

The effect of the nurse

The nurse as therapeutic agent may become the focus of sexual interest for the client. This may be demonstrated in a number of ways, from overt assault, as in parts of the body being grabbed, or a client exposing his genitals, to verbal suggestions or propositions and looks which may be experienced as lecherous or uncomfortable. Such advances will often be impersonal, in the sense that the client is acting out sexual frustration on the nearest available target, but may be experienced as threatening. Moreover, as in any therapeutic work, if the nurse is unable to deal with the client's sexuality, then ultimately the client is denied an avenue for therapeutic help. Several factors need to be considered here.

Personal safety

If a nurse is visiting a client at home, then it is reasonable to expect a degree of safety. If sexual advances are being made that the nurse feels unable to deal with, then support and supervision will be necessary to explore other possibilities, e.g. only working with the client in an organizational setting or, ultimately, referral if the threat impedes the therapeutic process. This is the extreme, but should not be ignored if it is necessary.

Clear contracting and boundaries

It is important to contract with the client, where possible, in terms of personal boundaries, to be overt in stating that this will not be a relationship of friendship or sexual relationship. It is incumbent on the nurse to be able to respond clearly and honestly to any suggestion from the client that it might be otherwise.

Assertive–empathic response

A skilled way to deflect sexual advance involves acknowledging the sexual issues while being assertive enough to clarify the boundaries and to self-protect where necessary. Two different scenarios come to mind as examples. One is within a therapeutic relationship where there are contracted sessions. If the client expresses sexual attraction in this setting, then the goal of the nurse must be to clarify the issues without deterring the client from exploring his sexuality if this is relevant. So the scenario may go something like the following:

Client: 'I'd love to take you out, nurse, for a good night out.'

Nurse: 'So you feel attracted to me. You also know that I will not act on that attraction and that we are working together on your feelings of isolation and shyness. It must have taken you some courage to say what you have, and I wonder how we could use this to help you be more open outside this relationship.'

Here the nurse empathically acknowledges the statement, clarifies the boundaries and relates the issue to the overall issues of the client. Obviously the precise response will vary depending on the problem area and the relationship between nurse and client, but generally speaking, the more immediate the nurse can be in the situation, the better.

Where the nurse is involved in a more general therapeutic setting, the scenario may be different. For example, a client may grab at the nurse's bottom as she is making a bed. In this case the response still calls for empathy and clarity, but will have a different focus and might be along the lines of: 'While I can understand that you might be frustrated, I don't want you to grab me like that. It makes me feel uncomfortable and makes it hard to work with you professionally. I must ask you not to do that.' In this way the nurse is able to protect herself and reject the behaviour while not putting the client down. Hopefully, this approach will enable a therapeutic relationship to develop or continue along the lines of mutual respect. At the end of the day, the response will depend on the degree of experience and skill of the nurse, but it must be emphasized that she is entitled to support from peers and managers on such issues so that her personal integrity is not threatened.

HIV/AIDS

Finally in this chapter, it is appropriate to look at HIV/AIDS, as this is a potential problem throughout life for anyone who indulges in at-risk behaviour. The treatment of those with sexually transmitted disease is far from new to nursing, but the challenge posed by HIV seems to have sharpened the focus of issues that nurses face. It also reflects our own vulnerability and can be frightening to contemplate. A clear understanding of how the disease spreads, and the issues for nurses and clients, can help. So can addressing some of the common myths which have been associated with HIV.

What is HIV?

HIV stands for human immunodeficiency virus. The virus works by attacking the immune system and destroying the immune cells, the T4 lymphocytes. As a retrovirus, it can insert itself into the host cell nucleus. It takes between 6 and 12 weeks from the initial exposure to the virus before antibodies to HIV can be detected through a blood test. Once a person is infected, it seems that the virus remains in the body for life.

It is as yet unknown conclusively whether HIV necessarily leads to AIDS (acquired immune deficiency syndrome), although the percentage of people developing AIDS is increasing. The body, having no resistance available, falls prey to opportunistic infections and viruses that eventually cause death, which can be slow and painful.

HIV seems all the more frightening because there is as yet no known cure, despite current research efforts. The most successful treatment so far is the use of AZT, and many HIV-positive people benefit greatly from making positive changes in lifestyle to maximize their health. An HIV-positive diagnosis does not mean imminent death – people can survive for many years.

How HIV is transmitted

Much of the fear concerning HIV is due to ignorance about how it is transmitted. Early medical responses were almost inhuman in this fear, with medical staff donning over-the-top protective clothing – as one HIV-positive client reported, 'it was like being treated by spacemen'. Now that we know more about the condition, such overreaction is curbed, but there are still areas of confusion as to how HIV is transmitted.

The only known way for HIV to be transmitted is through the exchange of bodily fluids. This is mainly through sexual activity; exposure to blood and blood products; perinatally from mother to unborn child; and through needle sharing among intravenous drug users.

HIV is not transmitted through sharing lavatory seats, cups or other objects. Nor is it endemic to particular groups of people. Although it was first identified publicly as affecting gay men, heterosexual people are just as much at risk, depending on their lifestyle. Issues of HIV also affect lesbian women, although so far it seems that the infection rate is low. The risk of being exposed to HIV depends on the risk factor attached to a particular activity, not on social identity. High-risk sexual behaviour is any unprotected sexual encounter with people of unknown or positive HIV status, where bodily fluids are exchanged.

Needs of clients

People who are HIV-positive, and those who develop AIDS, need care in three areas, physical, psychological and social. Whatever can be done to alleviate, prevent or minimize physical suffering and discomfort must be available to the client. All workers should be aware of social factors which may affect the client's quality of life, such as housing needs and perhaps support needs, such as the buddying system pioneered by the Terence Higgins Trust. It is useful and supportive to at least show an understanding of social needs, and optimally to be able to give information about appropriate resources.

The psychological needs of clients are of particular relevance here. These will vary according to the client's situation at any one time, and may be roughly classified as follows.

Pretest counselling

Pretest counselling involves exploring the knowledge base of the client and giving appropriate and accurate information in a manner which empathizes with his concerns and apprehensions. Thus the client may be enabled to make an informed choice about whether or not to have a test. It may also involve advising clients on safe practice, so as not to put themselves or other at risk while waiting for results, or indeed if they decide not to have a test.

Getting the results

If the test is negative, clients may still need support with concerns and some educative input on minimizing risk. They will also need to know that a negative result cannot be confirmed until a repeat test three months after the last at-risk behaviour. If the test is positive, the client may be shocked and distressed. Immediate issues seem to concern questions such as who to tell, how to tell them and what the medical implications are.

Coming to terms

The HIV-positive client will need help with accepting their status and exploring ways of living with the diagnosis. This will involve offering support and information so that all possible resources which will be useful to them now and in the future can be explored.

Living with HIV

Clients' needs at this stage will vary depending on whether they are asymptomatic or symptomatic. Information, appropriate medical care, health education and good-quality counselling all have their part to play.

While general points are worthy of the nurse's consideration, two points need underscoring. One is that each individual is precisely that, unique in their specific needs, fears and relationships. In other words, it is important to stay working with the whole person, and not just their HIV status. The second point is that attitude remains all-important. A recent research project identified that nurses were less likely to feel comfortable or willing to socialize with people with AIDS than with those suffering other life-threatening illnesses such as leukaemia, the alternative used in the research (Forrester and Murphy, 1992). Attitudes towards this group of people were generally more negative, confirming an earlier study on the attitudes of doctors. It seems that illogical fears and attitudes that clients are responsible for their own illness (blame) underpin this negativity. It is thus important that the nurse self-challenges on this area in order to deliver humane and effective service.

It must also be remembered that HIV is a highly stigmatized disease, and people of positive status often encounter prejudice in everyday situations. They may also be discriminated against, sometimes quite violently, for being gay or promiscuous. Responsible nursing care, then, should not add to the stigma which is already a part of the problem.

NEEDS OF NURSES

As stated earlier, the treatment and accommodation of people with sexually transmitted diseases is not new to the nursing profession. It seems that HIV, however, has thrown old issues into sharp relief in challenging nurses with their attitude to both sex and death – both societal taboos – at once. Experience suggests that there are four main areas which nurses may find difficult when they all come together.

Sexual attitudes

Nurses may have to challenge their own prejudices about the client's sexual identity or sexual behaviour. They may also be involved with relatives, for example parents who do not know their son is gay; heterosexual partners who did not know their partner had been unfaithful to them; gay partners who feel excluded from the care, and sometimes the death, of the client. Such issues may be taxing to the nurse, and again require an attitude of acceptance and warmth which will help them to use their skills appropriately in the situation.

Attitudes to death

As with any terminal illness, those dealing with AIDS clients will have to confront their own fears and help the clients deal with theirs (see Chapter 17).

Identification

Many people diagnosed as HIV-positive, and those who die of AIDS, are between the ages of 20 and 40. Nurses may identify such clients with themselves, or with their own offspring, and this may be personally challenging. Nurses may also identify with the mode of transmission of the disease. Most people have taken risks in their sexually active lives, and the HIV-positive client may stimulate feelings of 'It could so easily have been me'. It may also be difficult for the nurse working with HIV and AIDS to dissociate sex from fatality.

Ethical issues

Nurses may be challenged by the knowledge that one of their HIV-positive clients is putting others at risk through needle sharing or through unprotected sexual activity. This may stimulate the nurse into feelings of anxiety and inappropriate responsibility. Again, our suggestion is that it is useful for the nurse to have strategies in place which help her to respond as effectively as possible while respecting the confidentiality of the client and the ethical code of the profession. Once again, the importance of support and supervision for nurses working in a challenging area must be stressed (see Chapter 4).

SUMMARY

The area of sexuality is challenging for client and nurse alike. Sexuality involves more than acts of sex: it is an aspect of self with all the experience, fears and attitudes that this may entail. The nurse's major task in this area is to integrate skills and knowledge with self-awareness and self-challenge, in order to maximize client service.

This chapter suggests that sexuality is constructed according to the individual's life experiences. It will be influenced by physiological function and psychological and sociocultural issues. Most people are likely to experience some area of sexual difficulty at some point in their life, whether this is impaired functioning, adverse experience or simply a period of confusion. Specific potential problem areas are highlighted. HIV is introduced as a relatively new area of challenge. In the next chapter, a model of working with adult survivors of sexual abuse will be introduced.

FURTHER READING

Belliveau, F. and Richter, L. (1971) *Understanding Human Sexual Inadequacy*, Hodder and Stoughton, New York.

Bond, T. (1991) *HIV Counselling*, British Association for Counselling, Rugby.

English National Board (1989) *AIDS: Meeting the Challenge*, Ashford Press, London.

Green, J. and McCreaner, A. (1988) *Counselling in HIV and AIDS*, Blackwell, Oxford.

Glover, J. (1985) *Human Sexuality in Nursing Care*, Croom-Helm, London.

Heath, S. (1982) *The Sexual Fix*, Macmillan Press, London.

Kaplan, H. S. (1974) *The New Sex Therapy*, Brunner/Mazel, New York.

Lion, E. (1982) *Human Sexuality in Nursing Process*, John Wiley, Chichester.

Miller, R. and Bor, R. (1992) *Theory and Practice of HIV Counselling: a Systemic Approach*, Cassell, London.

Miller, R. and Bor, R. (1989) *AIDS: a Guide to Clinical Counselling*, Science Press, London.

Pratt, R. (1991) *AIDS – A Strategy for Nursing Care*, Edward Arnold, London.

Weeks, J. (1986) *Sexuality*, Ellis Horwood, London.

World Health Organization (1975) *Education and Treatment in Human Sexuality: the Training of Health Professionals*, Technical Report Series no 572, WHO, Geneva.

A model for working with sexual abuse

21

Janice M. Russell

This chapter presents an overview of a model for working with adult survivors of sexual abuse. As stated in Chapter 20, there is increasing awareness of the long-term psychological effects of sexual abuse, sexual abuse as a possible causal factor in some psychiatric conditions, and the prevalence of sexual abuse within the community at large. The model presented here (Figure 21.1) offers a method of working through this challenging area in a purposeful way, offering maximum safety and support to both client and mental health workers. The cautionary rider is that it is only as applicable to the client group as any other therapeutic technique which is grounded in counselling philosophy and skills. In other words, it will not 'cure' everybody but it has proved extremely useful to a wide client group and has been welcomed by a variety of helpers.

One or two clarifications are necessary at this point. The term 'sexual abuse' is used to denote any behaviour inflicted by one party (the perpetrator) in a position of trust or power over another (the victim), without the informed consent of the victim, for the sexual gratification of the perpetrator. This encompasses a whole range of behaviours, including verbal, non-verbal and viciously physical. It will include forced behaviour as well as inappropriate and coerced behaviour.

The term 'therapist' will be used here for convenience, in the sense of mental health nursing being a therapeutic activity. It is not used to mean a trained psychotherapist. The word 'victim' here refers to the person who has been sexually abused, be it a one-off episode or a long-term process. A 'survivor' is any person who has been abused and has survived the experience. This recognizes the courage and strengths of the individual who has coped thus far, even if some of the coping mechanisms have been inadequate and destructive, or are no longer useful. As a long-term label, however, the term 'survivor' has a downside. It is my personal belief that to identify oneself lifelong with reference to a particular event or set of experiences does not capture the richness of the human spirit when the events have been fully integrated. I know of no-one who refers to themselves as a bereavement survivor. Ultimately, the sexual abuse survivor may become a person who, as one strand of their experience, albeit a highly significant strand, has been sexually abused.

Finally, the term 'mentally debilitated' is used to describe a person who, for whatever reason, is not in a position to offer informed consent or to make responsible decisions. Although the term is clumsy, it would be unethical not to recognize that some people need advocacy, asylum and a certain amount of protection at particular times in their lives. This is where the mental health worker, hopefully with support, will at times make clinical judgements that temporarily assume responsibility for the client's wellbeing. Debilitation seems to me to be a useful description, and is not intended either as a medical or a derogatory label.

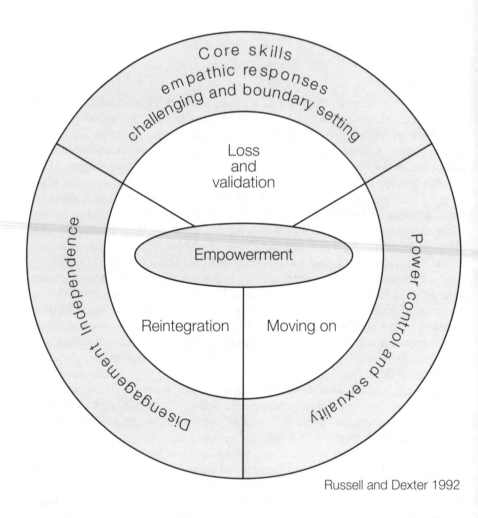

Russell and Dexter 1992

Figure 21.1 A model for working with sexual abuse

THE MODEL

The objective of the model is to offer a systematic framework through which the client and therapist together aim to achieve integration and movement in the client, within the client's own value system. For clients, this entails moving through recognition and validation of the loss experienced within or through the abuse; an understanding of where they are now; how they would like this to change; and a means of achieving the goals they set themselves. For therapists it entails an understanding of what the issues may be; their personal reactions to these; a commitment to clear contracting and boundary keeping; and access to appropriate support, supervision and training.

The model has two main underlying premises. One is that it is essential for the process to be one of empowerment for the client. Sexual abuse involves loss and disempowerment, so it is therefore imperative that the helping process is under the client's control and not mystical. As any process of this nature is complex, it can be best understood and operated by having a systematic approach which aids clarity and purpose.

The second premise is that the therapist may go through a parallel process with the client in terms of issues of boundary keeping, sexuality, control and power. In other words, just as the client may be experiencing feelings of shock, helplessness, anger, fear, disgust, or even levels of arousal, so may the therapist, who sometimes has to hear graphic details of intimate or violent events. Stories range from the client having seen an adult expose his genitals to them, for example, to children having their vagina or anus cut open with a razor blade to enable forced penetration. It is important to be able to hear such accounts with sensitivity and genuineness without compounding the client's feelings of shame or fear.

A useful exercise is, with a colleague or peer group, to brainstorm all the activities you can think of which might constitute sexual abuse, and name them as graphically as possible. Discuss your reactions to each activity – which is easier to hear than another, which seems unbelievable, are any frightening, are any arousing?

Using a framework reminds the therapist that they need clear self-awareness and appropriate supervision and support so that they do not complicate the effects of abuse by their own interventions. Rather, they are then able to draw on their own resources and skills to offer the most effective help for the client.

The model is fuelled by counselling skills, which need to be used throughout the helping process. The issues which arise for client and therapist may occur at any point. The model is divided into three parts to aid clarity and purpose. In practice there may be movement backwards and forwards, although the beginning and end remain constant. In some ways it is helpful to see it as a multilayered spiral, to be gone round again and again in some instances. The outer perimeter represents tasks, issues and skills for the worker, and the inner perimeter issues for the client.

Empowerment – the centre

The empowerment of the client within their own value system is the central aim. This may entail a change of attitude, feeling or behaviour, and must be of the client's choosing. While this applies to any counselling work, it has a particular relevance here because the sexually abused person has been actively robbed of their own power or control over themselves. Thus the more the client is able to understand and assimilate the helping process, the more they are able to use their energies and resources to empower themselves and exercise control over their own lives.

This applies to both adults and children, while recognizing that children are often not in a position to take full responsibility and control for their own lives and actions, and should not be expected to. This is also true of the mentally debilitated adult. The support of an empathic and skilled mentor is crucial here to help such groups empower themselves emotionally as much as possible, and to take responsibility for providing a safe environment where they will be believed and helped to recover.

Beginning the helping process

The client

The main issues for the client here are the recognition of the loss the abuse entailed, whether tangible or intangible, and for their story or feelings to be validated. Loss may entail the physical loss of a person, place or things, or the 'hidden' emotional loss of identity, safety, continuity, trust, self-respect, childhood and security (see Hopkins, 1984). Part of the therapeutic process within this model, then, is to recognize the client's need to grieve. This need and process will be akin to that in any loss experience, and it is likely that the client will be moving through the stages identified in classic grief work (see Chapter 17). These are:

- Shock
- Denial
- Disorganization
- Depression
- Guilt
- Anxiety
- Aggression
- Acceptance
- Reintegration.

One of the possible differences from other grief work is that, just as the loss been hidden, so the grief has been suppressed. This may affect the amount of counselling needed in terms of length of contract, or the degree of support and challenge that needs to be offered. The principles remain the same. Clients recognizing loss for the first time may want to discharge some powerful emotions. The therapist needs to be able to allow such emotion without fear, but while exercising judgement if it seems that the client needs help in containing the emotions or in dealing with them appropriately. This involves drawing on the clinical judgement normally available to the mental health worker.

Working with a client who has recently been abused offers tremendous scope for the helper to validate their experience before the pattern of suppression has been established. Research and practice indicates that the immediate response of the helper to a child who has been abused, or indeed to an adult victim who presents at the time of the abuse, is a key factor in the future development and recovery of that client. While this may seem to add further pressure to the helper, it also offers tremendous potential for rewarding therapeutic work.

The therapist

The therapist's responsibilities are first, to set clear boundaries with the client. This is a particularly important part of the counselling process, as one of the problems of abuse is that boundaries have been invaded and broken inappropriately. Thus it is incumbent on the therapist to be very clear and consistent on this point. It may be tempting for the therapist to feel protective when the client is feeling vulnerable, particularly when disclosure or exploration is accompanied by powerful emotions and/or confusion. Nevertheless, offering unclear boundaries is not usually helpful in the long term. Boundaries need to encompass limits of confidentiality, time, place, frequency and the relationship with the therapist. This last is of paramount importance. Therapists with statutory responsibilities and obligations need to be as clear as possible about who information will be shared with, so that a client does not feel unnecessarily betrayed.

When offering opportunities for clients to validate their loss, the therapist needs to offer support and challenge through empathic listening and acceptance without judgement. Acceptance is crucial as the client may have felt apprehensive in case they are not believed, or they may have made previous disclosures which have not been believed. I have worked with several clients who have gone through the mental health system with no validation to their experience. Thankfully, the climate is slowly changing and it seems that psychiatric nursing is increasingly recognizing this area of work.

Challenge is seen as constructive and is used in four main areas:

* The client's faulty thinking and irrational beliefs (I'll never get over this);
* Societal myths, i.e. more irrational beliefs (it's my fault, I asked for it);
* The client's resources and unacknowledged strengths;
* Self-challenge – do I see sexual abuse as mysterious, what do I avoid in this work etc?

The therapist may then aid the client to begin recovery through a process which resembles the classic stages of grieving.

Unless directly involved in the investigative process, there is no need for the therapist to hear a detailed account of abusive episodes for its own sake. Some clients need to share these as a therapeutic tool, some do not. The point is that validation can occur without an insistence on detail. Such insistence can become another pressure and thus disabling and, if fuelled by curiosity, may represent secondary abuse. By the same token, neither should therapists distance themselves from the events if shared. It is also important not to depersonalize the event or any feelings which are expressed.

The middle stage

The client

At this stage the client needs to be helped to explore the present scenario and to look at how they would like it to change. This will entail clear goal setting, and is often the turning point for the shift between powerlessness and loss of control to empowerment and exertion of control. This stage may entail the exploration and expression of strong feelings which may have been repressed for some time. The pivotal stage for recovery seems to be that of anger. Anger, used constructively, can be a highly potent energy force to fuel the process.

The therapist

The therapist may already be confronted with their own reactions, and it is often in the middle stage that these are less immediately identifiable than at the point of disclosure. However they work, they will be confronted by some powerful emotions and by their own issues of sexuality, power and control. They might feel the urge to suppress client's emotions, or to express their own anger or helplessness. They might be drawn to or repulsed by the client's material, or indeed by the client. They may wish to control the content of the client's work or, subconsciously, to exert power over the client through encouraging dependency. Therapists who manage this stage effectively are more often those who can put aside their own agendas and mobilize their own resources to facilitate those of the client. Where clients are locked into 'seductive' behaviour, it is an ideal opportunity for the therapist to help them find new ways of relating to people (see Russell, 1993). Interpersonal issues may be particularly relevant at this stage. Support and supervision for the therapist are crucial at this stage.

It is important to acknowledge that the therapist's reactions do not manifest only within the therapeutic encounter. Emotional reactions may show themselves in feelings of extra-protectivenes towards children, or other people they care for. It may be that their own sexual relationships are affected temporarily. Some people become angry at the perpetrator and may project such anger on to whole groups of people, e.g. where women begin to view male sexuality as suspicious. Others may question their own patterns of attraction and arousal, and ask whether they themselves are attracted to children, or speculate as to how people might be. They make take home feelings of disgust and offence at the nature of some of the events they know of, and may carry unpleasant pictures which invade their own sex life. For therapists who have themselves been sexually abused, personal issues may be aroused or revisited. Some therapists begin to search for sexual abuse in their own history, where they have not done so before. It is important for the professional support and supervisory service to recognize that these personal reactions are 'normal' and valid, and that help should be available where appropriate.

The final stage

The client

During this stage of the work, the client will be helped to find strategies to achieve the outcomes they want, and may be helped to deal with unfinished business. They may be aided in learning assertiveness skills, and will be helped to synthesize past, present and future events. This may entail coming to terms with mixed or ambivalent feelings towards the offender or other significant people. Here the client becomes fully empowered and is able to recover their identity and to exercise control over their own lives.

It may be that strategies involve revisiting the grieving process. For example, a client may decide that symbolic confrontation of the perpetrator will be useful to them. They may do this through a gestalt approach, say, in using 'empty chair' work. They may then wish to grieve the loss of the perpetrator if this had been a significant figure in their life. This is what is meant by going round the spiral – it is not a backward step but a part of the enabling process.

The therapist

The therapist's task here is to help mobilize the client's resources towards the stated goals. Again, it is important not to exercise judgement on the outcomes. Some therapists find it difficult to accept a client's love for a perpetrator where this exists. One client I have worked with found it difficult to conceptualize her father's repeated sexual acts with her from the age of nine as at all abusive. It is difficult sometimes to be non-judgemental of such a client while having to exercise professional judgement where other children are exposed to that same perpetrator.

It is the therapist's responsibility to enable separation and independence for the client, and to be mindful that this may engender their own issues around these themes. The therapist needs to be able to trust the client and to deal with their own feelings at this stage. For example, the therapist may feel sad at ending the relationship, and encounter their own sense of loss. When working with children, or adults who are not fully independent, it becomes important to be able to trust the child's carer, and this may involve helping them with their own feelings or strategies, as well as issues of professional judgement. Again, support and supervision are important here.

CONCLUSION

I have found this model to be useful and suggest it as a framework rather than a rigid structure. Its value is dependent upon skilful use and allows for a variety of approaches within it. One of the major issues it reminds us of is that therapists will need to empower themselves through skilled practice, self-awareness, support and supervision in order to facilitate the empowerment of clients. In practice, client and therapist will probably move around within the model rather than follow it through in a rigid fashion. The model was originally developed through working with adults and young adults, and has also been used to help children and their carers.

We need also to remember that the client must be in control of their own outcome, as far as possible. It may be that some individuals want to make limited changes: this may be all that they can accept or act on at this time. Some clients may want further help at a later point. Meaningful change can be a slow process as insight develops, and the client's value system must be observed.

In practice, clients may come for help at any point within the model or within the grieving process. Having this conceptualization at hand helps the therapist to make the appropriate intervention and to clarify the goals of the work.

The model is presented as a one-to-one relationship, but can also be used with groups. We have referred to the client as 'they' for convenience, but generally speaking more women than men present in the typical therapeutic context. This is probably because we live in a patriarchal society where men are in many ways more powerful than women, and where sexuality is constructed in ways which offer men a 'right' to women's bodies as pleasure tools (either literally, or through media representation, pornography etc.).

It should be acknowledged, however, that boys and men are sexually abused too. There are specifically researched contexts of male abuse, e.g. within institutions or within the sex industry (pornography, exploitative prostitution), and it is known that males are abused within other contexts. It seems that adult males have a lower reporting rate than females. The psychological effects parallel those of female abuse, but the manifestations may be different as male and female sexuality are constructed differently, i.e. male as active and female as passive. Recent research and practice suggests that many men find it difficult to disclose abuse by other men in case they are labelled as gay or, if they are gay, in case their sexual preference is seen as a 'symptom' of the abuse. Where they have been abused by older women, it seems to be difficult to report because it is supposed to be seen as a 'privilege' to be seduced by an older woman (see Draucker, 1992). Traditional models of masculinity suggest that men may be more likely to be aggressive rather than self-destructive or passive, and may find it difficult to ask for help as this may be seen as weak.

This model of working can be followed using any approach with which you are familiar and which may comfortably work with your client. My own belief is that basic and advanced counselling skills are the bedrock of clear work practice. I also encourage you to be as creative and wide-thinking as possible, and to use any materials or techniques which might help your particular client.

There are also many different methods available to help the client access and vent their feelings, and these might include:

- Art and drawing
- Gestalt work
- Working with metaphors
- Regressive work
- Writing
- Clay or plasticine modelling
- Play therapy
- Behavioural approaches.

Any approach which you are competent to use with your client will be an effective aid to counselling the sexually abused, provided that they are also comfortable with it and develop insight through its use.

Finally, another useful exercise is to consider your reaction to the following statements and discuss them with a colleague or peer group.

Abuse by boys (girls) is not as bad as that by adults.

Women and children ask for it.

It only happens to young women with conventionally 'good looks'.

Those who have been abused become perpetrators.

It only happens to girls and women.

Women and children make things up.

Children are seductive/provocative.

Sexual activity with adults is good for children.

Sexual abuse only happens in the working class/in the north/in certain cultures...everywhere else but here.

Professionals do not abuse.

It is pure enjoyment for a male child to be made to have sex with a woman.

Only men abuse.

Sexual abuse causes permanent and irreversible damage.

Reporting and intervention causes more harm than good.

We can define exactly what sexual abuse is and develop neat theories that explain it.

Sexual abuse is usually perpetrated by strangers.

Disabled children are not at risk.

The hope is that this chapter will have demystified the process of working with the sexually abused, and to have raised awareness. Although the subject may be difficult, sexual abuse happens to 'ordinary people' who, at the end of the day, need to be seen as whole people who need the very 'normal' skills and sensitivity that the nurse employs every day.

FURTHER READING

Axline, V. M. (1981) Dibs: *In Search of Self. Personality Development in Play Therapy*, Penguin Books, Harmondsworth.

Bain, O. and Sanders, M. (1990) *Out in the Open*, Virago Press, London.

Bass, E. and Davis, L. (1989) *The Courage to Heal*, Cedar Press, London.

Bass, E. and Davis, L. (1993) *Beginning to Heal*, Cedar Press, London.

Danica, E. (1989) *Don't*, Women's Press, London.

Draucker, C. B. (1992) *Counselling Survivors of Childhood Sexual Abuse*, Sage, London.

Driver, E. and Droisen, A. (eds) (1989) *Child Sexual Abuse*, Macmillan, London.

Elliot, M. (1985) *Preventing Child Sexual Assault*, Bedford Square Press, London.

Ernst, S. and Goodison, L. (1981) *In Our Own Hands*, Women's Press, London.

Feminist Review (1988) (Special issue, Spring) Family Secrets: child sexual abuse.

Friedrich, W. (1991) *Casebook of Sexual Abuse Treatment*, Norton, New York.

Green, L. (1992) Ordinary Wonders, Women's Press, London.

Hopkins, J. (ed) (1984) *Perspectives on Rape and Sexual Assault*, Harper and Row, London.

Nelson-Jones, R. (1982) *The Theory and Practice of Counselling Psychology*, Cassell, London.

Russell, J. (1993) Out of Bounds: *Sexual Exploitation in Counselling and Therapy*, Sage, London.

Westerlund, E. (1992) *Women's Sexuality after Childhood Incest*, Norton, New York.

Creative approaches 22

This chapter seeks to offer a wider perspective on ways of working with mental health clients. It is important for the nurse to recognize that verbal communication is not the only way of making contact with a client, and that various forms of approach can be helpful other than the traditional 'talk' therapies. We offer no definitive work here, just a hope that this mild stimulation will motivate the reader's interest in further exploration.

ART

Art work is often considered to be a very specialized area, and many mental health nurses may well think it completely outside the normal scope of their skills. Although we would not wish to oversimplify, or in any way to demean the skill and expertise of the trained and practising art therapist, we do believe that this is an area where nurses may profit from the pioneering work of other professionals. It is our belief that this approach would be more widely available to enhance the treatment of mental health problems if some simple aspects of art therapy were more universally adopted by skilled and thoughtful nurses.

At the risk of repeating ourselves, we would say that the mental health nurse is uniquely placed to offer this type of activity; she has almost constant contact, she has the trust of the client and she has the resources of time, energy and potential skill. There is a wide range of needy people who would undoubtedly benefit from these techniques. If simple rules are followed it is a safe but different communication method between the client and his emotions and, as a corollary, the nurse. However, we recommend that before any such therapy is attempted, the nurse should be quite sure of what she is doing. Consequently we offer the following brief guidelines:

1. Wherever possible, allow any art work to be introduced to the client in a non-threatening way. In residential, day hospital or group settings a simple 'Would anyone care to do some painting/modelling/ drawing?' should suffice. It may not be prudent to suggest that this is 'therapy' in the sense that it will involve some deep meaningful analysis of their innermost secrets.
2. There should be no compulsion or unnecessary 'encouragement', especially in the initial introduction. Most sessions will attract volunteers gradually when the more timid clients begin to realize that the sessions are 'fun'.

3. Remember that you are not an art therapist, and therefore no interpretation of the content of the session should be made. It is sufficient for the participants to enjoy the work, and when they feel comfortable you may be able to facilitate some discussion. This may subsequently lead to some sharing of meaning, feelings and themes that is helpful in an appropriately 'therapeutic' way. Here the skills of listening and empathic responses will be an invaluable ally.

4. During sessions clients may become anxious about what they should be doing, especially if they feel they are competing. Be there to support them and answer their questions.

5. A few useful hints about running an art group:
   - First explain quite clearly what you require of participants, and specify from the beginning what will happen to the art work afterwards. Is it just for fun? To stimulate discussion in the group? For the client to take away and think about? Or bring back later to an individual counselling session to 'talk through'? In all cases try to be specific and take out any mystery or possible foreboding that apprehensive clients may feel.
   - It may be better to offer coloured paper, as white paper staring back at people can often have an intimidating effect.
   - Explain that it is not necessary to fill the whole paper.
   - Explain that no-one will be expected to talk about their work if they do not want to, and what they do with their painting/model/drawing afterwards will be up to them.
   - Participate yourself if possible, as by modelling and demonstrating you may be able to break the ice naturally in later discussions, so that no anxieties are raised.
   - If you do participate, and are very able, it may be a good idea not to produce an exquisite piece of work that may discourage the less artistic in the group.
   - Explain that it is not a competition and that clients do not have to be artists to participate.

The latter holds equally true for the nurse. The benefits of art groups are manyfold, but few are to do with the content of the art itself.

No doubt by now you are intrigued to know what this is all about? We have suggested that the nurse/therapist should not interpret or analyse the work, so what is the purpose of the group? For many people with mental health problems the main benefits are as follows:

- The art group is an activity that is fun. At worst it will help alleviate boredom; at best it will be an absorbing and stimulating part of the client's life that he will anticipate with great pleasure.
- 'Through spontaneous painting, the client expresses himself, frees himself from repressed wishes and drives, fulfils desires, and creates a bridge between himself and the outside world' (Assael, 1978).
- Art therapy is a powerful form of non-verbal communication, and facilitates an increase in the empathic relationship between the nurse/therapist and the client.

- Emotions previously unseen or unrecognized may be expressed through art work, and more easily discussed.
- Self-awareness and insights are often raised for both client and nurse/therapist, especially in areas of their own relationship.
- If nurse/therapists are observant, they will use their observational skills during art groups to discover many facts about their clients, and their interactions with their peers.
- Sometimes the art work can be a sort of 'containment' device for the client, e.g. 'I can express some of my emotions on this paper, but then decide not to do anything with them yet. I can if I want put the paper away and go back to it when I want to, or feel ready to.'
- Lastly there is, in our opinion, a very definite therapeutic value in art work, which by its very nature is creative and expressive. It may facilitate lost skills of movement, concentration and purpose. Certainly through a planned and coordinated programme it can create group cohesion and enhance social skills for all participants.

Art therapy is used extensively in all fields of mental health work, but nurse/therapists, usually quick to catch on to a new theme or idea, seem to have been rather slow to include it in their skills repertoire. We offer this short review of the areas where it has proved useful in an attempt to illustrate what may be achieved.

Donnenberg (1978) used art therapy in a community of adolescent drug offenders, and concludes that its use enhanced group cohesion, helped identify the stages of development during treatment, and increased mutuality and expression within the group. Halbreich (1978) used painting as a complete dialogue between therapist and schizophrenic clients by simply painting something in one colour and encouraging the client to add or respond to it by painting on the same paper in another colour. The interchange in this situation was therefore entirely non-verbal, and it is suggested that this technique enhances the nurse's empathy with the client. It can certainly be seen that it may well be extremely useful for the more mute and inaccessible clients, who may refuse to speak but who may enjoy the distraction of art.

In what was a very specialized area, Carozza and Hiersteiner (1982) used art therapy for their work with incest victims. In one particular case, very highly emotive, frightening and embarrassing feelings were expressed through an art group, when verbal descriptions were out of the question. Since 1982, there has been more and more speculation about links between sexual abuse and adult mental health problems. Mental health nurses are now quite likely to be faced with disclosed sexual abuse than was the case then, and art work appears to be an extremely practical and effective tool to help clients explore past incidents of abuse. Art work has now become almost a standard technique when working with the sexually abused (see Chapter 21).

Clearly, much potential good can be done by encouraging the expression of non-verbal behaviour through art. We advocate that mental health nurses research the area before contemplating any elaborate therapeutic programmes, but we are confident that by following the initial guidelines many nurses will be able to add another most powerful tool to their armoury of qualities and skills.

DRAMA THERAPY

Background

Much of the present drama therapy or psychodrama techniques in current use are derived from early work undertaken by Moreno, a Viennese psychiatrist, in the early part of this century, when it was by no means as fashionable as it is today. Moreno's pioneering work must be acknowledged, for many of the refreshing and 'new' approaches we meet in mental health work in this field are rooted within it, including many aspects of group psychotherapy. Some of the work of Carl Rogers, especially the concept of dealing with the 'here and now', was originally provided by Moreno (1946).

Much has been written about drama therapy and there are some fine books dealing with the subject. We cannot, and do not hope to, compete with this literature; our purpose in including a short section here is simply to put drama therapy into the context of mental health nursing skills.

Theory

In our opinion, drama therapy is an important resource which may be used as an independent therapy with suitable clients or as a complementary therapy for many other people when appropriate. Psychotherapy and psychoanalysis seek to explore the individual's thoughts and feelings by intensive listening and skilled responding, with psychoanalysis taking a more theoretical and interpretive account. Psychodrama or drama therapy seeks to study and provide insights to and for the client through actions and words. Often words and simple non-verbal behaviour do not give sufficient insight into the real problems, needs and issues surrounding the individual; drama therapy seeks to fill the gap in this information, and in certain situations may solve some problems in the process.

The uses of drama therapy and its application to mental health work

Drama therapy uses many techniques designed to construct or reconstruct situations and their associated feelings, and act them out in a safe and structured environment. The simplest form is perhaps the role-play reconstruction used in social skills training. Here a person who is anxious or unable to enter certain social situations can artificially reproduce the scene and be mentally and physically escorted through the process. The individual can explain the thoughts and emotions he feels step by step, and rehearse more effective ways of dealing with the negative aspects of the situation as they occur. It could realistically be argued that assertion training, desensitization, skills training and most experiential educational methods are all based on drama therapy. The essential difference in many of these examples is purely the accent of 'client-centredness'. In behavioural techniques, the therapist has in her mind a desired outcome and uses positive reinforcement and the shaping process to mould the client towards this goal. The drama therapist is generally more interested in the process of insight rather than the direction in which it takes the client.

Its applications to mental health work are perhaps obvious, but it may be stressed at this point that it is not suitable for all people with mental health problems. Any process as powerful in releasing repressed or suppressed emotions must carry with it certain dangers or potential problems. There are unfortunately some clients whose conditions are characterized, quite fortuitously perhaps, by a lack of insight. Any method of therapy which seeks to break down that lack of insight may well be damaging to that individual's wellbeing.

Clients categorized as 'psychotic', especially those suffering from schizophrenia, should only be involved in drama therapy, or for that matter group therapy, after very careful consideration of the possible consequences of such action by the team responsible for their care (see Langley and Langley, 1983, p. 59). Similarly, some clients may be temporarily unable to tolerate a close introspection of themselves, and should not be considered for a drama therapy group. It should be realized that even despite careful selection of clients, an undesired reaction may occasionally occur within a group session. It is for this reason that only trained drama therapists, or nurses who have undergone a thorough instructional course under the supervision of a drama therapist, should undertake such a group, especially if it is intended to conduct therapy as an independent method. There are, however, simple techniques that may be of great benefit, and some of these are described below.

Role play

This is perhaps the simplest technique, although it is extremely powerful. Usually the client will act out using any props he may need by improvising or imagining, and playing out a scene. The nurse's role is usually to play a counter part in the situation, and she is advised by the client on the type of response he would normally expect. For example, the alcohol-dependent person who has difficulty refusing an invitation from a friend to go to the pub may ask the nurse to play the friend while he rehearses saying no. This simple technique helps the person relieve the feelings he has to deal with in the situation which he fears may bring about his downfall. The nurse may well pick up useful information at the same time about the individual's ability to recognize and deal with his emotions. Some people criticize this technique as being artificial and somewhat ridiculous. Indeed, we would agree that it might well be a little embarrassing at first, but we know of very few people who have tried this method who can still wholeheartedly say that there is no value in it. Despite its artificiality and unreal atmosphere, very much of the content of the role play does become real. The emotions expressed within it are mostly very real to the person acting out his situation, and the information extracted from it is generally very useful for personal growth (see Warren, 1984). Wherever possible a third person should be used to observe the role play, as she can then make notes about the various ideas, feelings and behaviours that she sees as potentially significant. This is then fed back to the client in a tentative questioning manner, in order for him to try to make some sense of it all. For this to be effective, the feedback should be as objective as possible and we suggest that notes and verbal feedback take a literal format. For example: 'I noticed when you spoke, Mr X, your voice trembled....' 'I noticed you clenched your fist when...' 'I saw you....' 'You said...after....' 'I heard you say....'

Avoid statements such as 'You were obviously very puzzled when...' as the latter indicates an interpretation on the observer's part.

It is necessary, however, to enable the client to match up his non-verbal and verbal behaviours and actions to his emotions in some way. For this purpose it is suggested that open questions be asked, such as: 'I wonder how you were feeling when...' or 'Perhaps you could explain to me what you were feeling when....'

Following the role play and feedback, the nurse may follow either a behavioural or a counselling approach to bring about change, depending on which is most suitable for the individual.

Another simple technique that follows on from role play is **role reversal**. This is simply using the same format as above but with the client playing the part of the other person. This is designed to initiate some insight into how others may feel in a situation, and to provide further information that may help the person communicate more effectively. Role reversal can also be played out with the client playing both parts. This requires a little more versatility but can be extremely effective in providing meaningful insight into the process of the interchange and how others react immediately to the client's verbal message. It is a good idea, however, to help the client change roles, to insist that he changes chairs when playing both parts. The actual process of bodily movement into a different chair appears to facilitate a complete change of role. Role reversal is extremely useful in family therapy, e.g. to have a young adolescent actually try for the first time to imagine how his parents feel, what they would say and how they would say it, can be very beneficial. When this is coupled with the parent observing this and seeing how their son or daughter sees them, real insights can be achieved. It is, of course, vitally important that all parties involved have ample opportunity following any role-play situation to express their feelings and thoughts fully, and that the debrief is handled skilfully.

Empty chair and happy chair

These are two very simple techniques that can quite safely and easily be incorporated into the nurse's repertoire. The empty chair is in fact a very useful 'safety valve' technique. In group or individual therapy, if an individual feels that emotions are running high, either positively or negatively, then they may be encouraged to release them safely and swiftly by expressing them to an empty chair. Usually a particular chair is designated, and in group situations this is made known at the beginning of the session. Anyone may approach the chair at any time and express his feelings. It is recommended in early sessions that the identity of the subject of the feelings is not exposed, so that no-one's feelings are hurt or anyone embarrassed.

The happy chair is designated in much the same way, except that using this chair indicates to the group that the person is unhappy, feels rejected, embarrassed or has a negative feeling. This invites the group to respond positively to that individual in any predetermined acceptable way. Mostly this will be in an upsurge of clapping, whistling and shouts of 'good old....' The amount of demonstrative affection the group is able to give will be entirely up to the individuals within it, but the skilled facilitator is usually able to ensure that the experience of sitting in the happy chair is in fact a happy one. A side effect of this situation which generally helps the group is the trust it generates within itself. People forming a group usually care for and nurture the separate members, and this procedure helps to reinforce this fact.

Guided fantasy

This most popular technique in drama therapy allows the client to experience his own mental imagery in a very relaxed and positive fashion. It is for some individuals very close to a light hypnosis, and can be extremely useful in allowing a person to become closer to personal insights in his life which he may have been hiding from himself. The process begins with simple relaxation exercises, ensuring that all the participants are relaxed and comfortable. This can often be facilitated by immediately preceding the event with a very physically exerting warm-up exercise, or dancing. Once the group or individual is relaxed, soft music may be played in the background and the therapist begins to guide the participants through a journey. This may be to a particular place, through a particular time, or to see a particular person. The subject of the journey will be constructed in the context of the individual travellers. It is important not to go too quickly or the effect of the imagery will be lost; similarly, it is important not to be too specific in describing the journey, as this may conflict with an already constructed image and spoil the effect. To be loose in descriptive terms allows the potential symbolism of the journey to be client-centred. Useful devices within a simple journey may be for a client to meet someone 'significant to him', for him to 'say something to this person' and 'remember the most important thing this person says'. The client may be invited to receive a gift from the person and return with it, or the person may do something before he leaves. The things a client experiences on his journey, the people he sees and what he hears should not be unduly influenced by the guide, so that when the client recounts the journey it will be full of meaning for him from his mental imagery. Often, following the return trip, the client will be asked to share what he wishes with another person or a small group. The significance or symbolism he wishes to attach to the journey is for him to imply.

An example of a simple journey is as follows:

> 'I want you to imagine you are in a safe and warm place, I want you to remember that you will return to this place after your journey, this place is always here and you can come back to it at any time if you want to for any reason....Imagine you are facing a door. Look closely at the door, see the handle and lock – open the door and before you is a long corridor; proceed along the corridor, taking notice of what you see. At the end of the corridor is a light; as you get closer you can see more clearly. Even closer, you begin to smell familiar fragrances. You can feel the temperature outside, and now see quite clearly the scene before you. Continue walking – as you walk you are aware of all the sounds around you, you can feel the texture beneath your feet, and hear the sound of your footsteps. There appears to be a building of some kind in the distance. Can you make out what it is? I think you may just be able to see a figure beside the building; can you make out what they

look like? As you get closer you can see more clearly the building and the figure. The person seems to be holding something for you. You may take it if you wish. Examine it. The person seems to be saying something now. It appears to be important. You may feel you want to reply; there seems to be a need to express something between you.

It's almost time to return now, take another look around, smell the fragrances, feel the sensations surrounding this place, say goodbye to the person and prepare to return. Begin your journey back.

You may just be able to make out the corridor now. Enjoy the walk back, take note of what you can see. You're just about in the corridor now, proceed along it to the door. Open the door, recognize the room you're in and open your eyes when you feel ready.'

Some individuals will simply find this a relaxing experience, while others may find that it turns into a significant walk into their subconscious. In situations where the client may be frightened, or is likely to imagine a particularly unpleasant journey, the therapist may feel she has to build in simple safeguards. Some ideas here might be to suggest they take a very close and trusted friend with them; to reassure them continually that the place is friendly; to describe in clearer and specific detail a 'springtime' walk; and to build more pleasantness into the journey; the person is smiling and so on. The skilled therapist should know her client sufficiently well to be able to build in safeguards as appropriate.

There are, of course, many more techniques that may be used; we simply do not have space in this small volume to include them. We do, however, recommend most strongly that the interested reader pursues the excellent material available (see Further Reading).

MUSIC AND DANCE

Music and dance are often forgotten among the mass of interactive therapies now presently available to the nurse/practitioner. However, we feel that this book could not be complete without at least a short explanation of these two powerful influences upon human behaviour, and would like to offer you some practical insights which we have come to through our fleeting exposure to these therapies.

Movement and dance

Most healthy individuals have at some time been invited to, or participated in, dance activity. The wild frenzied 'letting it all hang out' type dance appears to be poles apart from the rather controlled and skilful conventional dance steps. Nevertheless, both of these share common factors with very similar activities such as gymnastics, or almost any type of physically active sport or recreation. Whichever is your particular favourite, dance gives an expression in physical behaviour of the mental process within you. No experienced mental health nurse would argue with the very practical nature of encouraging the frustrated or aggressive individual to participate in some socially accepted physical activity. Similarly, dance and movement therapy is designed and structured to enable the client to find suitable expressions for his emotions.

For most people, dancing becomes an extremely entertaining activity. It not only allows an expression of mood or personality, but may also facilitate the expression of certain skills. There can be no doubt that the accomplished dancer is credited with an enviable skill, yet the movements involved are, paradoxically, rather meaningless. Perhaps even more noticeable is the fact that although it is a pursuit requiring considerable energy, most people agree that dancing is a form of relaxation. This could be because it is such a basic form of communication that there is only a release of mental energy rather than a need to expend it. The subject simply acts what he feels in the dance rather than having to think of ways of expressing it. Generally all forms of dance are socially accepted, and consequently there are no cultural restraints on the expression of mood within dance, and no-one is likely to be offended. The nurse involved in dance therapy may be able to increase her insight into the client's emotional state by observing his non-verbal behaviour and posturing, and the client may be able to communicate his emotions much more easily in a non-threatening situation.

Music

Music and dance are difficult to separate as distinct therapies, but it may be beneficial to make one significant distinction. When the client chooses the type of music he wishes to dance to, he is using the music to accompany his feelings: the music he chooses will match his mood. Conversely, if music is chosen for the client, a quite different effect may be observed. The client who was previously irritated and might have chosen a rather loud and lively piece may become quiet and relaxed when asked to dance to a soft and gentle sound. The point we make is that music may be used either to potentiate the expression of the present mood or to facilitate possible changes in it. This can only be reinforced by individual experience. Imagine that you are listening to specific pieces of music; can you connect emotions very directly with them? Try some of the more dramatic film scores for instance, or some of the classical pieces, which can be soothing, stirring or dramatic, or delicately intricate and complex. They nearly all have the power to arouse strong feelings and, in many people, highly emotional thoughts. Choosing music to set a scene will invariably require music suitable for the occasion. The simple fact is that if you want to feel a particular emotion, say sadness, you will almost inevitably choose music that reminds you of a sad event or time. Conversely, if you are happy and wish to remain so, the music chosen will be associated with happiness to sustain that mood. In therapy this has several practical applications.

First, in reality orientation, playing records which help the person focus back to a particular time will stimulate memories associated with that time. War songs are perhaps an obvious example but, perhaps more subtly, the wedding march or the funeral march may equally strike very emotional memories. The use of music in positive conditioning (see Chapter 3) can be very powerful, and associating a specific piece of music with the person's calm state may induce relaxation if it is replayed when he becomes anxious.

In its simplest context music is just pleasant; it is entertaining, occasionally creative and potentially soothing. Without music our world would be deprived of a wonderful source of sensory stimulation that a lot of people consider joyful. (See Langley and Langley, 1983, for some useful aids to appropriate music selection.) In contrast, one final consideration we would like to point out is that nurses sometimes forget that it is possible to spoil the effect by overexposure. To be constantly bombarded with sound, no matter how beautiful, may irritate an individual to the extent that all sounds are perceived as unwelcome noise. In practical terms, for music to be linked with therapy or simple pleasure it is most important that it should be separated from everyday sounds. Preferably music rooms should be available where clients can choose what they hear, but at least music should not compete for attention with the television, conversation and domestic noise.

IMPLICATIONS FOR THE NURSE

The main implication for the nurse in music and dance therapy is to be aware of just how powerful these techniques can be. There is, we feel, a general feeling among nurses that these areas are not very exciting, or that they are surrounded in mystery and therefore not particularly appropriate to them. We wonder if some of this attitude comes from the nurse's reluctance to join in some of these therapeutic pursuits with clients. Music is reasonably dignified and most nurses would have few reservations about becoming involved; dance, on the other hand, may be a different matter. We can understand that for some nurses using dance as a therapeutic endeavour may be somewhat embarrassing. We can imagine you saying something like 'I can't do that, I'd feel daft'. We can even reflect back to our student days and perhaps sympathize. Nevertheless, embarrassment should be no disincentive to ensuring that the client has every opportunity to express himself. In the long run the client will respect the nurse who risks looking foolish to help him, far more than the nurse who steps back and by her example denies him an additional therapeutic experience.

We believe music and dance therapy will play a significant part in the treatment and rehabilitation of clients in the future, and it is therefore our hope that nurses will shed their anxieties and reluctance over something different, take an interest in it and use it positively for their clients' benefit.

FURTHER READING

Art

Dalley, T. (ed) (1984) *Art as Therapy*, Tavistock, London.

Donnenberg, D. (1978) Art therapy in a drug community. *Confinia Psychiatrica*, **21**(1–3), 37–44.

Feder, E. and Feder, B. (1981) *The Expressive Art Therapies*, Prentice-Hall, Englewood Cliffs, New Jersey.

Mitchell, A.R.K. (1982) *Art and Drama therapy as Part of a Multidisciplinary Team*. Conference Paper, College of Art and Design, St Albans.

Pavey, D. (1979) *Art Based Games*, Methuen, London.

Drama therapy

Blatner, H. A. (1973) *Acting In: Practical Applications of Psychodramatic Methods*, Springer, New York.

Hodgson, J. (1972) *The Uses of Drama: Acting as a Social and Educational Force*, Methuen, London.

James, N. (1979) *Introduction to Drama Therapy and the Role of Staff Members*, Napsbury Hospital, St Albans.

Jennings, S. (ed) (1979) *Remedial Drama: a Handbook for Teachers and Therapists*, Pitman, London.

Langley, D. M. and Langley, G. E. (1983) *Drama Therapy and Psychiatry*, Croom Helm, London. (Highly recommended)

Remocker, A. J. and Storch, E. T. (1982) *Action Speaks Louder*, Churchill Livingstone, London.

Scobie, S. (1978) Drama therapy with psychotic adults. *Journal of the British Association of Drama therapy*, **1**(4), 13–16.

Music and dance

Bernstein, P.L. (ed) (1979) *Eight Theoretical Approaches in Dance/Movement Therapy*, Kendal, Hunt, Dubuque, Toronto.

Bunt, L. (1994) *Music Therapy: An Art Beyond Words*, Routledge, London.

Davis, W. B., Gfeller, K. E. and Thaut, M. H. (1992) Introduction to Music Therapy, W. C. Brown,

Storms, G. (1981) *Handbook of Music and Games*, Hutchinson, London.

Warren, B. (ed) (1984) *Using the Creative Arts in Therapy*, Croom Helm, London.

General

Axline, V. M. (1981) *Dibs: In Search of Self. Personality Development in Play Therapy*, Penguin Books, Harmondsworth.

Jennings, S. (ed) (1975) *Creative Therapy*, Pitman, London.

23 Research

Janice M. Russell

It is a generalization to say that most nurses do not come into the profession to become either academics or researchers, although in our experience this is probably true. Equally it is a generalization to assert that most nurses are not expert mathematicians, yet again in our experience this is also true. These two generalizations are, however, probably the two 'facts' that make nurses somewhat reluctant to embrace research. Nurses in general tend to avoid research and be suspicious of it when it is cited or quoted; it seems that many are doubtful of the mystery of the process and of statistics.

In a way this is both understandable and unfortunate. In the current climate of the decentralization of the NHS and the ever-increasing establishment of 'trust' status which heralds the privatization of the health service, and with the professionalization of nursing as an academic discipline, research is becoming more and more influential. For example, managers are using research findings to justify and rationalize changes in service provision and to enable them to identify, plan and implement change. Moreover, nurses are increasingly being asked to demonstrate research skills on degree and diploma courses.

It is our view that in the 1990s nurses must have at least a basic grasp of research in order to enable their clients to obtain a fair deal in an increasingly competitive and commercial market. There is no doubt that research can be helpful in the pursuit of excellence, and it is essential for nurses if they are to support their practices as legitimate, and avoid being unduly influenced and manipulated by the spurious and misleading use of research findings by others.

In order to ensure that you are not being exploited or manipulated by people quoting research, it is important that you are able to read, understand and criticize at least the main elements of research. On a positive note, the world of research opens up a whole new area of study that can influence and enhance nursing practice once it becomes available to the practitioner. As a sharp example of this principle, take a common research- based assertion:

> Behavioural techniques are the best methods to secure effective treatment outcomes for psychiatric clients suffering 'neurotic' illness.

This is based on work done by Eysenck (1961, 1966), who used an experimental design and systematically 'proved' that neurotic patients responded better to behaviour therapy than to psychotherapeutic treatments. In addition to this he asserted that two-thirds of neurotic patients 'spontaneously remit', whether treated or not. Although in our opinion this was a very good piece of research, it raises questions for the discerning reader. For example, how many cases have to be studied before such generalized findings can be taken as 'true'?

As well as measuring outcomes in terms of anxiety ratings, depression scores and phobic response rates, is it not as important to measure some of the qualitative reactions within therapy? For instance, during the phase before 'spontaneous remission', how much trauma and distress is wreaked upon the individual? What are the costs of not treating this client in terms of divorce rate, unemployment, sexual activity, damage to interpersonal relationships, and general quality of life?

If the absolute logic of the findings were applied to service delivery, would it not be rational to say 'if they will get better anyway why do anything?' An astute 'cost-conscious' manager may be tempted to take this approach. The discerning and caring nurse needs at least to be armed with the 'answers' to this tack. Other research based on qualitative approaches rather than the objective 'number-crunching' statistical argument needs to emerge.

WHAT IS RESEARCH?

Some of the mystery of research needs to be unravelled. Basically when the process is laid bare it is simply finding rational and evidence-based answers to well thought-out questions. It also acts as a means of investigation and aids clarity in understanding the rich world of human behaviour, where often clear answers do not abound.

Many nurses take the attitude: 'I've been nursing long enough to know what I'm doing – what do I need research for? Anyway, research just boils down to common sense doesn't it?' To be honest, this is true: much research is about common sense, and a lot of nursing practice is based on tradition and custom, not requiring a research-based approach. However, there are long-established nursing practices that make no sense. Before Lister identified the need for antiseptics the practice of washing one's hands was thought to be unnecessary. We were taught that swabbing an injection site with ethyl alcohol, and treating pressure areas with spirit and oil, were essential procedures. Although both of these nursing practices were seen as 'common sense' at the time, research has undoubtedly disproved their value.

Mental health nursing has perhaps seen even more dubious practices. Electroplexy, hydrotherapy, deep narcosis, modified narcosis, insulin coma and modified insulin coma therapy are just a few practices which, thankfully, have had their mystical pseudoscientific rationales dented. On more psychological and sociological ground, feminist research has done much to challenge attitudes and beliefs about women, mental health norms and depressive illness (see Broverman and Broverman, 1970).

Testing the fashionable theories and therapies of the day is difficult when professionals have their ideas and beliefs set intractably in support of them. Research is an effective way of challenging their continuance, of demonstrating what is helpful to the client group, and of ever reviewing the basis of good practice.

At its best, research gives us definitive answers to questions such is which is better (given a particular set of circumstances), which is quicker, easiest, most cost-effective, least likely to cause harm, most long-lasting or simply expedient. It should provide wider options and enhance choices based on current knowledge and thinking, and occasionally raise further questions to be answered before we can rationally proceed. It can therefore help us have confidence in what we are doing, and equally raise doubts when necessary to prevent us 'rushing in where angels fear to tread'. It should prevent us from becoming infatuated with our personal preferences and thus becoming dogmatic and rigid. It should therefore provide us with a basis to know why and how we should practise our chosen profession with effectiveness instead of jargonistic rhetoric. At worst it provides us with statistical interpretations of data, calculated in such complex and misleading ways that the findings become blurred or, worse, manipulated to support the originator or financial stakeholder: 'There are three kinds of lies, lies, damned lies and statistics' (attrib. Mark Twain).

How then are we to sort out the helpful from the misleading? How can we trust any research? The answer, although not to everyone's taste, is that we must learn how to read, measure and evaluate research. The next section is a brief outline of the process of research. It is intended not as an exhaustive text but as an introduction to the reader who has some interest in the subject, to demystify it and make it more accessible.

GENERATING THE RESEARCH PROBLEM

We have discussed the probability that there is often a link between commonsense practice and research findings. When you are a nurse in training, you may need to take one step backwards from the commonsense perspective and consider how to generate a research problem. What kinds of issues might lend themselves to being rigorously reviewed under the umbrella of research? What might interest you, the researcher, and stimulate interest and usefulness in the audience to whom you present your findings? At the end of the day, the interest of the researcher ideally underpins the research process – in the words of C. Wright Mills (1959), it should capture the 'sociological imagination'. Indeed, the process of research, while lending itself to structure and vigorous testing, is creative and imaginative. It is often begun by the researcher chasing the particular 'bee in their bonnet'.

In generating the research problem two central terms need clarifying, as they recur throughout the research process. The first term is **theory**. We follow Silverman (1993) in using this term to refer to a set of explanatory concepts relevant to a particular problem. It is relevant only so long as it has some degree of usefulness. For example, at one time society held the theory that young women who stopped eating for a period of time were possessed by the devil. In 17th century England, this theory was grounded in the concepts of possession and of good and evil, which reflected the way in which people made sense of their world, i.e. through theories of religion and magic. Its usefulness was in helping communities to find a way of coping with the starving woman in ways which helped her to recover, and which gave some sort of meaning to the experience.

Such theories are no longer useful to us because the explanatory concepts are not relevant to our culture. Currently, slow starvation would be explained by the concepts of eating disorder, control, aversion, inner struggle or whatever, all informed by **psychological** theories of behaviour. Theories underlie all research, as without them there is no impetus to get the process going.

Having identified a research problem in relation to the theory that informs it, it is common to define the research question in terms of a **hypothesis**. This means a testable proposition, and is only useful as long as it has some possibility of validity. So, we might propose the following hypotheses:

- Clients who have manic depressive episodes would respond better to behaviour therapy than to client-centred counselling.
- Our responses to the dangers of illegal drugs are dependent on ignorance and medical scares.
- There is a link between some depressive states and childhood sexual abuse.

These three statements are all hypotheses which can be tested for their validity. They all have some theoretical underpinning, e.g. depressive people can be helped by talking cures, sexual abuse can have long-term psychological effects. It is possible that they are all valid statements, and that there is a chance of proving them to be true.

In setting out a hypothesis, the student or researcher is beginning their own unique research process. At this stage, it is necessary to be as clear and specific as possible. If they follow their interests, it is likely that most professional nurses will have some questions that are raised by their practice. The knack is to turn the general question into the testable proposition.

To take an example already cited, you may set out wondering: 'Would clients suffering mania/depression respond better to a behavioural approach rather than the client-centred counselling approach which I have adopted?'. More generally: 'What is it I do that is really helping the client?'

In terms of more descriptive studies the question might be just:

'What is happening to the client throughout this process?' Even more vague might be questions such as:'Why do we do this or that? I wonder if I did that rather than this would the result be the same/better/worse?'

These examples are crude and so not researchable. Such general questions need to be made more precise and measurable. For example, for the question 'Would behaviour therapy be more effective than client-centred counselling with these clients?' to be researchable, terms would have to be specified. So, we would need to identify:

What do we mean meant by 'more effective'?

What is the precise nature of 'client-centred counselling'? What is the nature of 'behaviour therapy'?

What are the criteria for the clients to be termed 'manic–depressive'?

The research question then becomes more measurable, depending on the definitions proposed and the methodology adopted. So the original question might become a hypothesis which follows the 'hunch' of the researcher: 'Clients suffering from episodes of manic depression as defined by...respond more rapidly to behavioural programmes, in terms of identifiable behaviour and subjective appraisal, than they do to Rogerian counselling, where no direction is offered from the therapist.' This is still clumsy, but begins to elucidate the question. We can now start to break down the research into manageable component parts.

At this stage it will be useful to initiate a **literature search**, in other words, explore existing literature on the subject.

It is important that this is done thoroughly for several reasons:

- The research you are proposing may have already been done.
- The literature unveiled may well prove to be invaluable in clarifying the study further and informing your research design.
- The main concepts or ideas in the question or hypothesis will be informed by it in relation to current understanding and knowledge.

The literature search used to be the most arduous of tasks. Not too many years ago it involved the manual sorting of indexes, abstracts, lists of titles and piles of old journals. Most of these operations are now computerized, with CD-ROMs (Compact Disk Read Only Memory) and online searches of international databases, which makes the whole operation very quick and easy. The reader still baffled by this technology is referred to a wonderful, good-natured resource known as 'the librarian'. (Our grateful thanks goes to this professional group, whose knowledge, helpfulness and encouragement has been most gratefully received by us on many occasions.)

Once a literature search has been conducted, the salient articles and books need to be scanned for relevant material. Although time-consuming, this is necessary to ensure that the next step is well informed. From this reviewed knowledge and information it is likely that a hypothesis or several hypotheses will be formulated, and the researcher is ready to make a research design. Initially, they must choose their **methodology** and **methods** and identify the **variables** which need to be taken into account in the data collection phase of the research. It should be stated at this point that not all research questions have clear hypotheses. This is because more weight is increasingly being given to investigative research, e.g. finding out how people's situations or perspectives are experienced by them or how supervision might affect nursing practice, etc.

METHODOLOGY

Methodology is the general approach to studying the research topic. In other words, it addresses the question of how you will go about collecting useful data which will inform the analysis. There are two main types of methodology, **quantitative** and **qualitative**.

Quantitative

Quantitative methodology has its roots in positivism, an approach which seeks to discover social and psychological laws through the establishment of facts and numbers. The school of positivism claims that the study of people, how they function and how they interact, is the subject of scientific method; that we can be objective and unbiased about research into humankind.

Qualitative

Qualitative methodology accepts that research into people is subjective, and is more concerned with how people experience events than with providing a valid database. Qualitative methodology recognizes bias and limitations, but by no means gives the nod to sloppy or unrigorous approaches. Rather, it asks the researcher to recognize bias as a part of the research process.

Traditionally, there has been some dispute about which of these is most valid, but there is increasing recognition that both have something to offer and can complement rather than fight each other.

So for instance, in the example under review, we might decide to take a quantitative approach through observing the results of three sessions of behaviour therapy on six clients who are diagnosed as manic–depressive and comparing the results, in terms of observable behaviour, with six clients who receive client-centred counselling. The criteria for measurement would be decided by the researcher, e.g. spends more waking hours out of bed, makes fewer suicide attempts, washes more frequently etc. This would constitute a quantitative methodology – what factors can be reported under certain conditions, with how many subjects, and how many times.

A qualitative methodology might follow two clients, one in behaviour therapy and one in client-centred counselling, over a period of three months. They might devise a series of open-ended interview questions and leave much of the evaluation to the client's subjective account. Both approaches would have merit; one would illustrate a breadth of experiences and identify patterns, while the other might give more in-depth insights into the client's experience. At one time, positivists would have claimed that their methods were more objective. Although they might come up with slightly more objective tendencies, it must be remembered that the design of questions, experiments and analyses will always have some subjective influence. The researcher will have some influence depending on how he or she is perceived by the subject, i.e. in relation to status or power. The actual forms and questionnaires may not be 'user friendly' and thus the subject may be overwhelmed, become disinterested or confused. This latter point raises the issue of large-scale questionnaires: can they really be seen as representative of the general public or only for that portion of the population which is literate?

The general rule in designing the methodological approach is in trying to match it to the desired outcomes. The chances are that you will be researching something that interests you. Unless your livelihood depends on doing research, we suggest you let your interest lead you, and to be as clear as possible about what outcomes you would like within the resources available. These will include things such as time, money, space and the purpose of the research. A common mistake is to make 'good plans' well outside the scope of the researcher. A well-planned modest research project is of more use than a skimpy overambitious plan.

METHODS

Having decided on the methodological framework, the specific methods available within each one need to be considered. In qualitative research, it is generally suggested that there are four main methods available:

- Observation, e.g. case studies or group/culture observation;
- Textual analysis: analysing texts and documents;
- Interviews.
- Recording and transcribing, e.g. counselling sessions.

As Silverman (1993) notes, none of these methods is unique to qualitative methodology; indeed, they can all be used in quantitative methodology but with different emphases and purposes, so that, for example, large-scale surveys use fixed question techniques (interviews) with 'representative' sections of the population. They generate large numbers of responses, but we are not clear about the quality of the data in terms of validity and meaning (e.g. election polls). A qualitative methodology, however, might interview one small group of voters and try to elicit their thoughts and feelings about an election and identify the type of issue which might influence the voting tendency over the next 24 hours.

In quantitative research the major methods are:

- Surveys (e.g. market research, census, Kinsey reports, Hite report);
- Sociometrics (the measurement of preferences among members of a group, e.g. work teams, therapy groups);
- Experiments;
- 'Indirect' methods.

Experiments have been a traditional key method in psychology to date. These have included experiments on animals, where findings have then been used to generate theory to predict and shape human behaviour (e.g. Pavlov's dogs, Skinner's rats). They have also included using humans in test conditions to draw inferences about human behaviour (see Milgram, 1974). A third type of experiment which has informed theories of human behaviour has involved the measurement of physiological responses to stimuli (see Masters and Johnson, 1966).

'Indirect' methods are those that generate information which was not their primary object. So, for example, work with First World War veterans provided us with information about the psychological reactions known as 'shell shock', which would now be known as 'post-traumatic stress disorder'. Similarly, tests used in recruitment for the Second World War generated unforeseen information about the physical and mental health of a generation. IQ testing may be seen as an indirect method, where a test designed to provide information about an individual for a specific reason may then provide statistics for a larger picture.

SAMPLES

There are basically two kinds of sampling, 'random' or 'selected', also referred to as 'probability sampling', or 'non-probability sampling', respectively.

Random or probability sampling

This makes the claim that it samples and thus represents whole populations. The claim is supported because every member of the population to be researched is equally likely to be picked out. There are sophisticated techniques associated with finding 'random' samples which go beyond the scope of this chapter. This method is usually used for large-scale research. It is possible to make simple sampling techniques, however, which offer a degree of randomness. For example, you might choose every third client on your list, or all those with the letter p in their name, or throw twenty names into a hat and pick out eight. It should be noted that many researchers would argue that a true random sample is a logistical impossibility (for a clear exposition of random sampling techniques, see Sarantakos, 1993).

Selected or non-probability sampling

Non-probability sampling is less rigid and is left to the subjective choice of the researcher. This is where it becomes important to note carefully the characteristics and relevant history of the participants to see what other factors might influence findings. It is often associated with qualitative research, where the purpose is investigative rather than concerned to produce 'scientific laws'. Non-probability sampling includes the snowball technique, where one piece of the research suggests other potential participants, or where one participant puts others in touch with the researcher; the advert on the wall or in the paper; or theory sampling. Theory sampling means adding to the research process new individuals or groups who are deemed to be useful on the basis of the evidence so far. The sample lays no claims to representativeness, but may claim to offer a 'typical' cross-section of the community under review.

Any form of sample may produce a **non-response** rate, and the researcher will need to offer informed speculation as to why this might be and what implications it might have. Some researchers like to prevent high non-response rates as far as possible, and so take action such as supplying stamped addressed envelopes, making follow-up phone calls, even entering respondents' names into prize draws. There is some dispute as to how important the non-respondents may be (e.g. is it one particular type of respondent, whom the sample now misses), but researchers must make up their own minds on this. We suggest that, at the least, non-response is noted, with any evident patterns which seem relevant to it.

VARIABLES

Having chosen a specific method, the researcher needs to include all relevant information about the participant group. So, in the hypothesis above, i.e. the exploration into the effectiveness of two types of therapy with a particular client group, it is useful to know the variables which may differ from subject to subject and those which may influence the process.

Client details

- Gender, age, ethnic group, marital status;
- How long the condition has been diagnosed;
- Age of onset of the condition;
- What previous therapies have been offered.

Therapist details

- Gender, age, ethnic group, marital status;
- How experienced, how trained;
- How experienced with this client group.

There may be more. The point is to collect any information which may influence the effectiveness of the therapy in the particular conditions and situation. Such information will inform data analysis. For example, if 'unsuccessful' therapy coincides with all clients being female and all therapists male, then it would be wise to consider the implications of this finding and not just assume that the therapeutic approach is at fault. In other words, gender will become a significant variable.

COLLECTING DATA

The precise method of data collection will depend on methodological approach and the specific method being used. If information is being collected in a written form, it will be useful to develop a coding system to decipher it once collected. Specific systems will be designed for the particular research, depending on whether there are open-ended questions, closed questions, or whether some predetermined activity is being observed.

In an observational study, the researcher will need to make as specific a record as possible. This may entail the immediate writing up of field notes, or the use of other recording media, such as tapes, or the use of a 'rapporteur' who acts as a note-taking aide. Participants may be asked to submit written accounts of what is happening, or has happened, for them, and there is an increasing literature on the use of accounts in social research.

EVALUATION: RELIABILITY AND VALIDITY

The interpretation of data will then depend on the research design and the variables identified. You may wish to make simple observations of what you see happening, e.g. five out of six clients who received therapy reported feeling much better and identified a feeling of more energy, increase in appetite, more ease with sleeping etc. Such observations would be made at a cautious level and may conclude with identifying further research needs.

You may wish to make an interpretation which offers a causal analysis, e.g. behaviour therapy cures depression in nine out of ten clients. Here the behaviour therapy is the cause, the 'cured depression' the effect. Causal explanations are, of course, rife within human psychology, and must be subjected to rigorous exploration of the variables before making hard and fast claims. Perhaps Freudian theory is a useful example of how potential explanatory theories become used as rigid blueprints, and in the end may not be based on any tangible evidence. For example, Freud's ideas on incest and the Electra and Oedipus complexes were in the past taken as serious explanations for parental sexual abuse. Contemporary theorists are notably much more sceptical!

If causal links are established, the research may be used to make predictions about human behaviour and about the effectiveness of particular treatments or approaches. Again, this has been useful in 'hard' scientific research, e.g on the development of medicines, but it is slightly harder to be dogmatic about human behaviour. Apparent findings need to be subjected to tests of **reliability** and **validity**.

Reliability

Reliability means the degree of consistency with which the same research would elicit the same results, either by different researchers or by the same researcher over time. So we can fairly safely say that a body temperature of 104°F is potentially dangerous, on the basis of repeated observation over time by different observers.

Validity

Validity means the truth of the findings. The researcher must be sure that they are testing and measuring what they think they are testing and measuring. You may imagine that this is not a problem, but in practice ensuring validity is extremely difficult. For example, the researcher testing IQ may believe that they are testing and measuring intelligence, when what they may be testing is **mood**. It could be argued that children tested on standard IQ tests do better or worse in different circumstances on different days. If the child is unwell, has had an argument with a friend before the test, is depressed because of some significant event in their life, or something similar, they are likely to manifest scores that do not reflect their actual ability. Therefore the test is measuring mood, not ability or performance. Similarly, aptitude tests given to a group with a fixed time period may expect to measure ability, but in fact measure speed. School examinations, which are intended to test pupils' intellectual ability, often only measure their memory and immunity from or response to anxiety.

Variables that need to be considered when investigating the validity of results are numerous, but motivation, personality, distractability/concentration, physical health, mental health, cultural compatibility with the test and educational experience are a significant beginning. Therefore, in assessing validity it is centrally important to consider variables, and to remain fairly sceptical about what the results 'prove'. For example, at one time it was stated in Britain that black people had a higher incidence of schizophrenia than white people. When this was challenged in the light of cultural practice and meanings, and by the identification of elements of racism and ignorance in mental health practice, the claim could no longer be seen as valid.

Reliability and validity may never be absolute. They may be disproved at any time through further research, which is good news for the practitioner if we see new findings as offering us a richer and wider understanding of how people function, and of how we might help those who need mental health care. Silverman (1993) suggests that the best we can hope for in research is plausibility and credibility.

CONCLUSIONS AND IMPLICATIONS FOR THE NURSE

We hope that this chapter offers a coherent introduction to the task of carrying out research, and will stimulate the reader to further reading. Although it has been difficult to capture the intricacies of research in such a short space, we hope also that we have gone some way towards taking some of the mystery out of the process. With care and application, most people can carry out a small piece of research without too much trouble, using a mixture of observation, experience, common sense and skill.

Perhaps the most optimistic aspect of introducing research to the nursing practitioner is that demystifying the process enables the discerning nurse to read other people's research with a critical eye. So that when you hear statements like 'Four out of five HIV-positive patients in Xmoor hospital are gay men', you can consider the reliability, validity, sampling and variable checking of the research before accepting the results at face value.

Consider questions such as: 'Who was the sample to be tested?' (random or selected?); 'Is there more awareness of risk in the gay community which encourages people to be tested?' (validity? Did it measure levels of the virus in a group or the willingness of people to be tested?); 'Were only five people tested?' (does it represent the population?); 'How many 'straight' people agreed to be tested?' (have the variables gay/straight been adequately considered?)

If the population to be tested was 80% gay, then the findings mean nothing. If the gay community are more aware of risk, this means that they will be more likely to be tested, and the implications of the findings may reveal nothing more than this. Such questioning avoids the temptation to jump to the conclusion that 'HIV is a gay plague'. Ultimately, this approach and reflection leads to clearer knowledge, more accurate information, more self-awareness and better client care. In the end, this is what it is all about.

SUMMARY

The key features of the research process are suggested as follows:

- Generating the research problem. Key concepts here are that the problem under review should hold interest for the researcher and have some usefulness. All research problems are underpinned by theory.
- Forming the hypothesis. This entails putting the research question into some form of statement that can be tested, e.g. that one form of therapeutic intervention is better than another. This necessitates making the question as specific as possible. Sometimes, in investigative research, the hypothesis is defined during the process of research.
- Literature search. Having defined the problem, a literature search informs the researcher on possibilities and limitations.
- Choosing a methodology. Two methodologies exist, qualitative and quantitative. Qualitative research is more concerned to discover the meaning of participants' responses, whereas quantitative research is more concerned to offer statistical analyses and claim representative findings and predictions. The two can complement and inform each other. The methodology should be appropriate to the desired outcomes of the research.
- Research design. Having decided on the methodology, the researcher has a range of methods to choose from, e.g interview, survey, group observation. The method should be appropriate to the desired outcome, the size of the research study and the resources available.
- Sampling. Sampling can be done at random, so that it can claim to demonstrate some representation of a cross-section of people, or it can be focused and this be taken into account in the writing up.
- Variables. Variables are all those factors which might influence the findings. They may be characteristics of the research participants or researchers, e.g. class, race and gender, or of the conditions, e.g participants in the community, being in residential care, the researcher's experience.
- Collecting and recording data. This should be done as thoroughly as possible using whatever means are appropriate, e.g writing field notes, audiovisual recording, coding questionnaires. Central themes and issues are then identified.
- Findings are then evaluated in terms of validity and reliability. Validity means the truth of the findings – can we find explanations which refute this? Reliability is the degree of consistency with which the same research repeated would generate the same results.

FURTHER READING

Burnard, P. and Morrison, P. (1990) *Nursing Research in Action: Developing Basic Skills*, McMillan, London.

Couchman, W. and Dawson, J. (1991) *Nursing and Health Care Research: a Practical Guide: the Use and Application of Reseach for Nurses and Other Health Care Professionals*, Scutari Press, Harrow.

Field, P. A. and Morse, J. M. (1985) *Nursing Research: the Application of Qualitative Research*, Chapman & Hall, London.

Magdelena, A. M. and Karin, T. K. (1990) *Conducting and Using Nursing Research in the Clinical Setting*, Williams and Wilkins, Baltimore.

Mills, C. Wright (1959) *The Sociological Imagination*, Oxford University Press, Oxford.

Morse, J. M. (ed) (1991) *Qualitative Nursing Research: a Contemporary Dialogue*, Sage, London.

Nieswiadomy, R. M. (1992) *Foundations of Nursing Research*, 2nd edn, Appleton and Lange, Norwalk, Conn.

Powers, B. and Knapp, T. (1990) *A Dictionary of Nursing Theory and Research*, Sage, London.

Sarantakos, S. (1993) *Social Research*, MacMillan, Basingstoke.

Silverman, D. (1993) *Interpreting Qualitative Data*, Sage, London.

Working with groups 24

Andy Betts

Caroline is a single parent of two girls aged five and two. Since the birth of her second daughter life has seemed a struggle. She has lost much of her self-confidence, feels anxious in social situations and has periods of depression when it takes all her effort just to keep the family routine going each day. Caroline has had some individual counselling from a community mental health nurse. This has helped to an extent, but the CMHN's suggestion that she joins a new group at the local Community Mental Health Centre seems a good, if somewhat daunting, opportunity. Caroline arranges for a relative to look after the children once a week and agrees to attend the sessions, which last for two hours over a period of six months.

The group is a closed group consisting of ten members of both genders and two co-leaders. All the other members have similar kinds of difficulties to Caroline. Initially she finds the group to be a little frightening and exposing, but she gradually feels able to trust the others and surprises herself by some of the things she discloses in the sessions. In particular, she begins to understand her relationships with significant others in her life. The skilled facilitators prompt her to make associations between how she behaves with her parents and how she behaves in the group. These insights are very powerful for Caroline, and help her to understand her early experiences and how they relate to her current difficulties in relationships. The group context brought the issues to the surface with a therapeutic impact that individual counselling was unable to achieve.

Nurses often express an attitude of ambivalence towards groups. It is as if they are to be both feared and revered. The image of groupwork seems to be veiled in an aura of mystique and hidden forces that are too complex to begin to understand. It is as if the group has some kind of life or energy of its own that is distinct from the collection of individuals that compose it. These perceptions may be founded in the nurses' own experiences as members of various groups, or may just be what they imagine goes on in groups. It is possible that this attitude has contributed to the lack of substantive input on groups in nursing curricula, and also to the apparent willingness of mental health nurses to relinquish the responsibility of leading therapeutic groups to other health care workers. To discount groupwork is to ignore the potential of groups to make a significant qualitative difference to peoples' lives. The aim of this chapter is to both confirm the notion that therapeutic groups are complex encounters and also to demystify some of the processes that typically manifest themselves in groupwork. The following questions will be addressed within the context of the mental health nurse as group leader:

What is a group ?

What are the potential benefits of groups?

How do groups change over time?

How do therapeutic groups work?

What is group process?

What is involved in setting up and leading groups effectively?

WHAT IS A GROUP?

From the moment we are born we are members of a group – the family – and growing up involves being socialized into the ways of thinking, feeling and behaving which collectively define the nature of this group. At different times in our lives we join and leave various groups, which are all unique in the sense that they consist of different combinations of members. Our roles and behaviour are likely to vary depending on the respective tasks and composition of each group. Nurses do not work in total isolation but are typically members of a number of work groups e.g. multidisciplinary teams, nurse groups, working groups, committees, professional bodies, supervision groups, support groups, quality circles, educational groups.

Thompson and Khan (1970) note that proximity alone is not enough to turn a number of people into a group, but that there has to be some point of common concern and a relationship that unites the different individuals together as a single entity. This relationship serves to provide a shared conception of a unit distinguishable from other collections of people. In lay terms groups are larger than a couple and smaller than a crowd, but a therapeutic group typically consists of between six and fourteen people, with eight to ten considered to be the optimum number. The larger the group the more complex the potential interactions between members (see Figure 24.1). The common concern which 'glues' these individuals together as a group is the expressed intention to come together to address a common focus, which may be educational, social or personal. This focus becomes the task of the group. Therapeutic groups do not only invest time and energy into their task but also attend to the emotional life or group process. Smith (1980) defines groupwork as: 'an activity set up with the publicly stated intention of creating some change in members' own behaviour or feelings.'

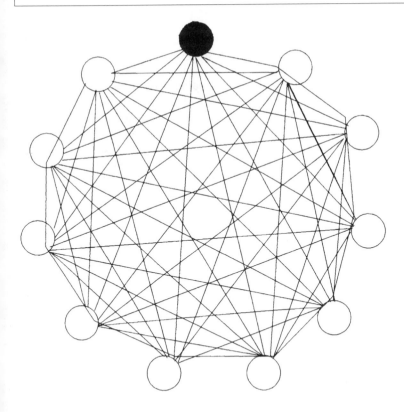

Figure 24.1　The possible range of interactions in a group of 10 plus a leader

HOW DO GROUPS CHANGE OVER TIME?

Groups are dynamic in the sense that they change over time. The experience of coming together as a group for the first time is clearly different from that of attending a group which has met regularly for many sessions. Likewise, the very last group meeting is likely to stand out as significantly different from previous sessions. Although each group will vary according to the membership and the theoretical approach of the leader, there does seem to be a typical generalized pattern in the evolution of all groups (Corey, 1990). It is important that the group leader has an understanding of the various stages involved in this process because they form the backcloth upon which all subsequent issues are thrown into relief. The leader must be aware that the group situation is constantly shifting in an identifiable pattern (Stock-Whitaker and Lieberman, 1964). One way of focusing on the development of a group is to describe it as a series of stages, although in reality it is not experienced as precise self-contained phases following a neat progression.

Many frameworks have been suggested to describe group development and their similarity seems to confirm that some common general trends do become apparent in groups over time (Mahler, 1969; Rogers, 1970; Schutz, 1973;

Gazda, 1989). Tuckman (1967) identified four stages, which he called forming, storming, norming and performing. Each of these stages is characterized by shared focal issues which, although the group members are not usually fully conscious of them, significantly influence what happens in the group and how different members respond. For the group leader an additional phase occurs before the first session, and will significantly influence how the group progresses. In the following description this stage is termed the pregroup stage. In recognition that all groups one day come to an end, a sixth stage is added to Tuckman's progression, namely endings. These six stages are: pregroup, forming, storming, norming, performing and ending.

Pregroup

The success of any group will depend to some degree on the planning stage. Corey (1990) suggests that the following points need to be considered:

- The basic purpose of the group;
- The population to be served;
- A clear rationale for the group;
- Ways to announce the group and recruit members;
- The screening and selection of members;
- The size and duration of the group;
- The frequency and time of meetings;
- The group structure and format;
- The methods of preparing members;
- Whether the group will be open or closed;
- The degree of consent;
- The follow-up and evaluation procedures.

The purpose of the group is strongly associated with the population to be served, and consequently the recruitment of members. For example, a Community Mental Health Nurse (CMHN) working from a mental health centre may notice that a high proportion of recent referrals consists of women experiencing lack of confidence associated with anxiety. Other members of the team also have a number of clients with similar difficulties. Discussions lead to the formation of a group to be run weekly at the mental health centre. The idea for the group emerges from the population and a perceived need. The homogenous factors for this particular group are women and anxiety. By targeting the population in this way the management of the group becomes more focused. Other groups may benefit from a wider cross-section of the population across gender, age and life difficulty. Houston (1984) recommends discussions with colleagues you think will enrich your thinking at this pregroup stage.

Announcing or advertising for the group should include clear information about its rationale and aims; the time, frequency and venue; how to join; and criteria for who is suitable. The selection of members will be determined by the degree to which their needs and goals are compatible with the identified goals of the group, and whether their contribution is likely to be productive or counterproductive. To an extent this will be determined by the nature of the group. The CMHN in the previous example may make the decision that selecting a woman who meets the criteria but who is also alcohol dependent would be counterproductive to the potential progress of the group. Of course, in a different group her inclusion may be totally appropriate. It can be seen, then, that selection is not based purely on the needs of the individual but on an assessment of how that individual's inclusion is likely to affect the group process. Ideally the group leader will interview each prospective member for the purpose of screening and orientation. This screening is a two-way process, providing the opportunity for prospective members to make informed decisions as to whether the group is likely to be suitable for them. Hopefully the decision is arrived at mutually, but if there is a discrepancy between the client and the leader it is the ultimate responsibility of the leader to make the final decision (Corey, 1990).

Figure 24.2 illustrates two important continua regarding the nature of groups. The degree of structure within a group will depend on the theoretical approach and leadership style of the group leader. A highly structured group is one characterized by the directed activities suggested by the leader. Examples of this might be educational meetings or a social skills group using directed role play. At the other end of the continuum is the unstructured group which has minimal organized activities, with the leader making fewer demonstrably active interventions.

The decision concerning open or closed groups is highly significant. A closed group does not accept new members once it has started, whereas open groups allow new members to join, usually as replacements for people who leave. According to Beach (1987), closed groups are more stable and promote

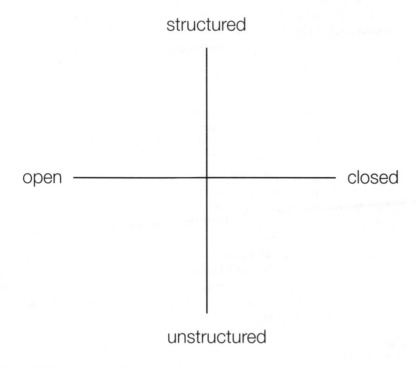

Figure 24.2 Group continuums

loyalty and reciprocity, but open groups have an inbuilt instability due to the changes in membership. In these days of limited resources it may be that the decision whether to have open or closed groups is influenced by economic arguments. Open groups may provide the opportunity to retain the maximum number of participants, although the progression of the group is likely to be slowed down.

Ideally all members make the choice to participate of their own free will. Yalom (1985) regards motivation as the most important criterion for inclusion in a group. Some of the reticence that prospective members may express can often be profitably addressed in the pregroup interview.

If this pregroup planning is done well, then all the conditions are in place to establish what Oatley (1980) describes as a cultural island characterized by 'finite time, specific place, isolated from the outside world and free of interruptions. The participants commit themselves to stay on the island for the course of the group.'

Forming

Yalom (1985) likens the initial stage of a group to the social code illustrative of a cocktail party. Conversation tends to be polite, rather superficial and of little substantive interest to any of the participants. The early sessions are characterized by uncertainty, anxiety and dependency on the leader as the members search for meaning, endeavour to find out who the other people are and decide on what commitment they will make to the group. The behaviour in the group is influenced by the search for a response to why we are here, what is it we want to do and how do we want to go about it? In this search the group members typically behave as if they were helpless, and look to the leader for guidelines. The leader's response to these questions will depend on their theoretical orientation. Leaders must judge for themselves to what degree they will attempt to meet the unrealistic expectations placed on them by the members. Their response may range from an initial brief statement addressing the bare essentials to highly structured and informative interventions. In a long-term closed psychotherapy group the leader's intervention is likely to be at the former end of the scale. The leader of a short-term assertiveness training group is likely to respond more actively to the group's expectations. The less structured the group the greater the anxiety and ambiguity as to how members are to behave, but it is this anxiety which may be the facilitative factor in bringing to the surface the conflicts that need to be addressed. Yalom (1985) suggests that too much leader direction tends to limit the growth of the members, and too little results in aimless groups.

Whatever the theoretical orientation of the leader and the type of group, it is probable that the initial session will include some discussion about what is to be allowed and what is not. The negotiation of ground rules at the beginning helps to create the boundaries of the therapeutic space. Typically this negotiation will include the following:

- Confidentiality
- Attendance and absence
- Lateness.

Storming

This exploratory stage is concerned with members attempting to find their places in the group. The issue is whether a member will be included or excluded. The polite conversation of the forming stage is exchanged for the expression of more primitive feelings such as jealousy and hostility. The issues which come to the surface are concerned with competition, rivalry, power, status, scapegoating, dominance and rebellion. In particular, the group ceases to behave as if it was helpless and dependent on the leader. It is not uncommon for the leader to be challenged, criticized or to have her suggestions rejected. It is important that the leader views this experience in the context of group process, rather than taking it as a personal attack. At this stage those who are quiet in the group tend to become even more silent, and those that are vocal contribute even more. Gradually the members' centre of reference shifts from the leader to addressing each other more directly (Foulkes, 1984).

Norming

The norming stage is a period of developing cohesion. There is a feeling of bonding and a sense of group spirit. Relationships in the group are organized around liking and affection. People feel safe enough to become increasingly frank with each other and express their feelings more openly. Members typically experience a sense of wellbeing and belonging. The talk is of 'us, we, our' and represents a group identity and union against the 'outside world'.

Performing

This is the working stage of the group, when the cohesion which has emerged is translated into action. The group is well prepared to carry out its task, with individuals showing commitment to the aims of the group. It is as if the group as a whole is less confused and troubled by the interpersonal conflicts going on. Any conflicts which do surface between members are generally handled in a productive manner. Leadership and initiative is spread around the membership more than at previous stages.

Ending

All groups come to an end and group members are sometimes surprised by their degree of emotive reaction to this. The end of the group often evokes strong feelings of separation, which seem exaggerated when viewed in the context of the meaning of the group to the individual. This may be because of old unresolved feelings of loss and separation being triggered by the here-and-now experience. The discussion usually focuses on the past experience together and suggestions for meeting again. This represents a psychological preparation for the loss and a denial of the end. This stage is not always handled well, and may be the weak link in the therapeutic chain (Abse, 1974). It is essential that the group leader views these conflicts as part of the normal group evolutionary process. They represent opportunities for the group to make progress and any attempts to stifle or deny them are counterproductive.

POTENTIAL BENEFITS OF GROUPS

Potentially, groups offer some advantages over one-to-one interventions. Bloch and Crouch (1985), acknowledging the work of Yalom (1985), identified ten possible therapeutic factors within groups. They define a therapeutic factor as: 'an element of group therapy that contributes to improvement in a client's condition and is a function of the actions of the group therapist, the other group members and the client himself' (Bloch and Crouch, 1985, p.4). These ten therapeutic factors are:

1. *Acceptance or group cohesion.* Feeling accepted by the other group members gives a sense of belonging and support. Cohesive groups represent an island of emotional comfort and general acceptance which is in itself a healing factor. Dickoff and Lakin (1963) found a strong correlation between group cohesiveness and client outcome.
2. *Universality.* The feeling that 'we are all in the same boat' serves to reduce the sense of isolation and uniqueness which individuals may experience. This seems particularly helpful in the early stages of a group.
3. *Altruism.* Contributing to a group may improve a member's self-image through discovering his potential to help others in the group.
4. *Instillation of hope.* Witnessing others improve over time may lead to an increased sense of optimism regarding one's own potential progress. Yalom (1985) suggests that a group which includes members at different levels of progress has the effect of raising members' hopes.
5. *Guidance.* At times information giving may be of use to members. To a greater or lesser extent group work usually includes an educational component, e.g. the teaching of assertiveness techniques.
6. *Vicarious learning.* Groups offer opportunities to observe others working through their own particular difficulties. In this way a group member who does not overtly participate at a certain stage may be actively reflecting and learning from observing others.
7. *Self-understanding.* Discovering and accepting previously unknown or unacceptable things about oneself, for instance, learning that current reactions to people or situations in the group are associated with earlier periods in life.
8. *Learning from interpersonal action.* The group offers an opportunity for members to try out different forms of interpersonal behaviour within a safe setting, and to reflect on the responses of others.
9. *Self-disclosure.* Jourard (1971) highlights the therapeutic effect of revealing personal information to the group. Although this involves taking risks, because we can never predict with certainty the response of other group members, it appears that the act of revealing oneself to others enables us to know ourselves in a deeper sense.
10. *Catharsis.* The expression of strong emotions within the group setting is strongly encouraged in most groups. The process of discharging these feelings appears to have a therapeutic effect, although Bloch and Crouch (1985) warn against overreliance on this factor as a lasting cure.

Different combinations of these therapeutic factors will be significant at the various stages in the life of the group. The theoretical approach of the group leader will also determine the focus and prominence of these factors.

GROUP-AS-A-WHOLE

It is not uncommon to hear comments which refer to the group as if it was a single living entity, with its own moods, attitudes and feelings. In supervision a group leader may state that 'the group was angry today'. In a particular session all the contributions may be experienced as variations on a theme, even though they are made by different members. Foulkes and Anthony (1973) observed that the group-as-a-whole is different from the sum of its parts. They viewed the group as a complex matrix in which the spaces between people are not empty.

> If we hear an orchestra playing a piece of music all the individual noises are produced each on one particular instrument. Yet what we hear is the orchestra playing. In the same way group processes reach us in a concerted whole – what we experience in the first place is the group as a whole (Foulkes, 1984).

THE GROUP LEADER

The effective group leader is proficient in three main domains (Figure 24.3). She is able to form therapeutic relationships based on the core conditions described in Chapter 2; she is interpersonally skilled and able to use those skills appropriately and wisely; and she has a sound knowledge of group

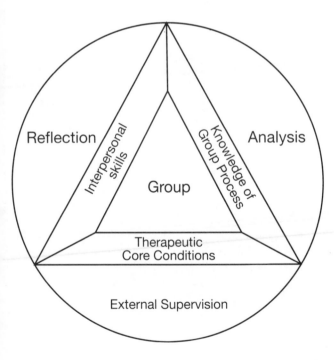

Figure 24.3   The effective group facilitator

processes which serves to inform her interventions. The art of facilitating groups is demonstrated by the ability to interact with group members at the same time as attending to an internal reflective analysis of the group process. To a large degree this comes with experience and external supervision.

FURTHER READING

Bloch, S. and Crouch, E. (1985) *Therapeutic Factors in Group Psychotherapy*, Oxford University Press, Oxford.

Corey, G. (1990) *The Theory and Practice of Group Counselling*, Brookes/ Cole, Belmont, California.

Gazda, G. M. (1989) *Group Counselling: a Developmental Approach*, 4th edn, Allyn and Bacon, Boston.

Rogers, C. R. (1970) *Carl Rogers on Encounter Groups*, Harper and Row, New York.

Yalom, I.D. (1985) *The Theory and Practice of Group Psychotherapy*, 3rd edn, Basic Books, New York.

Management principles and skills

Many nurses tend to believe that nurse management is the same as administration, and state quite openly that they trained to be a nurse not an administrator. We firmly believe that all nurses would benefit from learning management principles and skills, even if very few will ever become nurse managers.

Administration is a part of management studies which helps senior nurses formulate policies, calculate manpower, devise plans and collect data. This is not, however, what we wish to discuss here. Management as applied to nursing involves the skilled use of resources to effect a high degree of nursing care. This is the area where nurses of all grades should be skilled if they are to maximize the therapeutic potential for their clients.

This chapter seeks to identify the resources available, principles for their use and strategies particular to nursing situations. We end with a short section on leadership, which we hope will be useful to those nurses responsible for teams.

RESOURCES

It is necessary to identify resources as they are often hidden, and if the nurse is unable to see what is available to her she will inevitably fail to maximize them. Resources can be broken down into people, time, equipment, environment and finance. In order to see the elements in more detail, let us take each separately.

People

There are often more people involved in the care of clients than was originally thought. For instance, in a hospital environment laundry workers, porters, cooks, seamstresses, domestics and storemen may seem insignificant to the ward nurse, but in terms of influence and power these people have the potential both to enhance and to sabotage nursing care. Good relationships, thoughtful appreciation and sound communication are basic principles to bear in mind when considering people resources.

Close to the client, the nurse may see herself in isolation as the person who knows their wishes, hopes and expectations best. This is as it should be, but she will be able to help the individual fulfil only some of these at best. Doctors, physiotherapists, occupational therapists and psychologists are but a few of a constant file of professionals, also skilled and specialized in fulfilling particular aspects of the client's needs. To understand the role of each professional and non-professional helper should be the aim of all nurses who wish to manage their clients' care effectively. Looking at people resources even further, two other factors emerge. The first is to acknowledge that the specialist who offers a particular resource is also a person. She has a unique interpersonal relationship style, and consequently each person has a personality potential as well as a special knowledge. The skilled nurse will try not only to find the best specialist, but also the best personality match whenever possible. The second factor to acknowledge is the timing of the person resource. Each person who may potentiate a therapeutic effect will do so only if the timing is right. A social worker invited to discuss aftercare with a client is only an appropriate resource if the client is ready to accept the idea of discharge at that moment. Even more subtle timing may be seen with the terminally ill client. Religious or spiritual advisers may be very powerful people resources, but if their use is poorly timed the results may be seriously harmful to the client's progress.

Occasionally the sex of the person is significant: a few years ago both of us were involved in the care of a client who from time to time became very deluded. His delusion normally took the form of a religious persecution, and within it he held the belief that all male nurses were homosexual and conspiring to persecute him for his religious beliefs. Although at most other times we had a good relationship with him, it would have been foolhardy for either of us to attempt to persuade him to accept an intramuscular injection during these periods. Even though he occasionally became violent and aggressive during these deluded periods, the most appropriate person resource was a female nurse. More often than not she was successful without any untoward incident, where we would undoubtedly have failed.

Availability of manpower is of course a major factor in people resources. So often in UK hospitals staff are overworked and thin on the ground. For this reason alone, the nurse should be skilled at managing people resources. During periods of manpower shortage, the maximum effectiveness of individuals should surely be the principle to the forefront of our minds. If each person is operating at maximum efficiency in areas where she is effective, the task – in this case client care – will be achieved. If it is not, this proves only that resources are insufficient and not that management is poor.

To summarize briefly, people resource management is identifying the right person to help the client at the right time, bearing in mind personal skill, knowledge, personality, gender and availability.

Time

Time is seldom considered as a resource with anything other than a cursory examination. In fact, time is one of the most squandered of all resources. The nurse who learns how to manage her time effectively will have the advantage of being seen to be in control and never in a flap. Once it is accepted that time can be accounted for, allocated and controlled, the nurse will run out of it less often.

Drucker (1967) suggests that time is such a valuable resource that we should control it more carefully than physical resources. More materials can always be found, but time cannot be manufactured – once it has been expended it is lost forever. We suggest that the most practical way of controlling your time is first to measure it. Take account of what you spent it on today: be totally honest and make a list. Better still, take a notepad to work, divide it into half-hour periods and note down exactly what you have spent time on. It is likely that your list will include many periods sitting scratching your head wondering what's next. Ordering your priorities will take even more time, and talking to colleagues and planning care another large slice. Using the telephone will undoubtedly crop up frequently, sometimes to give information and other times to pass it on. In most organizations there will be some statutory slot for a 'handover', some system of shift changeover or organized communication. Somewhere on the list will be writing reports, filling in forms and evaluating nursing care and client progress. These areas, we are fairly sure, will figure prominently in your lists.

We are not suggesting that anything on your list is a complete waste of time, but what we are suggesting is that it may be organized more efficiently. If you take your time seriously, and make a list, then we are confident that the conclusions drawn will be helpful. We are convinced that most nurses will organize their time effectively once its waste is drawn to their attention. Additionally, we suggest that you also consider the following questions as thought provokers:

- Did I spend that long because it needed time or because I like doing that?
- Was that time spent effective for good client care?
- If I put all those little bits of time spent on the same thing together, would it have been quicker/more efficient? (e.g. ten telephone calls to various departments throughout a shift, as opposed to ten minutes all together).
- Could I have combined these two jobs together to save time?
- What are my priorities in the list?
- How much time did I spend during the day on each priority?
- What time have I spent on low priorities that I could transfer to high priorities?
- Is there something on the list that crops up again and again and yet seems to achieve nothing?
- Which items rob me of valuable time?
- What do I want to change?

Equipment

Equipment is a valuable resource which is often abused by nurses of all grades. Items of equipment in a ward area tend to fall into the following categories:

- Necessary – without it the nurse would not be able to function, e.g. items such as tables, chairs, beds and kitchen equipment.
- General medical – this equipment would probably be found only in a hospital, but is considered necessary for most areas: oxygen/resuscitation equipment, sphygmomanometer/syringes, needles.
- Special therapeutic – this is the equipment that makes the difference between an area that houses clients and one that has a therapeutic value – items such as paints, paper, record player, games etc.

These categories are simply to aid the nurse in evaluating how important each item of equipment is to her. Each item we have suggested may be put into a different category for different people. What is important is that all nurses have a clear idea of which piece of equipment falls into which category. We believe that without such a clear idea, very wasteful equipment collection policies are soon implemented. To illustrate this, all the observant nurse needs to do is to look in store cupboards and determined how much previously valued equipment is lying unused. All these items may be 'on order' in other units, and desperately needed. It is very easy to become 'I'll order it just in case'-minded.

When recommending the ordering or purchasing of equipment, the skilled nurse who is aware of resource scarcity asks herself the following questions:

*   Is it necessary, special or general?
*   Can it be borrowed when required, or is it vital that it is owned by the unit?
*   Will it be used?
*   Is there something more valuable we need first?
*   Can it wait?

Once these questions are answered thoughtfully, a more logical case to purchase or order may be evident. Any item of equipment may be considered a luxury by someone who does not value it. A heart–lung machine is a necessity to a thoracic surgeon, but may be seen as extravagant by a patient on a waiting list for a walking frame. Before leaving this section we feel it should be stressed that we are not advising mental health nurses to 'make do and mend'. In fact, it is our experience that nurses are perhaps too good at this – we are simply saying that careful judgement is required. This should not deter the nurse from insisting on equipment that she requires, but it should certainly sober her judgement when requesting expensive items.

Environment

Resources within our environment are often missed. Sometimes the simple conversion exercise is overlooked in the struggle for perfection. Examples of this are numerous: one charge nurse stated that he could not take female clients on his unit because he did not have the correct facilities. By reorganizing a dormitory area and making one toilet block female only, integration was able to take place without any structural changes being made. Linen cupboards can be changed into offices to free space for music or therapy rooms. It is not necessary to be constrained by the physical environment. In most units there are areas not in constant use that can be used for activities that take space. Recreation halls, occupational therapy departments and gymnasia are seldom in use all the time. Moving clients into these alternative environments creates additional stimulation, and gives space for such creative therapies as drama, music and movement, yoga and keep fit.

Alcohol and drug dependency units await large financial commitment from bureaucratic sources. Millions of pounds are spent creating new 'glossy' units to help these particular individuals. Is this because without these special environmental facilities they cannot be helped? Essentially, the only difference between these units and the present arrangements is that similarly diagnosed individuals will spend whole days together. Surely, then, with some thought, alternative group meeting places could be found within existing structures? We are not suggesting that new units should not be built, not that they are not worthwhile projects, as they do have many advantages. The point we seek to make is that there are many environmental resources untapped, if the nurse looks for them. Nurses should not be straitjacketed into waiting for 'the new unit to open'; if a need exists it should be served as quickly as possible, and this means seeking resources that exist already. We have seen admission units create mother and baby units with no more resources than a 'desire to serve'; therapeutic communities set up in run-down old houses; and alcohol specialties in side wards and dormitories. Will and imagination are the only management tools required to manipulate the environment.

Finance

There remains a myth that without money no progress is possible. We use the word 'myth' because it is our experience that commitment, positive attitudes and personal skills are far more important to progress than money ever will be. It is unfortunately a fact of life that money is required to purchase staff, equipment and premises. The availability of finance, however, is in most cases dependent upon the original premise that staff involved need to show commitment to the enterprise requiring support. Most nurses the UK are now beginning to realize that finance will not always – and in some cases seldom – be supplied by central government. Voluntary agencies, charities and bene-factors are a source of income that remains largely untapped. If these people and organizations are impressed by a need, an idea or an enterprise that is by its very nature highly altruistic, funds are usually forthcoming. In smaller, possibly even more frustrating, areas of financial insufficiencies, a more imaginative tactic is required. In the past few years, one of the authors had the task of managing a rehabilitation unit of four wards. The most active of the four, involved in predischarge work, continually submitted requests for an electric cooker. This was by no means unreasonable, as clients about to go back into the community should at least have some practice at cooking their own meals. The problem was not so much the cost of buying a cooker, but the necessary electrical installation work required. The solution to the problem was found by asking what the clients were actually going to cook on it. In discussions it appeared that breakfasts and suppers were the main need. This was quickly catered for, not by the purchase of a cooker, but by the purchase of a toaster and an electric ring. All they required to cook could be easily achieved without expensive wiring. Although this example may seem trite, it does illustrate how divergent thinking can sometimes circumnavigate the need for additional finance. Management is, after all, about managing with what is available. A clothesline across the bathroom is not as appealing as a tumble drier, and a bicycle is not as comfortable as a limousine, but if we each cut our cloth according to our needs, a prime principle of management is achieved.

MANAGEMENT CONTRASTS

Task versus client

Systems organization in nursing currently operates on two main principles, 'task-orientated' systems, and the more widely accepted 'client-orientated' system.

The task system has several advantages for the management of a unit. It is generally efficient and succeeds in completing the work schedule; everyone knows what they are responsible for and they are easily identified should substandard or unfinished work be discovered. The system operates on a task list, and nurses are delegated to a series of duties, e.g.:

Staff Nurse Jones
Take report
Check O_2 and resuscitation equipment, including aspirators
Give out medicines
Doctors' round
Group therapy
Handover

Student Nurse Brown,
Supervise clients' dressing

Student Nurses White and Black
Supervise clients' washing
Give out breakfast
Escort clients to occupational therapy

Enrolled Nurse Green
Supervise students early morning
Assist S/N Jones with drugs
Prepare clients for ECT
Escort to ECT
On return assist S/N Jones with doctors' round and group.

This is a very simple management system which has inbuilt communication, supervision and accountability. Its great disadvantage, which makes it largely unacceptable for current practice, is its lack of continuity and the dehumanizing effect it may have on nurses operating within it. The nurse delegated a task to carry out may well not understand why she is doing it, and may not relate personally to the clients involved in the process. It is largely mechanistic, valuable interactional processes may be ignored, information specific to individuals may be missed and, more importantly, the nurse's interpersonal skills are largely wasted.

Client-orientated systems are now widely used, and take as their basis a more continual and humanistic approach. Based on a nursing process system, each nurse is allocated a number of clients and it is her responsibility to respond to the needs of these individual throughout her contact with them. An organized plan of care is decided and written in a Kardex system, so that accurate information is always available. Untrained nurses are allocated to teams so that their progress can be monitored and their work supervised by a trained nurse, the team leader. This system has many advantages: it is easy to divide clients into high-, medium- and low-dependency and allocate staff accordingly; nurses are involved with a smaller group of clients and have a continual input into total client care. Rather than doing a whole task for all the clients, they are involved in all the care for a group of clients.

The disadvantages are of a practical nature. In periods of staff shortage, the groups of clients become so large that some tasks may be missed or forgotten. This is no 'grand design' strategy, so individual care is largely left to the initiative of each supervising nurse. A criticism levelled at this system is that it is wasteful of resources: on a surgical ward every nurse may need a dressing trolley at the same time. In the mental health setting, its potential effect can disintegrate if individual care plans send clients from a nurse's group in different directions: Nurse Brown is responsible for total care of clients A, B, C and D. Clients A and B require ECT; client C is scheduled to go to the Occupational Therapy Department and client D is to attend the Psychology Department.

It may occur to you that, as in all systems, advantages and disadvantages can be potentiated and minimized respectively only if the manager is versatile and flexible. Any system has inherent faults; the intelligent and skilled nurse takes from each what she needs for her circumstances.

Positives versus negatives

Contrast the nurse who constantly voices her indignation at her colleagues who are always late, sloppily dressed, uncaring, untidy, unprepared, lazy, ill-tempered and boring, with the nurse who compliments her colleagues for their positive attributes. How many times have you been 'caught' doing something wrong and chastised for it, but can you remember being 'caught' doing something really well? The principle is simple. It is unlikely that you will change someone's faults very quickly if at all, although you may stop them doing something, but what do you replace that something with? Taking the contrasting view, most nurses have some positive strengths. They are good at something, they show a talent, a flair for a particular task – is it not more productive to potentiate this than to condemn the negatives?

The ideal nurse, we suppose, is perfect at everything, but in reality nurses are like every other individual, with skills ranging from below to above average ability. The skilled manager will identify all these and maximize the above-average ones and largely ignore the below average. If a nurse is encouraged, rewarded and commended for valuable service, she will continue to improve and work hard. If she is continually harassed, punished and reprimanded for the inadequacies she largely cannot control, her entire work performance will suffer. An acquaintance of ours illustrates this point quite clearly. He was considered rather slow, showed little initiative and was generally dissatisfied with his job. It was only when he was asked whether he knew a suitable venue for the staff Christmas party that he volunteered to organize it and subsequently showed his brilliant talent for social and recreational organization. When this talent was recognized, rewarded and potentiated, his work improved generally, his initiative was considerably increased and his commitment to the unit became total. His ability was generalized into areas within the rehabilitation team, organizing day trips, bazaars, holidays, shopping trips and such. The learning exercise for everyone is that if you do not use people's talents you lose them; if you ignore people's potential, they cease to function altogether.

Decision making versus problem solving

An ability to make decisions is an attribute most nurses would wish to own. Indecisiveness in the nurse is a difficulty that may call into question her other skills. However, making decisions is not a difficult process provided there are at least two possible courses of action. To shave or not, to go out or stay in, to buy a car or a bicycle, are hardly difficult or earth-shattering decisions. More serious choices involving more complex issues may take longer, and deserve more thoughtful consideration. It would not be appropriate to decide whether to sue for divorce with the same cursory thought as it would take to decide whether to eat at 8 or 9 o'clock. Making these decisions becomes more difficult when the choice has to be accurate. These more complex issues fall within the realms of problem solving, for decision making is only a small part of this.

To take a familiar model of problem solving as an illustration of the process, we shall look at a management problem with Gerry.

> The unit officer has to decide what action to take about Gerry's persistent lateness. Although he is always very apologetic, he continues to come late. Sometimes ten minutes, sometimes half an hour, but on some occasions he's been as late as two hours. It has been decided that some action has to be taken.

Decision choices

1. Formal discipline; a series of these will result in termination of employment.
2. Transfer him to another unit; this will simply get him out of your hair.
3. Continue to reprimand him; this has proved to be ineffective.
4. Ignore it; the ostrich strategy tends to breed resentment or even encourage modelling behaviour within other staff.

The choices appear difficult until we apply a problem-solving approach:

Problem:	Gerry's lateness.
Goal:	Gerry reporting for on duty on time.
Assessment:	Factors affecting Gerry's lateness: buses don't run early morning; stays up too late at night; girlfriend works late hours; very tired in morning.
Plan:	Adjust hours to accommodate difficulties: i.e. Gerry works late shifts permanently.
Implementation:	Monitor punctuality.
Evaluation:	Solves problem. Gerry reports for duty on time. The organization is satisfied. How does Gerry feel about it?

Gerry was a particularly bright young man with lots of ideas and a very caring nature, and he was a skilled nurse. Taking any decision from (1) to (4) above would have solved very little and possibly resulted in losing Gerry's expertise. Looking closely at what the problems were and what outcomes were needed made the original preselected decision obsolete and the final decision more effective. Note that in the evaluation stage some feedback is needed from Gerry, too. In reality Gerry became very unhappy about working constant late shifts and eventually returned to normal shifts, but by this time his punctuality had greatly improved.

To summarize: for decision making to be effective, it has to occur within a problem-solving framework. Decisions themselves can be good, bad or indifferent. When the decisions that are taken address the problems accurately, and provide realistic and workable solutions, then and only then can we congratulate ourselves and claim to have the quality of a good decision maker.

Delegation

'If you want a job done well, do it yourself' and 'There's no point having a dog and barking yourself' are contradictory in content. They do, however, represent two generally accepted viewpoints which are central to the issue of delegation.

One of the most difficult things a nurse in a team has to learn is that there is neither the time nor the necessity to conduct all nursing practice herself. She has learned through her training and by making endless mistakes that she is reliable and competent and she has no difficulty in trusting herself. In the event that she does make an error, it is hers to own and deal with. Once she is an established professional in a team, even when working autonomously in the community, a time comes when the nurse has to accept that some of her workload needs to be relinquished if she is to remain effective. Charge nurses and ward sisters who continue to operate independently of others breed resentment, inadequacy and frustration. Difficult as it may be to delegate tasks that you feel competent to perform yourself, it is important to understand how others feel when you continue to show no trust in their abilities.

The skill of delegation is not to divorce yourself from responsibility, nor to accept all responsibility with no control. The skill is to be able to assess the ability of others, to select appropriate tasks that they can competently complete, and to monitor and supervise the implementation of your directions. In situations where nurses are expected to delegate tasks, they are temporarily becoming trainers and supervisors as well as practitioners. It is a compliment that their judgement is appreciated, that they are considered not only as competent professionals, but also as having the insight and personal resources to accept additional responsibility for someone else's performance.

This responsibility may hang heavy, but this is how it should be, for a good delegator needs to balance her judgement and trust and her suspicion and control finely. Bad delegators commonly ask the impossible of their subordinates, putting them under intolerable pressure and consequently putting themselves at risk when things go wrong. Equally, poor delegators direct too little towards others and reduce their own effectiveness by trying to do everything themselves. The effective delegator is the person who finds herself and the team constantly occupied in a purposeful way. Everyone's talents are being used to the full without risk to the client.

Contingencies

Every good manager knows that no matter how good her plans are, 'sod's law' still decrees that anything that possibly can go wrong will go wrong. It is for this reason that when a plan is about to be implemented, a contingency plan should be set up alongside it. The skilled nurse tends to do this almost automatically, mostly because in the process of becoming skilled an awful lot of mistakes have been made. It is through these past mistakes that a repertoire of contingency plans is accumulated. The experienced nurse may say that it is just common sense to plan for the possible eventuality, but although common sense is sometimes a rare commodity, it is what management is mostly about.

Contingencies are the well thought-out 'what ifs?' If Joe vomits on the coach, what can be done? If Arthur gets lost at the fair, what action is available? Who shall I report to? What should I do first? What are my back-up plans – the contingencies? In education, every teacher knows she must always have contingency plans for the material that runs out too quickly, the unexpected question from the class or the last-minute rescheduling of a timetable. Behind every seemingly faultless implementation of a plan there is a manager with an endless supply of well thought- through contingency plans. When they are at their most effective, no-one is aware they have been used. A ship does not sail without liferafts; a fighter pilot does not fly without his parachute; and likewise a plan should never be implemented without the contingencies being worked out.

Leadership

The successful leader should have the ability, qualities and skills previously discussed. She should be aware of resources available to her, know the strengths and weaknesses of her team, be able to make sound decisions that help solve problems that arise, and be able to delegate prudently. Having said all this, many people have these abilities but do not make good leaders. If these are the basic ingredients, what else is necessary? It is our view that the successful leader has, in addition, all the following qualities in various percentages.

She is a planner; she sees the whole nature and direction of the tasks and gradually moves forward towards what she sees as the overall goal of the team. She is intuitive in this planning, having experience, awareness and intelligent insight, and she is able to judge accurately what will and will not work. Intuitive is the only appropriate word to describe this ability, because it is a natural quality: it is not hard work for her to judge, foresee and plan. As if this is not enough, we see many other essential ingredients in this successful leader, for it is probably even more important that she is a brilliant communicator. There is no one in her team who is not aware of what she should be doing. Everyone knows what the overall outcome will be, and a complete trust in the leader is established. This communication skill is not unidirectional, for the wise leader knows that each one of her team not only has good ideas but has a need to share them. Furthermore, even the ideas that are not so good have a kernel of quality which may be valuable if sifted out.

The leader will have ideas from many sources: her team, herself, other groups, individuals and her clients. It is her job to sort these out, to direct them appropriately into strategies that help the movement towards shared goals. She must be able to modify them and make them acceptable and usable both to the organization and to her team. She must be consistent in her approach and correct in her decision making, or else her credibility as leader will suffer. This applies just as much to the 'democratic' leader as it does to the autocrat, for there is always someone who will need to apportion blame whenever things go wrong. Finally, she must be seen to be strong, reliable and fair.

How can each of us employ a systematized approach to becoming such a leader? First, we believe whether you adopt a democratic or an autocratic style of leadership will depend largely on your personality and temperament. We would suggest, however, that much greater pressure is applied to autocratic styles, as others in the team may feel more threatened and contribute less, and therefore the leader may be more easily scapegoated. Leadership by example, i.e. demonstrating in yourself all the skills and qualities you expect in your subordinates, is a very powerful model but it is also very demanding and fraught with danger. Any mistake, misdemeanour or substandard performance by the leader gives a precedent for subordinates to do the same. In a purely democratic style, the leader depends largely on her skills of oratory, logic and reason to demonstrate how each suggestion or idea could be used to fulfil the aim. Thus each member's intrinsic ability to be honest, work-orientated and sensible is necessary before this style can be initiated in its pure form. It is also interesting to note that many leaders believe themselves to be democratic until they are put to the test. Their style may then change to that of 'benevolent autocrat', where the leader knows what the course of action must be, takes it to the team and sells it to them. We recognize this particular device as one which we have both used on numerous occasions in the past; it is simply veiled autocracy.

If these are the main and most popular styles, we would suggest that neither is perfect. It seems better that each individual should take from each style as the occasion determines. We suggest that a reasonable compromise exists as follows.

Listen to all arguments and discussions without contaminating them with your own, and then introduce your own ideas to the discussion. Logically and rationally rule out the unacceptable, refine the promising and then communicate your intention to act on your findings. Your reasons for taking particular actions should be clearly stated to avoid confusion. Subsequently, it should be stressed that an idea will be tried as soon as possible, but within a prearranged time period it will be evaluated by free discussion and then adjusted. The advantages of this system are that it has an open approach, it takes ideas from many sources, it refines them, communicates intention, acts and has built-in safety in the form of evaluation and adjustment (see Figure 25.1)

It is important to have **shared objectives** if a leader is to be effective. For every member of the team to have the same firm idea of what they are trying to achieve will have a very powerful effect. When issues become vague, and

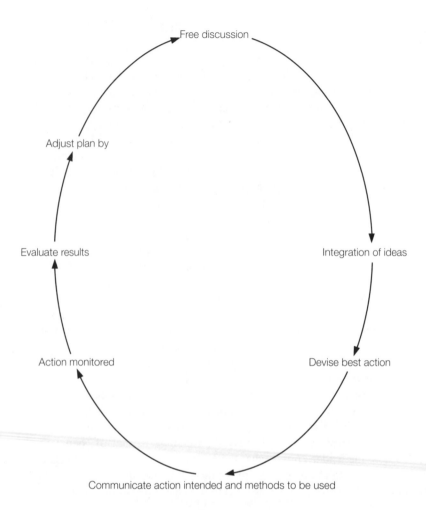

Figure 25.1 A circular model of communication and action in management

arguments and disagreements rage, the leader will be able to focus this energy productively on to the goal. Therefore, it would seem reasonable to have a series of set objectives to attain within a set period, to encourage observable task achievement. For example: The team at their weekly meeting decide the following objectives:

1. By next week – three teams will be set up to begin low-, medium- and high-dependency planning.
2. By the end of the month – each client will be dependency-assessed.
3. Within two months – individual care programmes will be in operation for each client within a framework of high/ medium/low dependency.
4. Broad aim – within six months each client will be actively engaged in an individual progressive rehabilitation programme. He will be continually monitored by his nursing team so as to operate at his optimum potential.

Once these types of objectives are set up, everyone knows where their efforts are to be directed. Progress can be measured and, in the light of progress, new objectives formulated or old ones modified. When difficulties arise, if these objectives are firmly fixed in the leader's mind she can use them as a focus to encourage positive action.

Methods of achieving objectives will be monitored and supervised by the leader using her discretion. Some members of the team will be effective in working towards objectives and some will be less effective. The leader's role here is to **observe**, **listen** and finally **demonstrate** when she is sure it is necessary. Leadership by example is very appropriate here. It is very powerful, as it shows the leader's skills as a practitioner as well as a manager. Equally its appropriateness must be valid, as interfering in the work of another professional must be well timed or it may breed resentment. If she is aware of how other members are successfully achieving objectives, the leader's role is to share this success with all the other members of the team. This will not only be helpful to the recipients, but will be praise and encouragement to the originators of the methods. The successful leader will be patient, rewarding, reassuring and stimulating.

By its very nature, leadership carries with it difficult components: correcting people's mistakes, maintaining standards and making difficult administrative decisions which may be unpopular. We would not advocate a whingeing, weak, apologetic style of admonishment, or bad news bearing, but neither would we say the cold calculating approach is necessary. It has been our experience that the effective leader, despite making 'hard' decisions, tends to remain respected and popular. This is because her decisions are based objectively and fairly on the task that has been agreed, and she is prepared to discuss, reason and, if necessary, justify her actions. It is not necessary for a good leader to pretend to be either super cool or super perfect: she will have emotions and these need to be disclosed on occasions. To share how unhappy she is, or how difficult it was to make a decision, is not a weakness and it does not hurt to show subordinates that she is human. Similarly, admitting mistakes and readily accepting criticism is not necessarily harmful. The technique of leadership in this area is to demonstrate how useful the criticism has been and how great an education was the mistake. This is not advising anyone to be ingenuine, simply to learn how to turn defeats into victories. We believe that most people would agree that individuals capable of retrieving something from a disaster are to be admired and looked up to – perhaps an apt description of a leader.

To summarize: the ideal leader/manager:

Demonstrates that she is consistent, patient, strong and fair.

Continually encourages and praises.

Listens, discusses and proposes.

Makes accurate problem-solving decisions.

Occasionally observes, evaluates and adjusts, reprimands and admonishes.

Is aware of resources in people, time, equipment, environment and finance.

Calculates the strengths and weaknesses of her team.

Accepts criticism, her mistakes, and that she is human, and uses each to its maximum potential.

Interferes only when necessary and does so by demonstrating a better way.

Shares her ideas, information and resources with her team.

Delegates appropriate tasks to competent personnel.

Does not become high-handed, big-headed, lazy, take her work home, or develop an ulcer.

Is neither an autocrat nor a democrat, but simply a person using her skills and qualities, intelligence and emotions to their maximum potential in a goal-orientated approach.

MAKING SENSE OF QUALITY

No doubt by the time you read this you will be seriously beginning to prepare yourself for the responsibility of 'taking charge' and all that this involves. You will, in your practice thus far, have come across an amalgam of approaches and issues that will be related to the world of quality. Taking charge also involves being clear about what you must achieve. This is aided by knowing what standards you are striving towards and how to measure progress in this direction. This aspect of quality applies to client care, unit and hospital management as well as self-management (which is often neglected).

How much do you know about the following and how many of them have anything to do with quality?

- Patients' Charter
- Standard setting
- Donabedian approach to standard setting
- Maxwell's dimension of quality
- Nursing audit
- Clinical audit
- Medical audit
- BS 5750
- Risk management
- Personal development.

An aspect of quality that incorporates all the above and more is organization-wide quality (NHSME EL (93)116). This is sometimes known as total quality management (TQM) or continuous quality improvement (CQI) or quality through leadership (Wash, 1991). We will deal briefly with this concept here and refer you to the Appendix for more technical aspects.

A definition that suits TQM is: 'Quality means continuously meeting agreed customer requirements at lowest cost by releasing the potential of all employees'. In your case the customer can be the client (sometimes referred to as the consumer) or it can be your internal customer, i.e. anyone who is at the receiving end of a service. Whether this is doctor, the next shift or nurse management, in this situation you are a supplier and they are customers.

By lowest cost, we mean in the most efficient manner, i.e. getting it right first time, every time. So much waste goes on in the health service and nurses should be trained in the concept of prudent cost consciousness, which does not necessarily mean using the cheapest material but is more to do with being on time, being organized, being clear in communication – many of the things described earlier in the chapter.

Where you may experience TQM is through your involvement in quality improvement teams, projects or circles. These are groups of staff brought together around a particular problem who, by using a variety of problem-solving techniques, attack the problem to create a more efficient and improved way of working. For a fuller description of TQM see Koch (1991, 1992), Atkinson (1990), Bull (1992) and Wash (1991).

However, there is one message with which we would like to end this book, and it is connected to both the values and philosophy underpinning TQM and our original aspirations for writing in the first place. The quality of organizational change and improvement in client care/management will depend largely on the personal drive of individuals to continuously strive for further personal development. In the past nurses have taken a lead in this area (and I suspect will continue to do so) and have significantly contributed to a health service where real health gain can be realized by everyone, physically, mentally and spiritually.

CONCLUSION

In this chapter we have tried to show that management principles and skills are important for every nurse. We have discussed aspects of resources that the nurse should be familiar with in order to be effective. Time, personnel, equipment, environment and finance are all resources that may be maximized if they are utilized efficiently, no matter how scarce they appear to be. Drawing together and comparing some contrasting approaches such as task/client orientation systems, positives/negatives, decision making/problem solving and delegation, was intended to provoke some thought on how you are currently operating, and whether other approaches might be helpful. Contingencies, quality and leadership are the final components of this chapter, as these are the tools of the implementor. The effective manager requires to plan contingencies and possess the qualities and skills of leadership if she is to be effective.

It has occurred to us that some of you may be puzzled that a book essentially about mental health nursing should end with a chapter on management, and we offer the following explanation. The nurse who has acquired knowledge and skills and is unable to focus and direct them appropriately is of limited use to the client. As this book was written to facilitate what we hope will be better care for the client, it seemed appropriate to end with a section on the skills required to potentiate such a noble desire, we end on the same note as we began, thinking of the people we seek to help - mental health clients.

Appendix:
The concept of quality

Eddie Byrnes, Aintree Hospitals

DEFINING QUALITY

Quality has been described as 'A notoriously difficult concept to come to grips with' (Nicklin and Lanksheer, 1990). This opinion is shared by Reerink (1990), who contends that, historically and currently, man has struggled to formulate and secure a definition of quality.

Donabedian (1980), also an expert on quality, describes three perspectives. He divides the first – the quality of medical care – into two domains: technical and interpersonal, defining quality of technical care in relation to risks and benefits.

> At the very least the quality of technical care consists of the application of medical science and technology in a manner that maximises its benefits to health without correspondingly increasing its risks (Donabedian, 1980, p.5).

He also stresses the importance of a client's personal definition of quality in relation to these benefits and risks by highlighting the individual client's decision as to whether or not medical intervention benefits their welfare holistically. What may be a quality intervention for one person may be worthless to another because of the effect on their lifestyle. Quality is therefore viewed by Donabedian as a balance between the care provided and the risks and benefits to the individual.

In attempting to define quality, Linsk (1990) identifies primary and secondary quality, describing primary quality for the competent physician as: 'Finding and treating the disease rapidly while at the same time forbearing unnecessary acts (Linsk, 1990, p.222). He goes on to describe secondary quality as:

- Efficient admission procedures;
- Polite personnel;
- Functioning elevators;

- One toilet for two clients rather than four clean floors;
- Responsiveness (to) dietary (needs);
- Prompt laboratory and X-ray turnround;
- Prompt response to the call sign [sic] call for assistance.

Although this appears to be a different view from Donabedian's, analysis of both definitions shows they share similar principles, namely:

- Appropriateness – of care
- Effectiveness – of care
- Accessibility – of care
- Efficiency – in delivery of care
- Acceptability – of care given.

Shaw (1986) describes these principles as 'elements of quality' and uses them and the element of 'equity' to clarify the nature and character of quality.

Maxwell (1991) suggests that in the context of health care provision there are six dimensions to quality. His criteria include:

- Access to service;
- Relevance to need;
- Effectiveness;
- Equity;
- Social acceptability;
- Efficiency and economy.

Although Shaw and Maxwell do not offer a precise definition of quality, they do provide a framework against which practitioners can attempt to specify and measure the quality of their service.

Quality assurance

Lang (1976) links the concept of quality with a quality assurance model. This model concentrates on bringing about change via assessment of current levels of nursing practice and movements towards improvement, and places the emphasis on assessment and changing practice. This emphasis can also be identified within many other definitions of quality assurance.

Lomas (1990) states: 'Quality assurance is the measurement of health care activity and the outcomes of that activity in order to identify whether the expected objectives of the activity are being achieved and when this is not the case to respond with effective action and reduce deviation from objectives.'

Securing measurement, evaluation and changing practice are implicit within many definitions of quality assurance (Vuori, 1989; Lewis, 1990; Milne and Drummond, 1990).

Donabedian describes the quality assurance process as consisting of three interrelated components:

- Structure - resources used to provide care;
- Process – the manner in which care is given;
- Outcome – the end result in terms of health and satisfaction for clients.

These components provide health workers with a useful framework for organizing quality assurance activities.

If nurses are to deliver high-quality care they need to develop systematic approaches to measuring the care they deliver. The Strategy for Nursing document (DHSS, 1989) says:

> There is no doubt that whatever the development in service and practice in which we become involved we are going to have to develop measurements of quality and effectiveness. No longer can we rely on intuition that nursing practice is effective. We are going to demonstrate that it is.

Therefore, to make the quality assurance process viable, the identification of standards and criteria is essential.

Mental health clients may have particular problems in participating in the evaluation of the quality of service and its outcome, due to illnesses which inhibit their ability to make rational decisions. Therefore it is vital to recognize that the appropriateness and effectiveness of service delivery requires careful review.

References

Abse, D. W. and Bristol, J. (1974) *Clinical Notes on Group Analytic Psychtherapy*, Wright, Bristol.

Akhtar, S., Crocker, E. and Dickey, W. (1977) Overt sexual behaviour among psychiatric inpatients. *Diseases of the Nervous System*, **38**, 359–61.

Altschul, A.T. (1977) Use of the nursing process in psychiatric nursing. *Nursing Times*, 8 September, 1412–14.

Altschul A.T. (1980) Team approach to psychiatric care. *Nursing Times*, 1 May, 797–9.

Argyle, M. (1975) *Bodily Communication*, Methuen, London.

Assael, M. (1978) Spontaneous painting: means of communication. *Confinia Psychiatrica*, **21**(1–3), 10–24.

Atkinson P. E. (1990) *Creating Culture Change: the Key to Successful Total Quality Management*, IFS Ltd, Bedford.

Barker, P.(1982) *Behaviour Therapy Nursing*, Croom Helm, London.

Barker, P. (1985) *Patient Assessment in Psychiatric Nursing*, Croom Helm, London.

Barker P. (1992) *Severe Depression*, Chapman and Hall, London.

Barton, R. (1959) *Institutional Neuroses*, John Wright, Bristol.

Beach, K. (1987) All together now. *Nursing Times*, 30 December, 38–40.

Beck, A.T. (1980) *Cognitive Therapy and the Emotional Disorders*, Meridian Books, New American Libary, New York.

Belliveau, F. and Richter, L. (1971) *Understanding Human Sexual Inadequacy*,

Bloch, S. and Crouch, E. (1985) *Therapeutic Factors in Group Psychotherapy*, Oxford University Press, Oxford.

Bohart, A.C. and Todd, J. (1988) *Foundations of Clinical and Counselling Psychology*, New York, Harper and Row.

Boyd, J. (1978) *Counselor Supervision: Approaches, Preparation, Practices*, Indiana, Accelerated Development.

British Association for Counselling (1992) *Code of Practice*, BAC, Rugby.

Broverman, I. K., Broverman, D. and Clarkson, F. E. (1970) Sex role stereotypes and clinical judgement of mental health. *Journal of Consulting and Clinical Psychology*, **34**(1), 1–7.

Bull, N. (1992) *Quality: For Those Who Care*, IFS Ltd, Bedford.

Burnard, P. (1989) *Counselling Skills for Health Professionals*, Chapman & Hall, London.

Carkhuff, R.R. and Truax, C.B. (1979) *Towards Effective Counselling and Psychotherapy: Training and Practice*, Aldine, New York.

Carozza, P. M. and Hiersteiner, C. L. (1982) Young female incest victims in treatment: stages of growth seen with a group art therapy model. *Clinical Social Work Journal*, **10**(3), 165–75.

Connor, M., Dexter, G. and Wash, M. (1984) *Listening and Responding: a Manual for Tutors*, College of Ripon and York St John, York.

Connor, M. (1986) *Listening and Responding*, Unpublished PhD thesis, Keele University.

Corey, G. (1990) *The Theory and Practice of Group Counseling*, Brookes/Cole, Belmont, California.

Dale, S. (1982) *Multiple Orgasms for Men*, Forum, London.

Davis, J. (1989) Issues in the evaluation of counsellors by supervisors. *Counselling,* August, 31–37.

Department of Health and Social Services (1989) *Strategy for Nursing*, DHSS, London.

Dexter, G. and Wash, M. (1986) *Psychiatric Nursing Skills: a Patient-Centred Approach*, Croom-Helm, London.

Dickoff, H. and Lakin, M. (1963) Patients' views of group psychotherapy. Retrospections and interpretations. *International Journal of Group Psychotherapy*, **13**, 61–73.

Donabedian, A. (1980) *The Definition of Quality and Approaches to its Assessment,* Health Administration Press, Ann Arbor, Michigan.

Donnenberg, D. (1978) Art therapy in a drug community. *Confinia Psychiatrica*, **21**(1–3), 37–44.

Drucker, P. F. (1967) *The Effective Executive*, Heinemann, London.

Egan, G. (1973) *Face to Face: the Small-Group Experience and Interpersonal Growth*, Brooks/Cole, California.

Egan, G. (1982) *The Skilled Helper: a Model for Systematic Helping and Interpersonal Relating*, 2nd edn, Brooks/Cole Publishing, Monterey, California.

Egan, G. (1986) *The Skilled Helper: a Systematic Approach to Effective Helping*, 3rd edn, Brooks/Cole, California.

Egan, G. (1994) *The Skilled Helper: a Problem-Management Approach To Helping*, Brooks/Cole Publishing, Pacific Grove, California.

Ellis, A. (1962) *Reason and Emotion in Psychotherapy*, Lyle and Short, New York.

English and Welsh National Boards for Nursing, Midwifery and Health Visiting. *Syllabus of Training*, Professional Register Part 3 (Registered Mental Nurse), London and Cardiff.

Eysenck, H. J. (ed) (1961) *Handbook of Abnormal Psychology*, Basic Books, New York.

Eysenck, H. J. (1966) *The Effects of Psychotherapy*, International Science Press, New York.

Fonseca, J. (1970) Editorial comment. *Nursing Outlook*, November.

Forrester, D. A. and Murphy, P. (1992) Nurses' attitudes towards patients with AIDS and SIDS-related risk factors. *Journal of Advanced Nursing*, **17**, 1260–66.

Foulkes S.H. (1984) *Group Psychotherapy: the Psychoanalytical Approach*, Maresfield, London.

Foulkes S. H. and Anthony, E. J. (1973) *Group Psychotherapy*, Penguin, Harmondsworth.

Freud, S. (1930) *Three Contributions to the Theory of Sex*, 4th edn, Nervous and Mental Disease Publishing, New York.

Freud, S. (1958) *The Complete Psychological Works of Sigmund Freud*, Hogarth Press and the Institute of Psychoanalysis, London.

Gazda, G. M. (1989) *Group Counseling: a Developmental Approach*, 4th edn, Allyn and Bacon, Boston.

Gentry, W. D. (ed) (1975) *Applied Behaviour Modification*, Mosby, St Louis.

Gilbert, P. (1992) *Counselling for Depression*, Sage, London.

Ginott, H.G. (1964) The theory and practice of therapeutic intervention in child treatment, in *Child Psychotherapy: Practice and Theory*, (ed M.R. Haworth), Basic Books, New York.

Halbreich, U. (1978) A non-verbal dialogue as a treatment of schizophrenic patients. *Confinia Psychiatrica*, **21**(1–3), 58–67.

Heath, J., Law, G. and Cross, I. (1982) *Nursing Process – What Is It?*, NHS Learning Resources Unit, Sheffield.

Hogan, R. (1980) *Human Sexuality – a Nursing Perspective*, Appleton-Century-Crofts, New York.

Houston, G. (1984) *The Red Book of Groups*, Rochester Foundation, London.

Houston, J.P., Bee, H. and Rimm, D.C. (1980) *Invitation to Psychology*, Academic Press, New York. (2nd edn 1983)

Jourard, S. (1971) *The Transparent Self*, Van Nostrand, New York.

Kaplan, H. S. (1981) *The New Sex Therapy*, Penguin Books, Harmondsworth.

Kinsey, A.C., Pomeroy, W.B., Martin, C.F. and Gebhard, P.C.H. (1944) *Sexual Behaviour in the Human Male*, W.B. Saunders, Philadelphia.

Kinsey, A.C., Pomeroy, W.B., Martin, C.F. and Gebhard, P.C.H. (1953) *Sexual Behaviour in the Human Female*, W.B. Saunders, Philadelphia.

Koch, H. (1991) *Total Quality Management in Health Care*, Longman, Harlow.

Koch, H. (1992) *Implementing and Sustaining Total Quality Management in Health Care*, Longman, Harlow.

Krumboltz, I.D. and Thoresen, C.E. (eds) (1969) *Behavioural Counselling*, Holt, Rinehart and Winston, New York.

Kubler-Ross, E. (1978) *To Live Until We Say Goodbye*, Prentice-Hall, Englewood Cliffs, New Jersey.

Lang, M. (1976) Quality assurance review in nursing. *American Journal of Maternal Child Nursing*, **1**(2), 75–79.

Langley, D. M. and Langley, G. E. (1983) *Dramatherapy and Psychiatry*, Croom Helm, London.

Lewis, M. (1990) Standards and nursing audit. *International Journal of Health Care Quality Assurance*, **3**(6), 21–32.

Linsk, J. A. (1990) The quality of health care: the practical and clinical view. *Quality Assurance in Health Care*, **2**(3/4), 219–225.

Littlewood, R. and Lipsedge, M. (1982) *Aliens and Alienists: Ethnic Minorities and Psychiatry*, Penguin, Harmondsworth.

Lomas, J. (1990) (Editorial) Quality assurance and effectiveness in health care: an overview. *Quality Assurance in Health Care*, **2**(1), 5–12.

Mace, D. R., Bravermann, R.H.O. and Burton, I. (1974) *Teaching of Human Sexuality in Schools for Health Professionals*, WHO, Geneva.

Macphail, D. (1988) *Family Therapy in the Community*, Heinemann, London.

Mahler, C. A. (1969) *Group Counseling in Schools*, Houghton Mifflin, Boston.

Maslow, A.H. (1970) *Motivation and Personality*, 2nd edn, Harper and Row, New York.

Maslow, A. H. (1971) *The Farther Reaches of Human Nature*, Viking, New York.

Masters, W.H. and Johnson, V.E. (1966) *Human Sexual Response*, Little, Brown, Boston.

Maxwell, R. J. (1991) Quality assessment in health. *British Medical Journal*, **288**, 147–1472.

Milgram, S. (1974) *Obedience to Authority*, Harper and Row, New York.

Milne, D. and Drummond, B. (1990) Quality assurance: implementation in nursing practice. *International Journal of Health Care Quality Assurance*, **3**(5), 10–18.

Mitchell, A.R.K. (1974) *The Nature of Depression*, NAMHO, Penguin Books, Harmondsworth.

Moreno, J. L. (1946) *Psychodrama 1*, Beacon House, New York.

Mowrer, O.H. (1960) *Learning Theory and Behaviour*, John Wiley, New York.

Murdoch, D. and Barker, P. (1991) *Basic Behaviour Therapy*, Blackwell Scientific, Oxford.

Murray-Parkes, C. (1976) *Bereavement: Studies of Grief in Adult Life*, Penguin, Harmondsworth.

Nicklin, P. and Lankster, A. (1990) Quality Matter. *Nursing Times*, 1 August, 59–60.

Norbeck, I.S. (1980) Psychiatric nursing with children, in *Psychiatric Nursing: a Basic Text,* (ed P.C. Pothier), Little, Brown, Boston.

Oakley, A. (1985) *Sex, Gender and Society*, Gower, Aldershot.

Oatley, K. (1980) Theories of personal learning, in *Small Groups and Personal Change*, (ed P.B. Smith), Methuen, London.

Pavlov, l.P. (1927) *Conditioned Reflexes*, Oxford University Press, Oxford.

Piaget, J. (1974) *Child Psychotherapy: Practice and Theory*, Basic Books, New York.

Poteet, J. A. (1978) *Behaviour Modification: a Practical Guide for Teachers*, Hodder and Stoughton, London.

Pothier, P.C. (ed) (1980) *Psychiatric Nursing: a Basic Text*, Little, Brown, Boston.

Ramsay, R. W. (1975) *Grief Therapy*, Sixty Minutes, CBS News, USA. (video)

Reerink, E. (1990) Defining quality of care: mission impossible. *Quality Assurance in Health Care*, **2**(3/4), 197–202.

Richards, B. (1982) *The Grafenburg spot and female ejaculation*. British Journal of Sexual Medicine, December.

Rogers, C. R. (1951) *Client Centred Therapy: Its Current Practice,* Implications and Theory, Constable, London.

Rogers, C. R. (1961) *On Becoming a Person: a Therapist's View of Psychotherapy*, Constable, London.

Rogers, C. R. (1970) *Carl Rogers on Encounter Groups*, Harper and Row, New York.

Rogers, C. R.(1977) *Carl Rogers on Personal Power: Inner Strength and its Revolutionary Impact*, Constable, London.

Rogers, C.R. and Stevens, B. (1967) *Person to Person: the Problem of Being Human*, Souvenir Press, London.

Roper, N., Logan, W. W. and Tierney, A.I. (1980) *The Elements of Nursing*, Churchill Livingstone, London.

Russel, J. (1993) Out of Bounds: *Sexual Exploitation in Counselling and Therapy*, Sage, London.

Sarantakos, S. (1994) *Social Research*, MacMillan, Basingstoke.

Schutz, W. (1973) Encounter, in *Current Psychotherapies*, (ed R. Corsini, F. E. Peacock, Itasca, Illinois.

Shaw C. D. (1986) *Introducing Quality Assurance*, Kings Fund Project, Paper No 64.

Silverman, D. (1993) *Interpreting Qualitative Data,* Sage, London.

Smith P. B. (ed) (1980) *Small Groups and Personal Change*, Methuen, London.

Schnarch, D. M. (1991) *Constructing the Sexual Crucible: an Integration of Sexual and Marital Therapy,* Norton and Co, New York.

Stock-Whitaker D. and Lieberman, M. A. (1964) *Psychotherapy Through the Group Process*, Aldine, New York.

Sundeen, S. J., Stuart, G. W., Rankin, E. D. and Cohen, S. A. (1976) *Nurse Client Interactions: Implementing the Nursing Process*, Mosby, St Louis.

Thompson, S. and Khan, J. H. (1970) *The Group Process as a Helping Technique,* Pergamon Press, Oxford.

Trower, P., Casey, A. and Dryden, W. (1989) *Cognitive Behavioural Counselling in Action*, Sage, London.

Tschudin, V. (1991) *Counselling Skills for Nurses*, 3rd edn, Baillière-Tindall, London.

Tuckman, B. (1967) Developmental sequence in small groups. *Psychology Bulletin*, **68**, 384.

Urbano, J. (1984) Supervision of counsellors: ingredients for effectiveness. *Counselling,* November, (50), 7–15.

Vuori, H. (1989) Research needs in quality assurance. *Quality Assurance in Health Care*, **1**(2/3), 147–59.

Warren, B. (ed) (1984) *Using the Creative Arts in Therapy*, Croom Helm, London.

Wash, M. (1993) Quality through leadership. *Managing Service Quality*, **1**(2).

Watzlawick, F., Beavin, J. and Jackson, D. (1968) *Pragmatics of Human Communication*, Faber, London.

Wolfe, J. and Lazarus, A. (1966) *Behaviour Therapy Techniques. A Guide to the Treatment of Neuroses*, Pergamon Press, Oxford.

Yalom, I.D. *The Theory and Practice of Group Psychotherapy*, 3rd edn, Basic Books, New York.

Index